A Text
By and For Audiologists

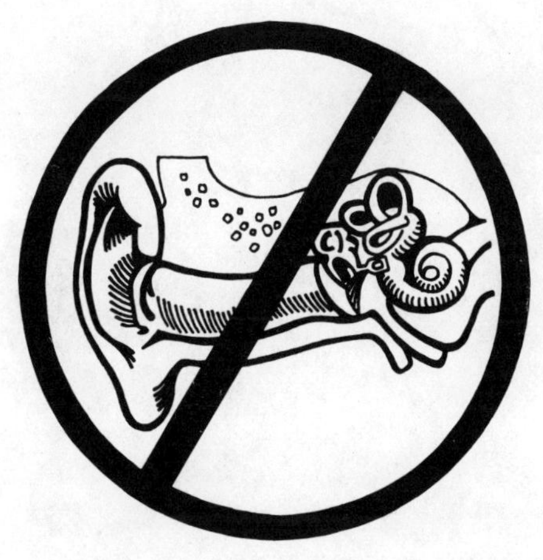

Auditory Dysfunction

A Text
By and For Audiologists

by

Sanford E. Gerber, Ph.D. FASHA
Professor of Audiology
Chairman, Department of Speech
University of California
Santa Barbara, California

and

George T. Mencher, Ph.D. FASHA
Director, Nova Scotia Hearing and Speech Clinic
Professor, School of Human Communication Disorders
Dalhousie University, Halifax, Nova Scotia

College-Hill Press • Houston, Texas

College-Hill Press
P.O. Box 35728
Houston, Texas 77035

Library of Congress Cataloging in Publication Data

Gerber, Sanford E.

    Auditory Dysfunction.
    Includes bibliographical references and indexes.
    1. Hearing disorders. 2. Ear—Diseases. 3. Auditory pathways—
Diseases. I. Mencher, George T., joint author. II. Title.
(DNLM: 1. Hearing disorders. WV270 G362a)
RF290.G48   617.8'86   80-17347

ISBN 0-933014-60-0

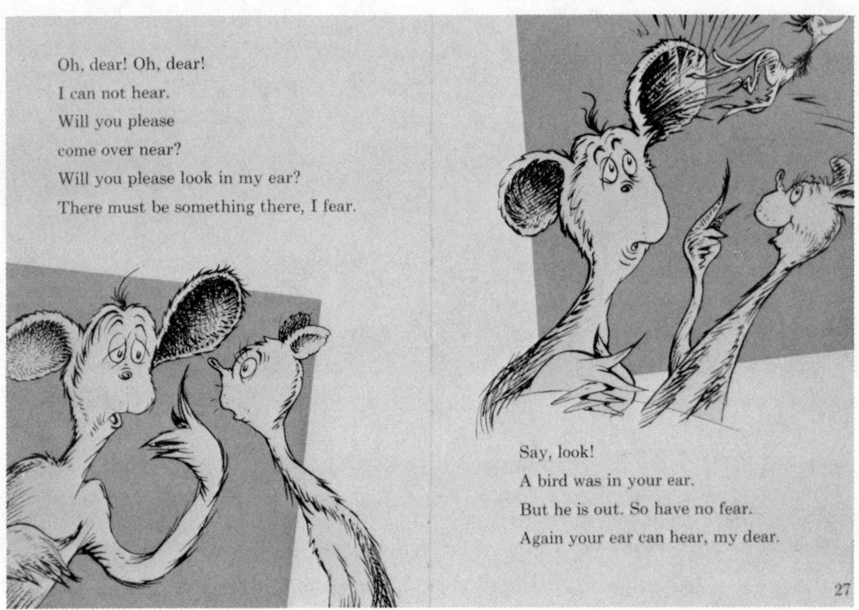

Reproduced with permission of Random House, Inc.

Dedicated to

L and L

Contents

FOREWORD

The authors have created a textbook which fulfills a need for the patient and the profession. This book is a synthesis of both the biological and psychophysical aspects of patients with auditory dysfunction. The current textbooks in this area deal primarily with only one aspect of auditory dysfunction. These can be either biological, in that they include medical, anatomical, pathological and physiological information, or they are only psychophysical in that they include audiometric and habilitative aspects of auditory dysfunction. This textbook synthesizes both aspects of the problems so that it can be used and understood by both students and professionals in all the areas of health care for patients with auditory dysfunction. This textbook will have its greatest impact in the care of patients with auditory dysfunction in that it will create a heightened understanding of auditory dysfunction through the synthesis of biological and psychophysical information which is clearly and accurately presented. A textbook with this format has been long overdue and serves to give the reader a total view of all the aspects of diseases and the interventions which comprise the complex area of auditory dysfunction.

Robert J. Ruben, M.D., F.A.A.O.
Professor and Chairman
Department of Otorhinolaryngology
Albert Einstein College of Medicine of
Yeshiva University and the Montefiore
Hospital and Medical Center
Bronx, New York

PREFACE

> Hearing loss today remains the most common physical disability in the United States—affecting more Americans than heart disease, cancer, blindness, tuberculosis, venereal disease, multiple sclerosis, and kidney disease put together. According to the U.S. Public Health Survey, there are approximately 236,000 deaf individuals of all ages and both sexes in the United States today. Among school-aged children, there are approximately 38,000 in schools for the deaf, about 100,000 more requiring intensive special management, and circa 250,000 more who are aurally handicapped to an important degree in the regular school environment. In the U.S. and other parts of the world for which we have figures, between 3½ and 5% of school-aged children have a hearing loss. Over eight million of the American population today suffer a partial hearing impairment of handicapping degree. Six million of these Americans have involvement in both ears.
>
> *(DiBartolomeo and Gerber, 1977)*

This is a book about diseases and disorders of hearing written by audiologists for audiologists. It is written with the philosophy that "contemporary otology and audiology are jointly responsible for the diagnosis and management of the ear and auditory system lesions" *(Goodhill, 1979)*. The otologist guides medical management; the audiologist guides communicative resources. Just as the otologist must understand audiological data, procedures, and rehabilitative methods, the audiologist must know and understand the otologist's procedures and methods.

Practicing otologists and audiologists recognize that the majority of hearing-impaired persons cannot expect medical intervention to restore hearing to normal, even though it may alleviate the disease process. For those patients, the audiologist becomes the primary source of rehabilitative care. In order to provide maximum restoration of a patient's ability to communicate aurally, the audiologist must have a comprehensive knowledge of the extent and nature of the handicap and what can be done about it. Fundamental to that knowledge is a general understanding of diseases and disorders of the ear; to recognize them, to understand what they are, to know what to expect from medical intervention, and to know what forms various medical and surgical treatment procedures may take.

The objective of this text is to offer to the beginning audiology student an introduction to hearing disorders, and to provide a basic framework from which the more advanced student may proceed. For this reason, it is also our hope that physicians and other hearing health care professionals will find this work interesting and useful. Contrary to most texts concerned with this topic, we have adopted the position that the patient is primary, the disorder is secondary. We have endeavored to be explicit about the humanistic concern. We are not dealing with hearing disorders; we are dealing with people who have hearing disorders. We hope that this attitude will be adopted by all of our readers. Herein we stress the ear for those who are interested primarily in hearing (clinical audiologists) and hearing for those who are interested primarily in ears (clinical otologists); but, most importantly we stress the problems of people.

The book is divided on an anatomical basis. Part 1 focuses on disorders of the sound conducting mechanism. Part 2 considers disorders of the sensory end organ. Part 3 reviews disorders of the neural transduction system. We progress, then, from the outside in. Part 4 deals with an assessment of the handicap.

Certain assumptions have been made in the preparation of this text. It is not a text about hearing testing or clinical audiology. We have assumed that the reader has taken another course on audiometry and/or has read a basic text on audiometry. We also assume that the reader has completed, or is completing, a course on aural anatomy and physiology. Therefore, we have not expanded our discussions to include testing methods or a study of the important anatomical landmarks.

As with all books and all authors, we have not been alone in this labor. We are grateful to many people for their guidance and assistance, but some must be especially recognized in print. Gregory S. Keller, M.D. read the entire manuscript to assure that we did not abuse otological accuracy; if we did, it is certainly our own fault. Ms. Mary Lory devoted long hours to preparing the bibliography. Ms. Sally Rizzolo assisted with the bibliography and figures, and prepared the case studies. Ms. Catherine McClean, M.S. contributed to chapter 5. We are indebted to Jack Katz, Ph.D., who read and commented on chapter 11. Our friend and colleague, Jeffrey L. Danhauer, Ph.D., read and commented upon the entire manuscript, not once but in three versions. The original drawings are by Louise Gerber. Our good friend, Robert J. Ruben, M.D., lent his great talent and enormous prestige to our labor by writing the Foreword.

And, most of all, again Louise and Lenore tolerated us being away from home, yelling at each other, and (maybe just once) yelling at them too. If we were they, we wouldn't put up with us.

SEG
GTM

References

DiBartolomeo, J.R. and Gerber, S.E. 1977. Pathology of hearing loss. In *Audiometry in infancy*, ed. S.E. Gerber. New York: Grune & Stratton, Inc.
Goodhill, V. 1979. Otologic relationships with audiology. In *Hearing and hearing impairment*, eds. L.J. Bradford and W.G. Hardy. New York: Grune & Stratton, Inc.

PART **1**

Conductive Hearing Impairment

The external and middle ears are intended anatomically and physiologically to conduct acoustic information to the sensory end organ, the cochlea. Any interruption of this function is described as a *conductive* hearing impairment. Hearing losses due to failure of conduction cannot be as handicapping as severe losses from failure of sensory or neural functions. One does not become deaf, in the popular sense of that word, from conductive impairment.

Conductive losses are quite common in childen. Although they are usually amenable to medical intervention, they may interfere with learning. If for no other reason, then, conductive impairments demand our understanding. The kinds of conductive losses which appear in adulthood are typically correctable, at least in part, by surgery. Knowledge of these disorders and the means for their correction is a mandate for the audiologist.

CHAPTER 1

Disorders

of the

External Ear

External ear problems are usually disorders or skin diseases caused by irritative reaction, fungus, or the presence of a foreign object. In general, a broad term incorporating most diseases of the external ear is *otitis externa*. The student is reminded that the prefixes "ot, oti, oto" refer to the ear; while the suffix "itis" refers to inflammation or infection, as in tonsilitis or appendicitis. Hence, otitis refers to any infection of the ear; and otitis externa, therefore, refers to an infection of the external ear (figure 1-1).

Problems that arise from pathology limited to the external ear usually have greater significance otologically than audiologically. That is to say, the extent (in frequency) and degree (in decibels) of a hearing loss which results from an external ear problem are usually limited. However, external ear disease is a problem that requires medical treatment. Furthermore, lack of treatment can lead to conditions which are more severe. For example, some forms of otitis externa have the potential to lead to otitis media (infection of the middle ear) or, by themselves, to do damage to the tympanic membrane and other nearby structures.

PATHOLOGY and ETIOLOGY

IRRITATIVE REACTIONS

Irritative reactions may be caused by constant rubbing, insect bites, contact with a chemical substance, or introduction of a foreign object. Irritation caused by improperly fitted ear defenders or ear molds is quite common. If the skin is broken, the risk of infection is markedly increased. Generally, the problem is rapidly relieved by treatment with a topical application of appropriate medication.

In general, hearing loss does not accompany irritations of the pinna

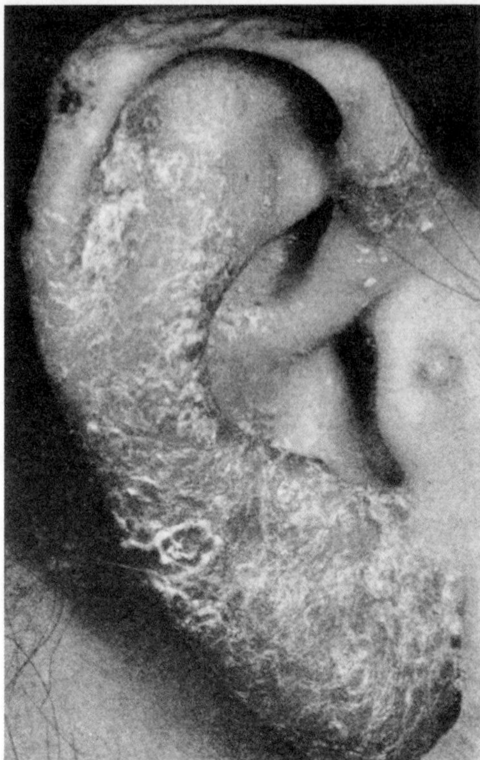

Figure 1-1. Lupus vulgaris, an example of otitis externa. *(Reproduced with permission of Edward Arnold Ltd.)*

and/or external auditory meatus. However, occasionally an irritation results in such a marked swelling that hearing may be minimally affected. When encountering such a patient, immediate referral to an otologist is essential.

TRAUMA

Once in a while, an audiologist will encounter a case of direct trauma to the external ear. This would include such things as a blow to the side of the head, a knife wound, even a human bite. In most cases, the surgeon's skill can restore a respectably normal appearance, and there should be no permanent effect on hearing.

FROSTBITE

Frostbite is a thermal injury to the pinna that occurs after long exposure to temperatures below freezing. It is characterized by a very painful swelling of the auricle, and, in the extreme, the pinna may become necrotic. Gradual warming and the use of antibiotics to prevent infection usually succeed in relieving this condition.

FUNGUS

Severe itching of the external ears is a common sign of the presence of a fungus. That symptom may also accompany eczema, insect bites, allergic reactions, and a host of other problems, including neurodermatitis, a psychologically based reaction which appears as a rash on the surface of the skin. The most common fungus infection is called otomycosis *(Gregson and LaTouche, 1961)*. Fungi tend to live in a warm, moist, dark environment; the middle ear and the ear canal offer a perfect breeding ground. A crusty appearance on the outside of the ear, the presence of a white flake-like epithelial debris, and constant itching are classical signs. Itching can result in scratching, which, in turn, can result in a further irritation of the skin of the ear canal. Treatment is purely medical, hearing loss is minimal, and immediate referral is required.

OBSTRUCTIONS

FOREIGN OBJECTS. What may occur more frequently than a disease of the external ear is an obstruction of the ear canal by a foreign object. Children especially are fond of putting things in the ear. But whether by child or adult, the introduction of a foreign object can result in an occlusion of the ear canal, perforation of the tympanic membrane, and/or an otitis externa. Buttons, beans, cigarette filters, and cotton balls are frequent offenders. Usually trapped at the narrow bony isthmus of the ear canal, they block the transmission of sound and accumulate cerumen, which compounds the problem. These objects often work their way along the canal until they lodge against the tympanic membrane, causing an increased hearing loss, as well as pain and discomfort. Sometimes objects become embedded under the skin of the ear canal and cause a slowly festering, low-grade infection or otitis externa.

Foreign objects in the ear produce a variety of problems ranging from simple discomfort, to occlusion of the external auditory meatus, to a scratching of the skin with a resulting introduction of undesirable bacteria which have the potential to damage the tympanic membrane and cause loss of hearing. Foreign objects need to be removed carefully and correctly. The audiologist must be able to recognize their presence and refer the patient for treatment.

EXOSTOSES. Sometimes bony growths, or localized hyperplasias, called *exostoses,* will arise from the tympanic ring due to an irritation or to some idiopathic cause (figure 1-2). These may take the form of multiple bony masses. One of the things which seems to lead to, or at least to aggravate, the growth of an exostosis, is what has been called "swimmer's ear." Persons who regularly swim in cold salt water repeatedly present an irritant to the lining of the ear canal which may develop into an exostosis. These growths are frequently bilateral, affecting both external auditory meati.

Patients rarely complain of pain or discomfort. DiBartolomeo (1979) reported that 40% of his cases presented a conductive hearing loss. He also reported that 80% of the cases initially seen had unilateral symptoms in the presence of bilateral disease. The symptoms included hearing loss, acute ear infections, pain, and tinnitus.

Treatment involves antibiotic therapy for ear canal infections and, when indicated, surgery for the exostosis. This surgery, a hospital procedure, generally involves cutting or grinding away the bony growth to provide a patent ear canal.

The audiologist must be alert to recognize an abnormality of the external ear canal when viewing the ear prior to audiometric testing.

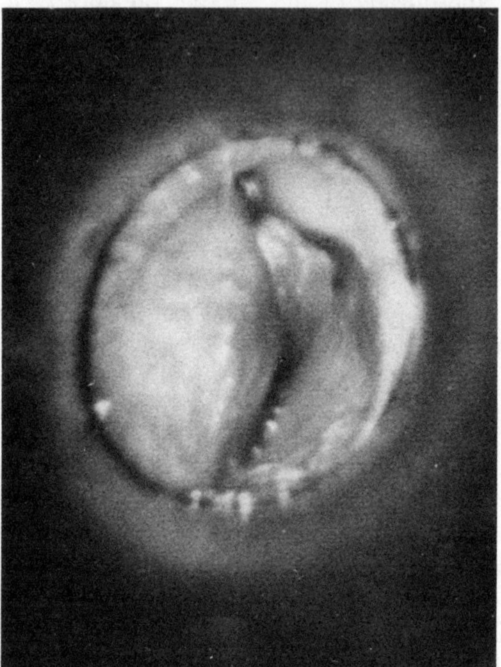

Figure 1-2. Otoscopic view of an exostosis of the external auditory meatus. *(Courtesy of Joseph R. DiBartolomeo, M.D.)*

TUMORS. Tumors of the head and neck may also invade the external ear and/or ear canal. Occasionally, hygroma (that is, a water-filled tumor as in figure 1-3) or hemangioma (that is, a blood-filled tumor) develop from part of the face and grow into the ear canal. Other conditions, such as carcinoma, may also invade the external ear (figure 1-4). According to Paparella (1973), 4% to 8% of all skin cancers appear on the pinna. These kinds of problems are not primarily audiologic and are usually not exclusively otologic either. They often require the services of an oncologist (a physician who specializes in tumors) and a maxillofacial surgeon. Any form of tumor which invades the ear canal may present with a hearing loss; therefore, the audiologist should be alerted to investigate the possibility that some type of growth may have invaded the external ear space and, if so, should immediately refer the patient for treatment.

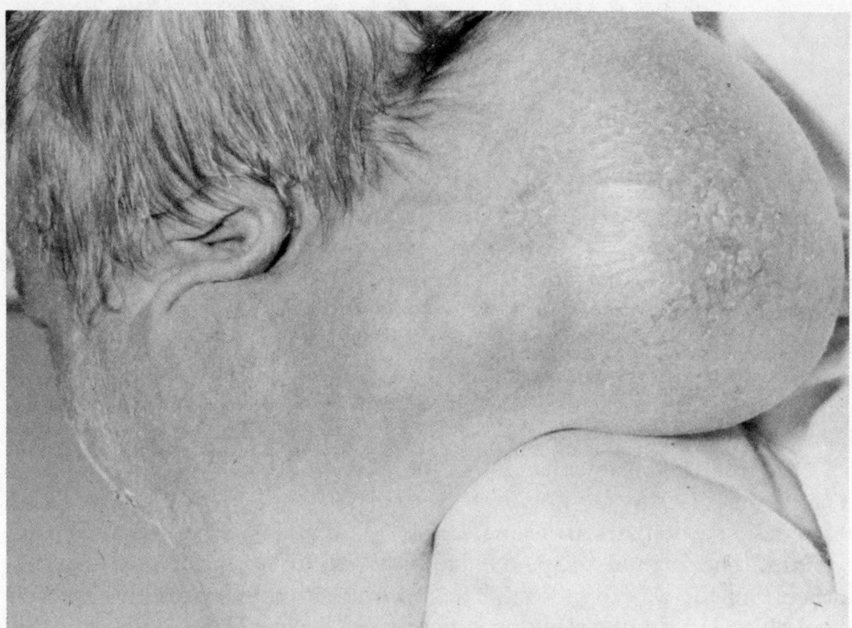

Figure 1-3. Hygroma (water-filled tumor) of the neck displacing the auditory peripheral organs.

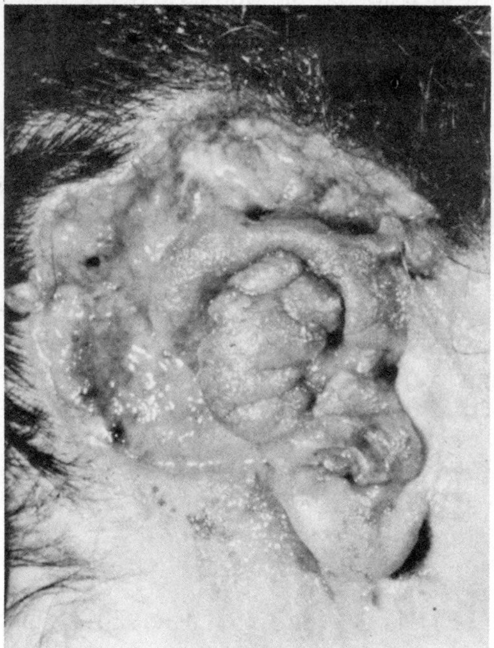

Figure 1-4. Carcinoma of right auricle and extension to adjacent soft tissue. *(Reproduced with permission of R.C. Bryarly, M.D.)*

IMPACTED CERUMEN

Cerumen, or ear wax, is produced normally by special glands under the skin of the external auditory meatus. In this sense, the surface of the meatus is unique; no other part of the body produces cerumen. The skin of the ear canal grows continuously and regularly at about the same rate as one's fingernails. It migrates outward and replaces itself approximately every three months. In most situations, the cerumen is carried out with it. In other words, for most of us, the wax produced by the skin of the ear canal falls out. Therefore, there is no valid reason for introducing a foreign object into the ear to remove it. In fact, quite the opposite is true. For example, cotton-tipped swabs do a splendid job of pushing the cerumen into (not out of) the ear canal. Undoubtedly, many cases of impacted wax are produced by well-intended and well-groomed persons who, thinking that they are cleaning their ears (or those of their babies), are actually pushing wax into the ear canal.

It is true, on the other hand, that some people do not easily shed cerumen. The reasons for this are not always apparent, but they would include such things as a particularly acute angle of the canal and/or an especially narrow isthmus. There could be some anatomical variation such that it would be difficult for the wax to fall out. These people should not treat this problem themselves. For routine cleaning, a family physician can be of assistance. But impacted cerumen should be removed by an otologist, a physician who specializes in the ear. It is a painless procedure which takes only a moment or so to do. Although there are people who have frequently recurring trouble with impacted cerumen and who must visit the otologist's office often, they are the exceptions. For most of us, the cerumen falls out and never becomes impacted.

One sign of impacted cerumen is a mild hearing loss of sudden onset. This is a surprising observation at first, but a moment's reflection reveals why the phenomenon is not so strange. As long as a sound wave can traverse the ear canal and reach the tympanic membrane causing it to vibrate, no hearing loss will ensue. Thus a gradual wax accumulation over time may go unnoticed. If, however, the accumulation becomes impacted and occludes the meatus so that sound waves can no longer reach the tympanic membrane, or if the impaction suddenly impedes the movement of the tympanic membrane, the patient may report a mild to moderate hearing loss of abrupt onset. Although the amount of hearing loss ultimately produced by impacted cerumen is usually small, there are other very serious causes leading to an abrupt hearing loss (see chapters 6 and 10). At the outset, the presenting symptom may be the same, and careful analysis is required. The audiologist is forewarned to check for impacted cerumen first.

MEDICAL CONSIDERATIONS

When a physician examines an ear with an otoscope, he is looking to see the color and mobility of the tympanic membrane. The drum membrane is normally grey in color. If there is a disease, especially of the middle ear, the membrane will mirror that in an alteration of its basic color or in its ability to reflect light. For example, the membrane may be pinkish or red from severe irritation. It may be purple or black from an old scar which has necrotized. In a rare situation, it may even appear to have white plaques due to tuberculosis, a disease which can occur in any part of the body except the teeth and nails. In short, the color of the tympanic membrane is an important clue in the diagnosis. And, if it is not visible at all, it may be obscured by cerumen or neoplasm.

In one otology clinic, the physician peered through the otoscope and discovered the tympanic membrane to be a beautiful shade of royal blue. An audiologist colleague concurred that that was indeed the color. Grey is normal; pink, red, yellow, and black all occur under various pathological conditions. Royal blue does not appear even in the ears at Buckingham Palace! The otologist asked the patient's mother if the family had been painting at the house. The affirmative reply indicated that the garage was being painted blue.

A great variety of foreign objects may be found in ears which require medical intervention. Foreign bodies usually can be removed by the use of a blunt hook or by simply syringing them out. If they do not come out easily—if, for example, they get wedged beyond the isthmus—it becomes necessary to remove them surgically via an endaural incision.

Some malignancies may appear first as a polyp in the ear canal. Shambaugh (1967) claimed that such polyps can be removed in the office, but careful and detailed inspection of the ear is required to locate their source. Furthermore, histological study must always be done to assure the absence of malignancy.

AUDIOLOGICAL CONSIDERATIONS

The audiologist's responsibility is to look at the outer ear and in the ear canal to do two basic things. First, a visual inspection and an otoscopic view are necessary to ensure that there is no obvious condition or disease requiring medical evaluation and treatment. Clearly, appropriate and prompt referral is an integral part of that responsibility. Secondly, the audiologist must ensure that nothing in the ear or on the ear will interfere with audiometric testing or compromise the health of the patient or the standards of the test facility.

The cleanliness of the audiological equipment and the safety of the patient are paramount. Whenever the possibility of ear infection arises, it is essential that the earphone cushions, ear inserts, and specula be sterilized to obviate contagion to other patients. In fact, many audiology clinics wisely disinfect equipment and instruments after every patient. This may be done by ultra-violet radiation or, even better, by chemical sprays (e.g. Staphene), However, the cushions need to be removed from the earphones if they are to be sprayed so that the spray does not contact the earphone diaphragm.

Collapsed Ear Canals

Because of unique differences in the structure of the ear, there are patients with enlarged tragi which are easily flattened when pressed. In the normal situation, the ear canal is opened and the tragus projects out, away from the opening of the ear canal. When a finger is pressed against the tragus, or more importantly, an earphone presses against the ear, the tragus is flattened across the opening of the ear canal. The result is an occluded ear canal, and, of course, an associated hearing loss, sometimes as much as 50dB.

A collapsed ear canal may occur due to an evacuation of air from the ear, which occurs when placing the earphones on a patient (especially a very young or very old person) who has an extremely narrow isthmus or highly compliant canal walls. A collapse will often account for significant differences between results obtained during testing in the sound field as compared to those obtained via earphones.

Sometimes a child with a suspected hearing loss will be referred from a school screening to an audiology center. This suspicion of hearing loss may be due to a flattened tragus or a collapsed ear canal. The audiologist should always be alert to that possibility.

If the patient has tragus or collapsed ear canal problems, the difficulty will usually be relieved by gently pulling upward and backward on the pinna as the earphone is placed over the ear. If that does not work, it may be necessary to hold the earphone against the head as opposed to fixing it in place with the headband. Ingenuity and caution are appropriate.

Audiometric Test Results

Audiometrically, one expects little or no threshold shift with disorders of the external ear, although exceptions have been noted. The audiometric contour would be flat or slightly rising. Speech discrimination should be normal. It would be inadvisable, if not foolish, to attempt tympanometry in the presence of pathology of the external ear.

Case Study 1-1:

External Ear Fungus

In March of 1976, Mr. C was seen for a hearing evaluation. At that time, test results indicated a bilateral high frequency hearing loss. Shortly after the evaluation, Mr. C was seen by Dr. O and was treated for a fungus infection in both ears. At the time of his initial test, it was suggested that he return within a year for a recheck. Pure tone tests at the second visit, following Dr. O's treatment, revealed normal hearing in both ears except for a slight notch at 4000Hz. His speech reception threshold was 5dB bilaterally, and speech discrimination was 100%. These tests showed improvement of Mr. C's hearing both for tones and for speech.

REFERENCES

Bryarly, R.C., Veach, S.R., and Kornblut, A.D. 1980. Metastasizing auricular basal cell carcinoma. *Otolaryngol. Head Neck Surg.* 88:40-43.

DiBartolomeo, J.R. 1979. Exostoses of the external auditory canal. *Ann. Otol. Rhinol. Laryngol.* Suppl. 61, 88:1-20.

Gregson, A.E. and LaTouche, C.J. 1961. Otomycosis: a neglected disease. *J. Laryngol. Otol.* 75:45-69.

Paparella, M.M. 1973. Cysts and tumors of the external ear. In *Otolaryngology*, vol. 2, eds. M.M. Paparella and D.A. Shumrick. Philadelphia: W.B. Saunders Co.

Shambaugh, G.E., Jr. 1967. *Surgery of the ear.* 2d ed. Philadelphia: W.B. Saunders Co.

CHAPTER 2

Anomalies of the External Ear

The human pinna, or auricle, seems to have lost — or maybe never had — the function it serves in most other animals. The clearest evidence supporting that argument is the fact that, in man, the pinna is on the side of the head. Observe the dog or cat. Two things are immediately noticeable: 1) the pinnae are on the top of the animal's head, and 2) the animal will move them when utilizing and fine-tuning the auditory system. The pinnae seem to perform the function of localizing antennae, used as a kind of early warning device, an assistance to the animal in locating the source of the sound. We homo sapiens, with a few humorous exceptions, cannot move our pinnae and, because of their location, usually find it necessary to turn our heads to locate the source of sound. There is a so-called "pinna effect": sounds reaching the head from behind strike the back of the pinnae and thus may be perceived as quieter than sounds reaching the pinnae from directly in front. However, any loudness difference is so small that it is not perceptible to most normal listeners. Apparently, the most useful functions of human pinnae are for support of eye glasses and the culturally centered decorative role of hanging earrings. They do not seem to play a significant role in hearing, although it has been suggested that they may serve as high frequency antennae *(Batteau, 1967)*.

PATHOLOGY and ETIOLOGY

A review of embryology tells us that the human auditory system develops in two parts. These parts are separated from one another by the incudo-stapedial joint. That is, the incus, the malleus, and the external ear develop from one group of primordial tissues. The stapes, the vestibular organs, and the inner ear structures develop from another group of primordial tissues.

Because the pinna and a portion of the middle ear are joined embryologically, if the patient demonstrates an anomaly of the external ear, the audiologist should be forewarned that there may be an anomaly of the malleus and/or incus as well.

Microtia and Atresia

Anomalies of the external ear may be classified under the general heading of aural *agenesis* or *dysgenesis* — a total or partial failure to develop. If it is the pinna which has failed to develop, the condition is described as *microtia*. If it is the external auditory meatus which has failed to develop, the appropriate term is *atresia*. An atresia is an absence of an opening. If the opening is present but abnormally small, it is called a *stenosis*.

Given what is known about embryology, it is reasonable to expect microtia and atresia to occur together. In point of fact, they usually do; but not always. Meatal atresia always occurs with severe microtia, but may also occur with a normal pinna *(Nager, 1973)*. There are several degrees of microtia, ranging from minor alteration of the pinna to complete absence of the auricle. The range is displayed in figure 2-1.

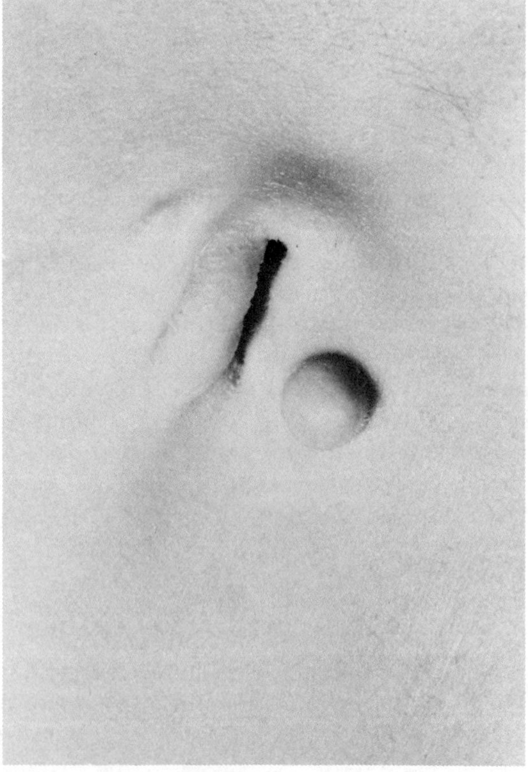

Figure 2-1a. Range of microtia.

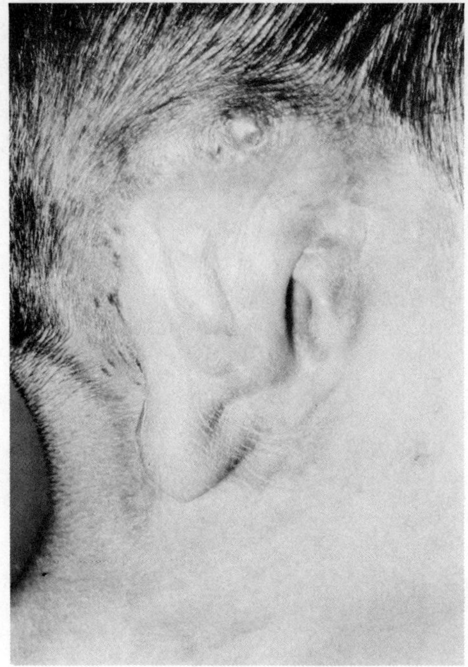

Figure 2-1b. Range of microtia.

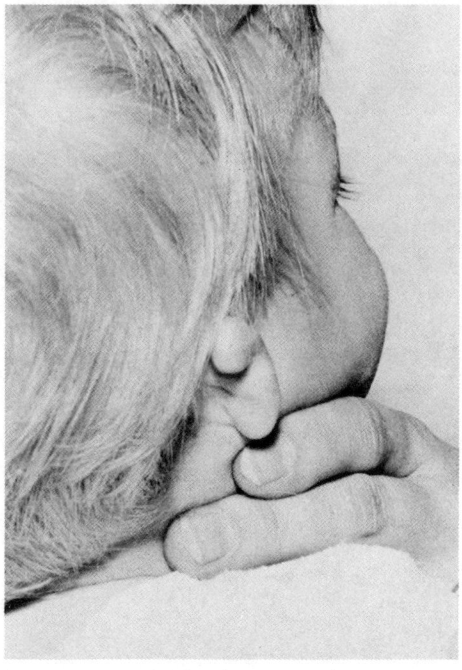

Figure 2-1c. Range of microtia.

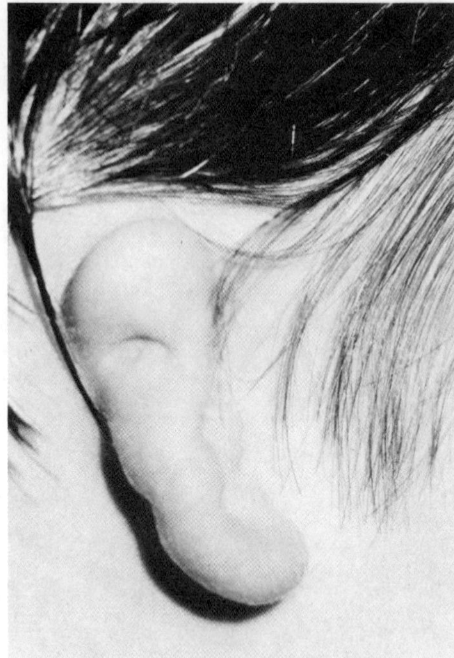

Figure 2-1d. Range of microtia.

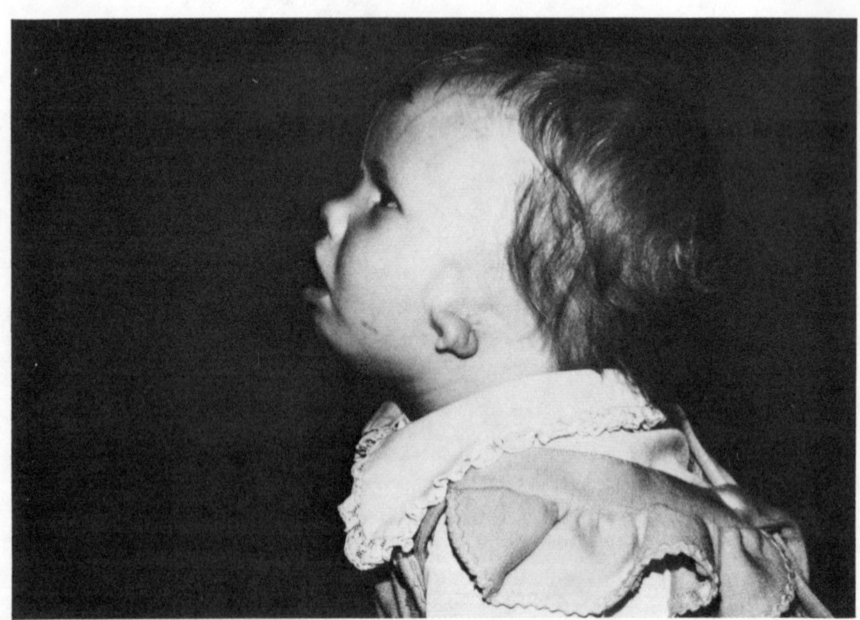

Figure 2-1e. Range of microtia.

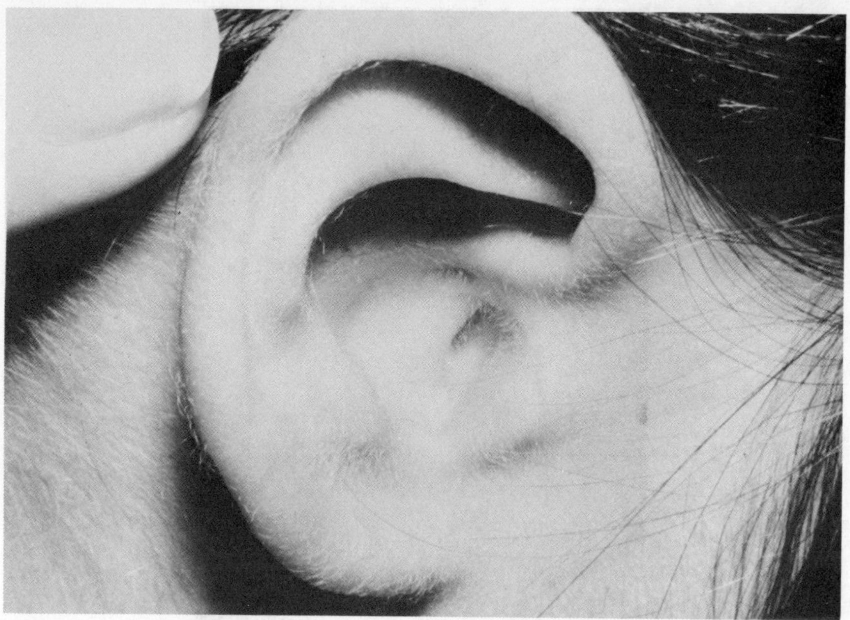

Figure 2-1f. Range of microtia.

There are some peculiar things known about microtia which are rather interesting and are not easily explained. Microtia is usually unilateral. It occurs twice as often on the right side of the face as it does on the left. It occurs twice as frequently in males as it does in females. Microtia may be due to some form of interruption of development which occurs at a vulnerable period in utero, or it may be an inherited disability.

A university clinic reported one family in which the mother and all three of her sons had congenital atresia without microtia. The members of that family all had moderate hearing losses due to the atresia; yet they had no immediately obvious signs (except upon close examination) of external ear anomaly. Clearly, the problem was a genetic disorder — one that had also occurred in the mother's sister. Curiously, though, the malformation did not occur in the grandparents, nor did it appear in the sister's children. One should assume, therefore, that the problem is due to a recessive mode of inheritance, a subject discussed in chapter 6.

OTHER ANOMALIES

Sometimes, patients have anomalies of the external ear and related structures that are not necessarily obvious. An extreme case would be the family described above in which there was atresia but no microtia. Other cases can be even more unusual, presenting with pre-auricular tags or an accessory auricle located near, or not so near, the pinna (figure 2-2); fistulae (pre-auricular pits) and cysts (figure 2-3). A fistula is a pit-like depression which may lead to a cyst, an epidermis-lined fistulous tract *(Paparella, 1973)*.

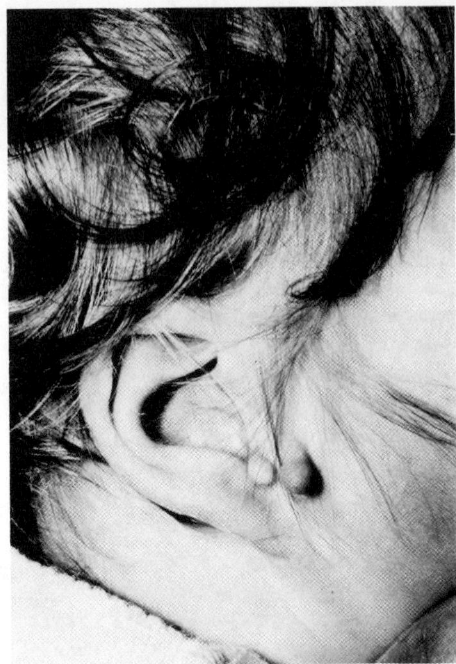

Figure 2-2. Accessory auricle.

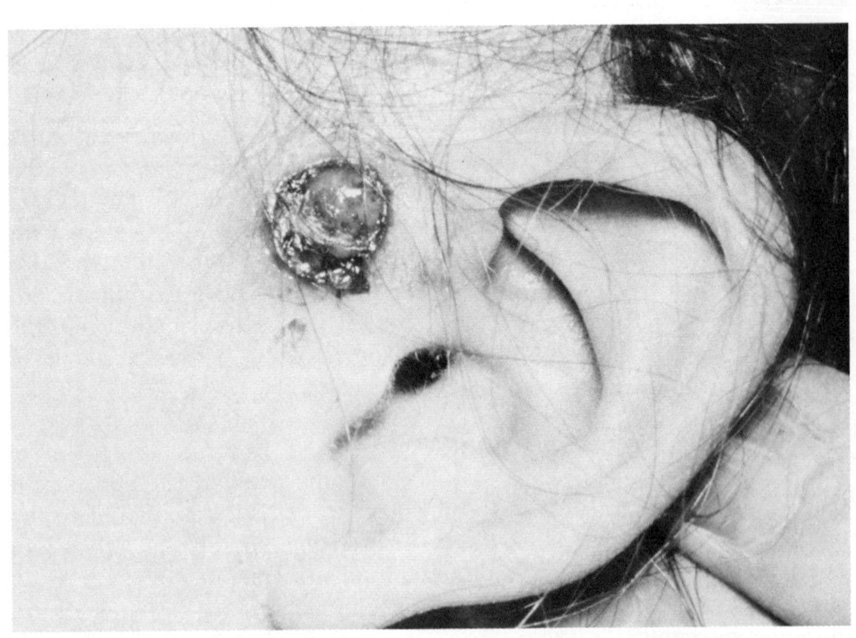

Figure 2-3. Pre-auricular pit with fistula.

At first thought, it might seem quite unimportant that a patient has a rudimentary pinna in addition to his normal ones, that he has a little tag or pit in front of his ear, or some sort of cartilaginous growth near the ear. In fact, it may not matter. In many cases, however, it does matter, as these things are frequently signs of other pathology. For example, one clinic reported the case of a pre-auricular pit on a grown woman who had always thought it was a type of dimple. The woman complained of a sudden hearing problem which had been related to her middle ear. Otological examination revealed that this pit was, in fact, a canal one and one-half inches long which was migrating into the middle ear. She was actually having severe middle ear problems because the canal had become infected and was allowing contaminants to reach the middle ear. Surgical correction was required.

Just as the pinnae may be too small or even missing, they can also be too large *(macrotia);* low set; or even placed at unusual angles *(lop ear)* on the head. The important concept is not specific placement, but rather that unusual placement can mean an associated malformation in the ear canal or middle ear, and that the patient should be carefully evaluated for hearing loss.

COMPLEX CRANIO-FACIAL ANOMALIES

Especially important anomalies of the external ear are those which are among the several stigmata of certain cranio-facial anomalies. The patient who has an anomaly of the external ear and of some other part of the face may have difficulties which are cosmetic, psychological, and/or sensorimotor, in addition to auditory dysfunction. For example, the patient who has a complex cranio-facial anomaly may first seek cosmetic treatment for appearance, and may then require the intervention of a speech pathologist for such things as velopharyngeal insufficiency and/or articulatory disorders. It is important that the audiologist be aware of speech disorders, and that speech pathologists be alert to the probability of a hearing impairment in such a patient. An encyclopedic discussion of the hundreds of complex cranio-facial anomalies is found in Konigsmark and Gorlin (1976); the reader is referred also to Mawson (1967), Gerber (1977), and Jaffe (1978).

As illustrations, two of the more common and apparent disorders are presented here. They are Treacher-Collins Syndrome and Crouzon's Disease.

TREACHER-COLLINS SYNDROME. Figure 2-4 is an example of Treacher-Collins Syndrome, properly called mandibulofacial dysostosis, which means a failure of bony development of the mandible and the face. It occurs in about 1.5% of congenital hearing losses. It results from a dominant, genetic mode of inheritance which means that it will be passed along to the offspring (see chapter 5). It is characterized by: 1) microtia (85%) and atresia (30%-40%) with accompanying conductive hearing impairment (although a sensory hearing loss has been noted in some patients); 2) a notch of the lower eye lid called coloboma; 3) a characteristic facial appearance caused by the maldevelopment of the bones of the face, especially those associated with the tempero-mandibular joint; 4) occurrence more often in males than in females.

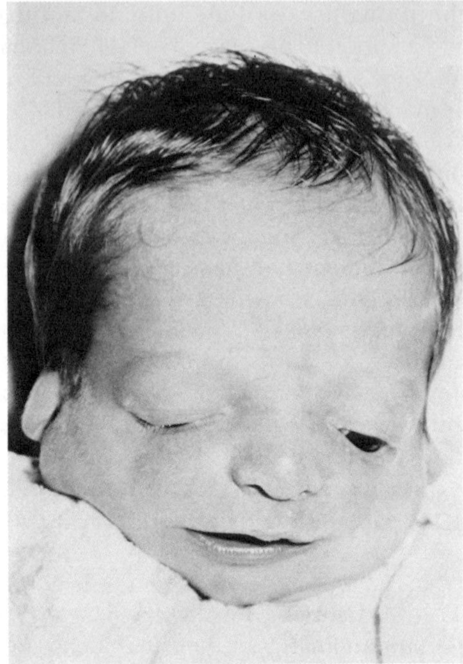

Figure 2-4a. Infant with Treacher-Collins Syndrome.

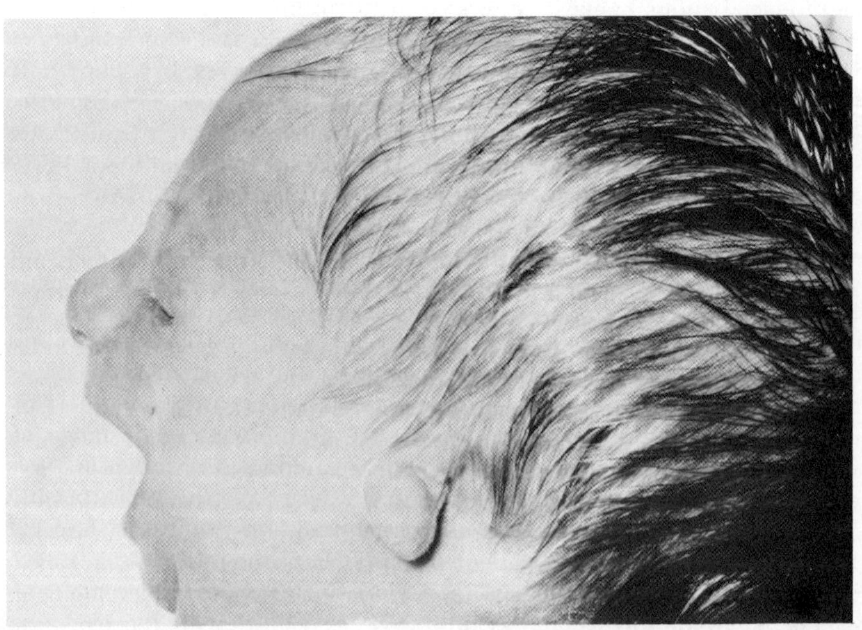

Figure 2-4b. Profile of same infant.

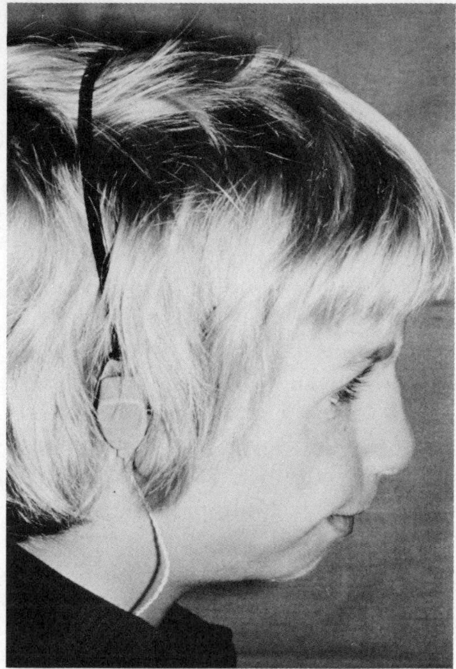

Figure 2-4c. Same child aged 10 years.

According to Konigsmark and Gorlin (1976) radiographic and surgical investigations have shown sclerosis of the middle and (rarely) inner ear, with poor delineation of structures; or there may be fixation, fusion, malformation, or absence of any one or all of the ossicles and/or the oval window. Furthermore, abnormalities of the labyrinth have been found in 25% of the patients. In short, conductive and/or sensory hearing loss, and a host of other sequelae, may be present. These all accompany, of course, an unusual facial structure.

Something of great importance needs to be introduced here. It is all too easy to see a child with Treacher-Collins Syndrome or some other cranio-facial anomaly, and come to an incorrect and dangerous conclusion. The harmful, old term "a funny looking kid" is a classic example. First, no one wants to be considered funny looking. Second, the fact that people may have a peculiar appearance should elicit great sympathy and not embarrassment in those of us who observe them. Third, and most importantly, the vast majority of patients with cranio-facial anomalies have normal intelligence and normal emotions. They know how they look, and they know how others look at them. It is essential to recognize that these patients are normal human beings who happen to have anomalies of the face which, by the way, can be improved by some rather marvelous surgical procedures. It is offensive to deal with such patients as though they suffer from profound mental retardation or severe emotional disturbance. They do not. They do suffer, however, from conductive hearing impairments. The audiologist assumes the full rehabilitative responsibility for such a patient as he must deal not only with the conductive hearing loss, but he must also be a counselor for a person with an anomalous face. If the audiologist is not able to be the counselor, he must refer the patient to a psychotherapist when that is required.

CROUZON'S DISEASE. Another relatively common example of a complex cranio-facial disorder is Crouzon's Disease. Patients with Crouzon's Disease, unlike those with Treacher-Collins Syndrome, usually do not have microtia or atresia, but are likely to have bony anomalies of the middle ear. The striking feature of Crouzon's Disease is an anomaly of the orbit which produces a characteristic bulging of the eyes known as *exophthalmos*. This is accompanied by other ocular deformities such as *hypertelorism* (increased distance between the eyes) and *strabismus* (cross eye). There are also anomalies of the nose and maxilla which contribute further to characteristic facies or facial appearance (figure 2-5). Such patients are likely to have normal intelligence and normal emotions, and must be treated accordingly. When the stigmata of Crouzon's Disease are accompanied by anomalies of the hands or feet (the so-called "lobster claw anomaly"), it is known as Apert's Syndrome.

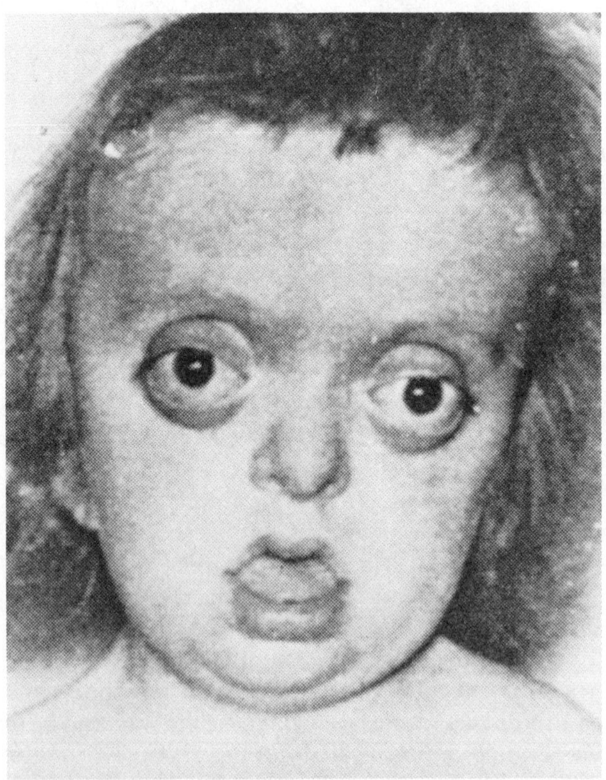

Figure 2-5a. Crouzon's Disease. *(Reproduced with permission of Laryngoscope).*

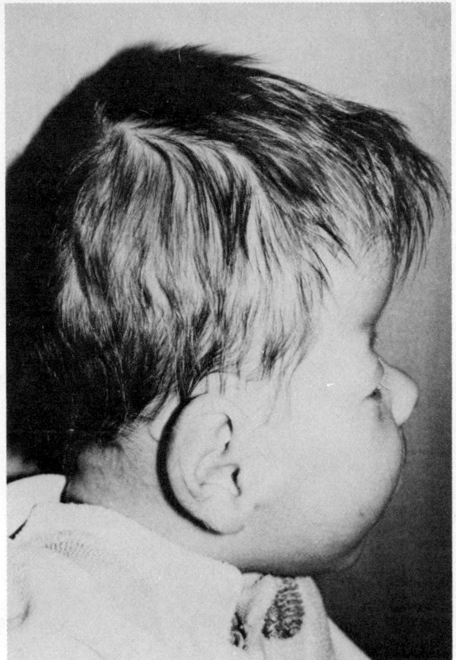

Figure 2-5b. Crouzon's Disease.

Most notable among the defects, associated with Crouzon's Disease, that affect hearing are an infrequent deformity of the acoustic meatus, ossicular ankylosis (fixation) or anomaly, and atresia of the ear canal. Occasionally the atresia is bilateral. Patients have been reported to have an absence of a tympanic membrane and middle ear structures. The most prevalent finding is fixation of the stapes to the promontory *(Konigsmark and Gorlin, 1976)*. In fact, Fraser (1976) reported a case in which Crouzon's Disease was mistaken for otosclerosis (see chapter 4).

Hearing loss is present in approximately one-third of the cases *(Boedts, 1967)*. The loss is conductive in the majority of the cases. It should be noted, however, that because microtia, or other similar anomaly of the pinna, rarely present in this disease, the patient may exhibit no overt or outward signs of ear anomaly but may still have a bilateral malformation of the ear canal and/or middle ear structures and demonstrate an associated hearing loss.

MEDICAL CONSIDERATIONS

What is to be done? Because microtia and atresia are usually unilateral, and hearing is not affected, frequently nothing is done. The problem is primarily cosmetic and will usually be dealt with by plastic surgery to provide a more normal looking pinna. Another approach would be the substitution of a prosthesis for the abnormal ear (figure 2-6). A still better solution might simply be long hair; although age, sex, and current fashions may influence that decision.

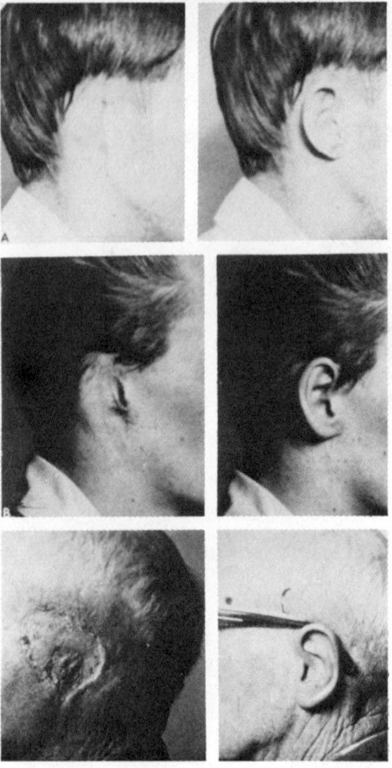

Figure 2-6. Prosthetic pinnae. *(Reproduced with permission of the W.B. Saunders Co.)*

There is no question that, in the case of cranio-facial anomaly, cosmetic surgery may be more important than anything else. When that procedure succeeds, it succeeds strikingly. For example, figure 2-7 illustrates the pre- and post-surgical appearance of a patient with extreme Apert's Syndrome. There will undoubtedly be unanimous agreement that, post-surgically, the young man is not beautiful by anyone's standards; but look at the change. Vive la difference!

Surgical intervention is usually not recommended to restore middle ear function. Occasionally, however, it is. Normally, of course, the operation would involve only one ear. The procedure is conceptually simple but, in fact, the surgery is difficult. It involves creating an ear canal where one does not exist. Many things must be done before surgery can take place. Remember that, developmentally, the ear canal arises from the same source as the tympanic annulus, malleus, and incus. Before creating a new meatus, the surgeon must know the extent of cochlear function, and what structures will be found within the middle ear cavity at the end of the new canal *(Nager, 1973)*. For this, simple skull X-rays are inadequate. What is required is a procedure called polytomography, which is a series of X-ray "slices" of tissue.

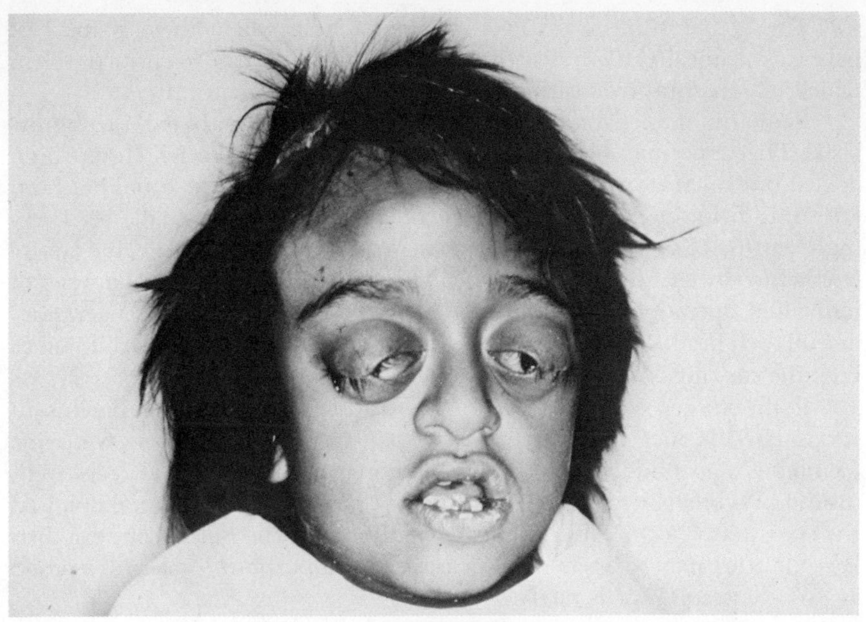

Figure 2-7a. Severe cranio-facial anomaly — pre-operative. *(Courtesy of George Chierici, D.D.S.)*

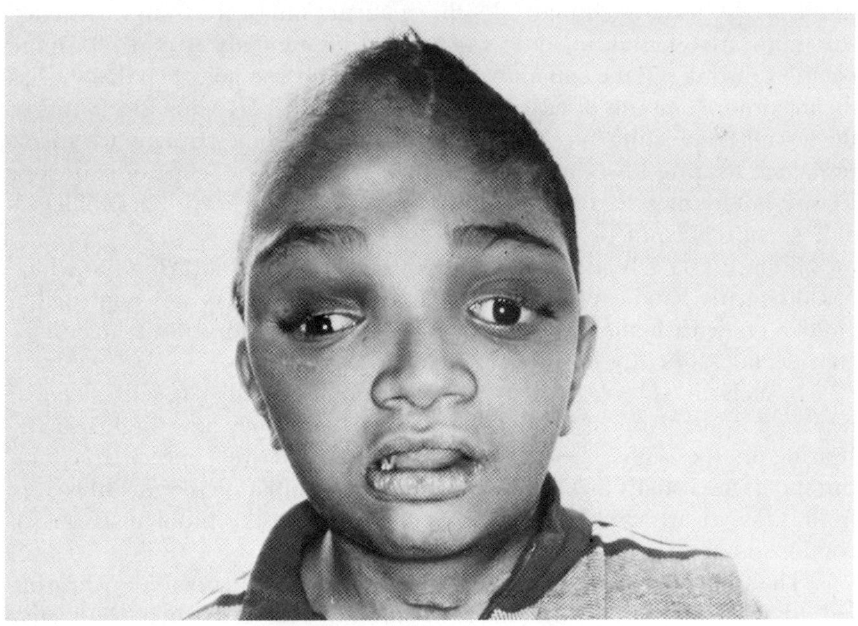

Figure 2-7b. Severe cranio-facial anomaly — post-operative. *(Courtesy of George Chierici, D.D.S.)*

The actual surgery involves drilling a hole where there is the best pathway. Ironically, it is a situation of going against nature to cure a problem which is unnatural by creating a natural structure, unnaturally.

If an arm or a leg, or any other bone in the body, is broken, it will grow back. The same may be true for the temporal bone tissue which has been drilled out to create an ear canal. Thus, a newly formed ear canal has been known to fill itself in. The failure rate of this surgery had actually been very high because of such a natural regenerative process. For example, the family referred to earlier, in which four members had atresia, underwent a series of individual operations to cure the problem. Four ears underwent operation, one on each head. Three of the four failed simply because it was so difficult to keep the ear canals open.

If the surgery does succeed, and because of recent developments in surgical techniques most do, then the patient will have a new tympanic membrane and middle ear sound conducting mechanism. If all goes well, instead of a bilateral moderate hearing loss, the result will be an individual with essentially normal hearing in one ear. If surgery succeeds for one ear, then later the other may be operated. Because, for most purposes, one ear is as good as two, the second ear is rarely done.

AUDIOLOGICAL CONSIDERATIONS

When dealing with a patient who has a microtia and/or an atresia, several things must be considered. First of all, it is important to stress that, since the problem is usually unilateral, the patient rarely has an associated communicative handicap, unless of course the anomaly is part of a more complex disorder. If the patient has no ear canal on one side, then that ear has the maximum amount of hearing loss possible (55dB HL) due to a failure of the sound conducting mechanism. It is true that some patients who have unilateral hearing losses may have trouble hearing in a theatre or church or lecture, but for most there is no significant auditory handicap. The problem is almost entirely cosmetic.

If the atresia is bilateral, then the patient will suffer a hearing loss which could be truly handicapping. In fact, since these disorders are congenital, a child born with bilateral atresia of the external auditory meati may have considerable difficulty learning spoken language.

In such cases the audiometric configuration is usually flat, with an equal hearing loss across most frequencies. Some patients may have slightly better hearing in the higher frequencies (2000Hz and above). Speech reception thresholds are usually at 45 to 55dB. Speech discrimination scores will be very high, often nearly 100%. This last is true because the problem is one of conduction and not of sensory function.

The audiologist will often recommend a bone conduction type of hearing aid for patients with cranio-facial syndromes and associated conductive hearing losses (figure 2-8). Such aids greatly assist the patient by providing signals which bypass the middle ear and which stimulate the cochlea directly.

These patients often require supportive services from speech pathology as well. Poor use of muscle structure, abnormal dentition, poor vision and hearing, and a host of other factors often result in speech and language delays which require treatment.

Modern medicine, surgery, and habilitative procedures have improved the lives of patients with complex cranio-facial disorders. Cosmetic surgery, hearing aids, and speech therapy often allow such individuals to lead normal lives.

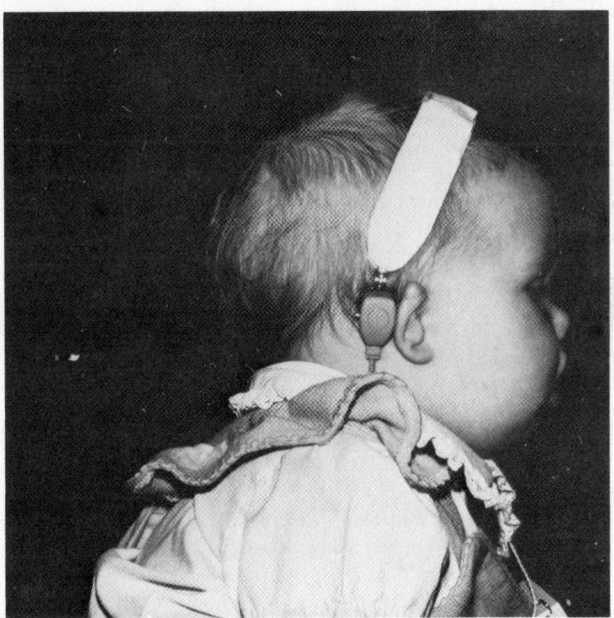

Figure 2-8. Bone conduction hearing aid.

CASE STUDY 2-1: ATRESIA

KM, aged 2 years, exhibits Goldenhaar's Syndrome. She had an initial evaluation in the office of Dr. D, and was referred to us for further testing. We found that she could localize to speech in the sound field at 55dB HTL with the signal on her right and at 50dB HTL with it on her left. A startle to speech was elicited at 70dB HTL. When a bone conduction vibrator was held to her mastoid area, and a signal of only 20dB HTL was presented, she stopped sucking on her bottle and lateralized appropriately. These data confirm the conductive nature of her hearing impairment. We have prescribed a hearing aid with a bone conduction vibrator and have begun a program of auditory habilitation.

CASE STUDY 2-2:

CRANIO-FACIAL ANOMALY

DC, now 13 years of age, presents with a congenital bilateral atresia of the ear canals concomitant with Treacher-Collins Syndrome. He was first seen at the age of 6 months, and at that time was fitted with a body-type hearing aid with bone conduction receiver. His mother and an older sister also display the stigmata of Treacher-Collins Syndrome. In addition, he has an isolated cleft of the palate. Palatal repair was completed when he was 15 months old; furthermore, he had additional facial surgery which included silicon implants, skin grafts, and dental restorations at the ages of 5 years and 5 years, 3 months. Radiological studies indicate that he has quite good palatal agility, although the speech pathologist reports that he has mild hyponasality and hypernasality. He does have some articulatory errors consistent with cleft palate, but generally his speech is intelligible.

When he was almost 7 years of age, an attempt was made to excise the atresia on the left side. The otologist, Dr. W, reported that he encountered thick solid bone after he had removed spongy bone. He decided to terminate the procedure to avoid endangering the inner ear which X-ray revealed to be normal. Unfortunately, the audiometric results which were reported did not indicate that contralateral masking had been used during the air conduction and bone conduction tests.

Now at 13 years of age, DC continues to display audiograms consistent with the conductive impairment of bilateral atresia. Speech audiometry was in correspondence with pure tone results; speech discrimination was 84% on the right and 92% on the left. He functions quite successfully, still wearing a body type aid with bone conduction receiver. It was recommended that he get a new aid of the same type.

(The symbol "A" on the audiogram indicates the aided sound field threshold.)

CASE STUDY 2-2: CRANIO-FACIAL ANOMALY

PURE TONE AUDIOGRAM

RIGHT EAR

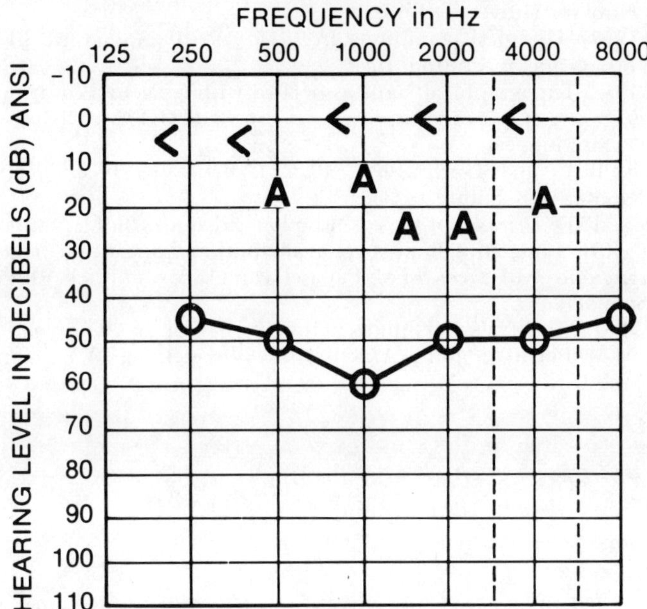

LEFT EAR

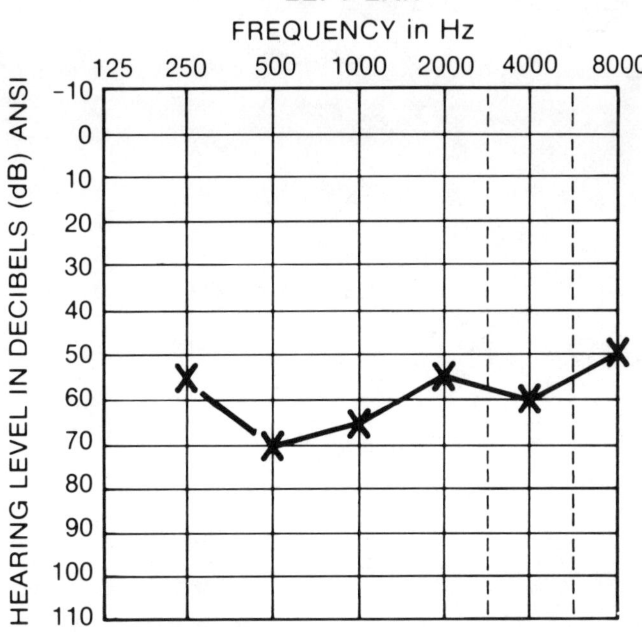

REFERENCES

Batteau, D.W. 1967. The role of the pinna in human localization. *Proceedings of the Royal Society* (London), Ser. B. 168: 158-180.

Boedts, D. 1967. La surdité dans la dysostose craniofaciale ou maladie de Crouzon. *Acta Otolaryngol. Belg.* 21:143-155.

Fraser, G.R. 1976. *The causes of profound deafness in childhood.* Baltimore: The Johns Hopkins University Press.

Gerber, S.E. 1977, High-risk conditions. In *Audiometry in infancy*, ed. S.E. Gerber. New York: Grune & Stratton, Inc.

Jaffe, B.F. 1978. Topographical signs associated with congenital hearing loss. In *Early diagnosis of hearing loss*, eds. S.E. Gerber and G.T. Mencher. New York: Grune & Stratton, Inc.

Konigsmark, B.W. and Gorlin, R.J. 1976. *Genetic and metabolic deafness.* Philadelphia: W.B. Saunders Co.

Mawson, S.R. 1967. *Diseases of the ear.* London: Edward Arnold.

Nager, G.T. 1973. Congenital aural atresia: anatomy and surgical management. In *Otolaryngology*, vol. 2, eds. M.M. Paparella and D.A. Shumrick. Philadelphia: W.B. Saunders Co.

Paparella, M.M. 1973. Cysts and tumors of the external ear. In *Otolaryngology*, vol. 2, eds. M.M. Paparella and D.A. Shumrick. Philadelphia: W.B. Saunders Co.

CHAPTER 3

Otitis Media

Otitis — meaning an infection or inflammation of the ear — is qualified in this case by the additional word "media" referring to the middle ear. Any inflammatory condition of the cavity of the middle ear, basically disease of the mucous membrane, is properly described as otitis media. It occurs far more frequently in children than in adults with its incidence decreasing after the age of six years *(Payne and Paparella, 1976)*. Shambaugh (1967) claimed an 80% incidence in children under three years of age. The severity of this disease's sequelae has only recently begun to be fully appreciated *(Hanson and Ulvestad, 1979)*.

The orientation of this chapter encompasses two themes. First, we adopt a new otological perspective, that of Goodhill (1979), that we are considering a continuum of disease processes all of which may be subsumed as *otomastoiditis*. Second, we view diseases of the middle ear from the audiologist's perspective of changes of the stiffness or the mass of the middle ear contents.

THE MIDDLE EAR TRANSFORMER

The primary purpose of the middle ear system in the human animal is to affect an impedance match between a gas medium (air) and a fluid medium (the cochlear fluids). A sound wave traveling through air and striking a liquid surface would be almost totally reflected. The middle ear mechanism affects an air-fluid interface by providing a mechanical amplifier which transduces the air-borne sound to the cochlea for fluid-borne transmission. Hence, the middle ear system "facilitates the transfer of sound in our environment to the cochlea" *(Feldman and Wilber, 1976)* and is, therefore, an impedance matching transformer.

When a sound wave travels the length of the ear canal and strikes the tympanic membrane, some of its energy will be transmitted to the ossicular chain and some will be reflected. This depends in part upon the frequency of the tone, but depends primarily upon the stiffness encountered at the drum membrane. Obviously, the stiffer the membrane, the greater the amount of the reflection, and the poorer will be the hearing for that ear. Hence, any pathological condition of the middle ear which increases the stiffness of the ossicular chain will be reflected in the form of increased resistance of the drum membrane to a sound wave striking it. The terminology in current use would describe such an ear as having a high impedance (i.e., the energy transfer is impeded) or a low admittance (i.e., little energy is admitted into the middle ear system). The opposite can occur also. If, for example, the incus were to become disarticulated from its connection to the stapes, the stiffness of the system would decrease markedly; this is a condition of low impedance or high admittance. Normally, the system's impedance lies between such extremes.

Stiffness is the principal component of the middle ear impedance. However, changes of the mass of the contents of the middle ear will also be reflected in changes of impedance. Clearly, the main source of the mass component is the ossicles themselves, and changes of their mass caused by disease or injury will also change the stiffness of the system. In general, changes of the mass will not be reflected as changes of impedance except for frequencies lower than 600Hz *(Simons, 1979)*.

Pathology and Etiology

Goodhill (1979) views *otomastoiditis* as a continuum of tubotympanitis-otitis-mastoiditis. All steps in this continuum do not necessarily occur, but the sequence is necessary. That is, not every one with tubotympanitis gets otitis media, and certainly not everyone with otitis gets mastoiditis, nor do they necessarily occur in rapid order; however, otitis follows tubotympanitis, and mastoiditis follows otitis. Table 3-1 (adapted from Goodhill) exhibits the sequence, and provides the outline for this section.

Table 3-1. Sequential Patterns of the
Tubotympanitis-Otomastoiditis Continuum*

1. Acute and Subacute Patterns
    A. Transitory tubotympanitis (mild mucositis, negative pressure, no middle ear fluid)
    B. Acute tubotympanitis (mucositis, negative pressure, clear serous or serosanguineous middle ear fluid)
    C. Acute purulent otitis media (tubotympanic mucositis, negative pressure, seropus, pus)
    D. Subacute or chronic secretory otitis media (tubotympanic mucositis, tubal blockade, sustained

---

adapted from pp. 295-6 Goodhill (1979) with permission of the author and Harper & Row Inc.

<ul style="list-style:none">
<li>negative pressure, seromucoid fluid — "glue" ear)</li>
</ul>

E. Acute otomastoiditis (tympanomastoid mucositis plus osteitis, mucopurulent middle ear and mastoid exudate)

F. Acute otomastoiditis with complications (labyrinthitis, lateral sinus thrombophlebitis, meningitis, etc.)

2. Chronic — Type A

A. Chronic otomastoiditis with tympanic fibrosis (healed osteitis, no middle ear fluid, middle ear and mastoid fibrosis, tympanic membrane perforations)

B. Chronic purulent otomastoiditis (otomastoiditis, mucosal polyposis, granulomatosis, osteitis, ossicular necrosis, purulent exudate, tympanic membrane perforation)

3. Chronic — Type B

A. Chronic purulent otomastoiditis with tympanosclerosis (otomastoiditis, osteitis, mucositis, tympanosclerosis, ossicular necrosis, and/or fixation, mucopurulent middle ear exudate, tympanic membrane perforation)

B. Chronic purulent otomastoiditis with keratoma (cholesteatoma), (otomastoiditis, osteitis, granulomatosis, polyposis, ossicular necrosis, keratoma in middle ear, mastoid, or both, and tympanic membrane perforation)

C. Chronic purulent otomastoiditis with tympanosclerosis and keratoma (cholesteatoma)

D. Chronic purulent otomastoiditis with keratoma (cholesteatoma), and/or tympanosclerosis, and complications (cranial nerve, meningitis, sigmoid sinus thrombophlebitis, brain abscess)

ACUTE AND SUBACUTE PATTERNS

During a period of an upper respiratory infection, especially in a child, there is a high probability of a transitory tubotympanitis. This arises from a closure of the Eustachian tube due to swelling, negative pressures, or infection from the nasopharynx. This transitory disease may become acute and lead to acute otitis media.

One expects to encounter otitis media in a child who is complaining of a sore throat and who has, or has just had, a cold or other upper respiratory infection. The respiratory mucous membrane contains an enzyme (lysozome) to fight bacterial invasion. In response to invasion, the production of mucous is increased, but "these epithelial tissues do not always distinguish between a dangerous live parasite and harmless inanimate protein" *(Shambaugh, 1967)*. Hence, the preceding condition may be allergenic.

This disease may go through a number of stages of varying severity.

Beginning with a subtle onset (i.e., transitory tubotympanitis), it flares to a powerful acute stage (acute tubotympanitis) and has a potential for leading to acute and then chronic otomastoiditis which can be both progressive and quite handicapping. Usually, parents become aware of acute tubotympanitis when it reaches the stage where their child complains of pain. Fortunately, the painful acute stage is of a rather short duration. The procedure at that stage is medical evaluation and drug therapy which usually resolves the infection.

Sometimes, when a patient has recovered from the initial infection (e.g., a cold), there is a possibility that the Eustachian tube may have become, or may remain, blocked. This is because of sloughing of epithelium and increased production of mucous. This tends to create a partial vacuum in the middle ear cavity. The inability to clear the middle ear and eliminate the partial vacuum triggers a response in which the mucosa exude a clear fluid which is devoid of pus and/or bacteria. Presumably, this fluid bath is designed to flush out the middle ear through the Eustachian drain. However, it doesn't always work, and frequently the fluid is not drained off and remains in the middle ear cavity. This condition is called *secretory otitis media,* meaning, simply, that there is a condition of the middle ear in which secretion is present. In this case, the secretion is a sterile fluid. However, the accumulation of sterile fluid may continue, resulting in swelling of the lining of the Eustachian tube and/or the middle ear cavity. This may be reflected as well in bulging of the tympanic membrane. The presence of the fluid in the middle ear gives rise, as it should, to a feeling of fullness. That feeling is often the principal complaint of the patient who has secretory otitis media. While it is possible for there to be a certain amount of pain with secretory otitis media, it is usually substantially less pain than occurs in acute otomastoiditis. Furthermore, Shambaugh (1967) has observed that "the virus, by destroying the ciliated epithelium, removes the first line of defense and permits bacterial invasion of the tissues . . ."

Goodhill (1979) states that "acute otomastoiditis and secretory otitis media are the most common antecedents of chronic otomastoiditis . . ." He reminds us that the pneumatic relations between the cavity of the middle ear and the air cells of the mastoid are complex. Consequently, there are various routes for the infection to travel to the mastoid air cells. Irrespective of the transport mechanism, Goodhill calls infection of any part of this air-cell system mastoiditis. Since acute mastoiditis is a result of acute otitis media, together they are called acute otomastoiditis.

If the sterile secretion does not drain or dissolve, but rather remains in the middle ear cavity, it is exposed to further infection and continued colds. Because the cavity is a warm, dark, moist place in which bacteria thrive, the serous fluid becomes a breeding ground for disease. The result is that the clear sterile fluid generated by the mucosal lining of the middle ear as a protective mechanism becomes just the opposite, a bacteria-laden pus, which can cause pain as it expands (in 12 to 24 hours) within the middle ear and presses against the tympanic membrane. Such a condition is called *acute purulent otitis media.* Sometimes the amount of fluid increases to the point that the tympanic membrane will rupture, resulting in a draining ear. At such a stage in the infection, the continued prescription of an antibiotic drug is essential to prevent the spread of bacterial disease. Bacterial (i.e., purulent) otitis media is more common than viral otitis media, and is the form usually seen in clinical otology.

Acute purulent otitis media is distinguishable from acute viral otitis media by several characteristics. Primary among them is that the disease is self-limiting, i.e., if there are no complications, it will go away. Furthermore, it is easily susceptible to antibiotic therapy which also relieves an accompanying fever. Antibiotics usually react against only those organisms which produce the disease, while having little or no effect on the subsequent symptoms such as serous exudate. Sometimes, then, the infection disappears because it has been cured; sometimes not. However, a serous residue may remain in the cavity of the middle ear.

Prolonged and/or recurrent serous otitis media may result in an accumulation of fluid which is so thick and viscid that a condition which is often called "glue ear" may appear. A more proper term for this condition is *adhesive otitis media,* a descriptive phrase indicating that the gluey fluid adheres to the ossicles.

Disease of the mastoid portion of the temporal bone, *mastoiditis,* may result from acute or chronic otitis media. At first, its symptoms are the same as those of the early stages of acute otitis media. But, according to Ruben (1972), an acute otitis media may result in acute mastoiditis within one to two weeks following the initial infection. As it continues, it will be revealed by a displacement of the pinna in the anterior direction due to the large amount of purulent swelling behind it (figure 3-1). This pus produces an abcess beneath the temporalis muscle. It must be treated both with antibiotics and with surgical drainage of the mastoid. Today this condition is rare with early and adequate antibiotic treatment of the acute otitis media.

Long-standing running ears (otorrhea) is a common symptom of chronic mastoiditis. In this case, it is rare to find clinical signs of active infection, but audiometry will reveal a conductive hearing loss. Chronic mastoiditis can lead to erosion of the temporal bone and eventually to inflammation of some of the cranial nerves. It can also lead to temporal lobe abcess or generalized meningitis. It must be treated surgically.

These prolonged acute and subacute conditions — whether serous, purulent, or adhesive — produce the various forms of chronic otomastoiditis.

Chronic Patterns

Goodhill (1979) divides chronic otomastoiditis into two types: Type A with reversible lesions, and Type B with irreversible pathology. Type A is further divided into two categories, namely, with and without purulence. On the other hand, the four categories which Goodhill included under Type B are all purulent.

Chronic non-purulent otomastoiditis (Type A) is characterized by tympanic fibrosis. In fact, progressive fibrosis "is a frequent sequel to secretory otitis." *(Goodhill and Brockman, 1979)* and takes many forms. It is

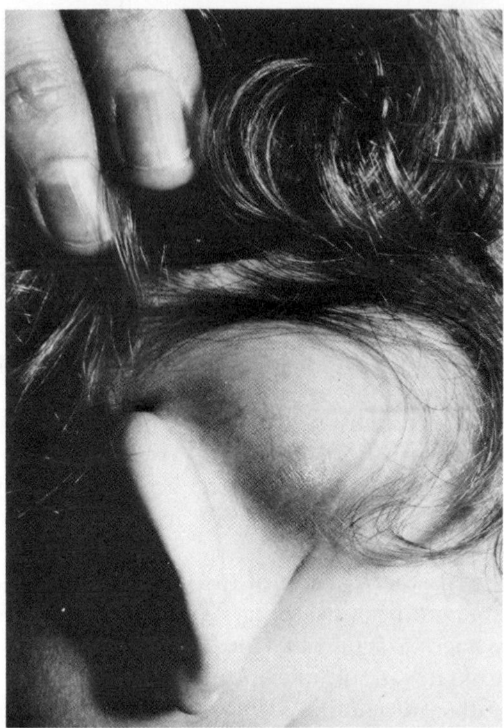

Figure 3-1a. Swelling accompanying acute mastoiditis.

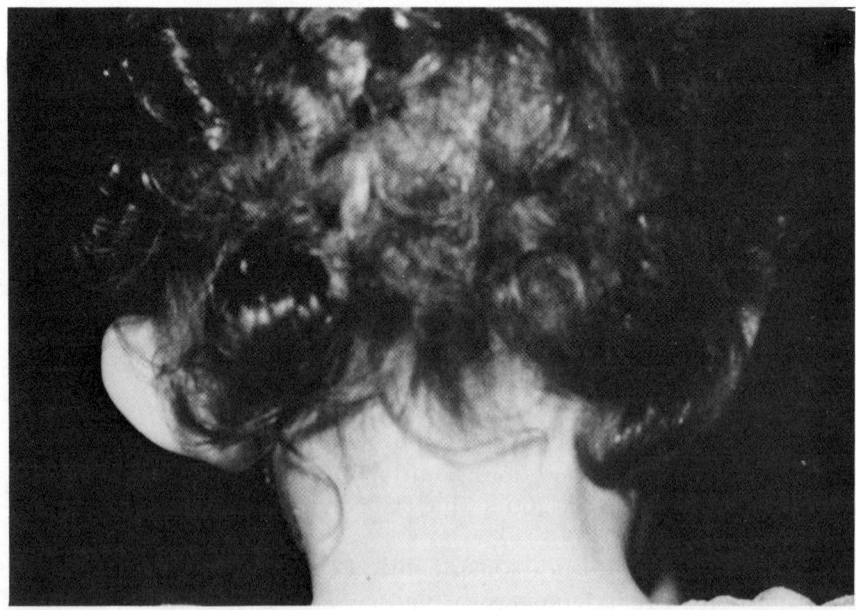

Figure 3-1b. Swelling accompanying acute mastoiditis.

distinguished by fibrous compartments or pockets in the mucosa of the tympanic cavity. One may find bands of scar tissue tying the ossicles to each other or to the tympanic membrane, and sometimes connecting the ossicles to the promontory.

The purulent form of Type A otomastoiditis may result in the growth of polyps in the mucosa and the development of granulomatosis and osteitis. There could be a purulent exudate through a ruptured tympanic membrane. In fact, Shambaugh (1967) claimed that perforation always occurs and the discharge is always mucoid. Frequently, the polypoid granuloma will fill the mastoid antrum; they may even extrude into the external meatus through the perforation. Osteitis of the mastoid is rare, but osteitis of the ossicles frequently occurs.

All classes of Type B chronic otomastoiditis are typified by purulence. The four classes are divided as 1) with tympanosclerosis, 2) with keratoma, 3) with tympanosclerosis and keratoma, and 4) any of the first three with complications.

Tympanosclerosis is marked by a variety of changes of the middle ear contents. The membranes become dense and inelastic from various chronic inflammations. There is a dense fibrosis which gives this disease its name of sclerosis. Secondarily, there may be destruction of bone and formation of new bone. Also, the lesions may be covered by different kinds of epithelium.

A keratoma (historically called cholesteatoma) is a pouch-like structure which may occur in any part of the temporal bone, but which characteristically occurs in the cavity of the middle ear. Unless infected by a secondary purulent otitis media, the patient with a keratoma rarely complains of pain. Thus, expansion of the mass — which may be as small as a seed or as large as a golf ball — may be insidious in nature and go unnoticed for many years. For example, one 71-year-old patient's keratoma probably had its etiology based on ear disease more than 50 years earlier.

Keratomas which are congenital are very rare, and they may occur anywhere in the cranial structures. Acquired keratomas are usually associated with long-standing perforations of the tympanic membrane. Keratomas are sometimes idiopathic, which means that they arise spontaneously; but usually they are caused by a long-standing disease or injury in the middle ear. For example, an old chronic otomastoiditis which resulted in a perforation of the tympanic membrane which healed poorly can give rise to a keratoma at the site of the old perforation. This is called secondary acquired keratoma. Shambaugh (1967) noted that "epidermis will enter the tympanic cavity" through a perforation. Similarly, scar tissue which may have developed on the tympanic membrane as a result of a perforation, and which itself then became an irritant, can give rise to a keratoma *(Mawson, 1967)*.

If the perforation is in the central portion of the tympanic membrane, the risk of keratoma is low. If the perforation extends to the posterior-superior pars tensa margin, there is a marked increase in the risk of a keratoma. Finally, if the perforation involves the attic and is in the pars flaccida, there is a serious risk of keratoma because of osteitis. The exact reason why these structures form is not really known. The method of formation is apparently related to the shedding of squamous epithelial tissue from around the surface of the perforation and into a trap-like pocket which develops. This material being shed is composed primarily of keratin, and is a favorable medium for culturing bacteria.

Goodhill (1979) claims that keratoma "of the temporal bone is the most common cause of persistent otomastoiditis with bone necrosis" and further that it "can produce tympanic membrane perforations, necrosis of the malleus, incus, and stapes, mastoid cell-wall destruction in any part of the temporal bone, and can involve the facial nerve, labyrinth, and temporal bone vessels." The bone erodes because "the pressure exerted by the accumulating layers of desquamating epidermal debris combines with the acid reaction produced by bacterial decomposition" *(Shambaugh, 1967)*.

A still more serious matter is the third form of Type B chronic otomastoiditis in which both tympanosclerosis and keratoma occur, and hence both sets of sequelae are possible. In such a case, the keratoma may invade the entire mastoid while the tympanosclerosis involves the contents of the tympanic cavity. Obviously, major conductive hearing losses would occur and there is a considerable risk of labyrinthine involvement with sensory hearing impairment.

The fourth and final class of Type B was just suggested: whether subsequent to tympanosclerosis, or to keratoma, or to both, significant sequelae may ensue. A frequent result is a labyrinthine fistula with concomitant vestibular problems. Paralysis of the VIIth cranial (facial) nerve occurs frequently.

MEDICAL CONSIDERATIONS

When should the primary health care provider refer the patient with ear disease to an otologist? Participants at the International Conference on Early Diagnosis of Hearing Loss *(Gerber and Mencher, 1978)* discussed that question and recommended the following guidelines:

WHEREAS, middle ear effusion can occur in the newborn and in infants; and

WHEREAS, middle ear effusion may persist chronically for months or years producing a mild bilateral hearing loss; and

WHEREAS, prolonged mild hearing loss may produce speech, language, educational, and behavioral problems,

RESOLVED: particular attention should be paid to those newborns likely to have sustained middle ear effusion . . . as with all children, these newborns should be closely followed, and the effusion be considered a problem if it is sustained (more than three months) or is recurrent (over 50% of the time for six months). Diagnosis should be based upon pneumatic otoscopy, tympanometry, and audiometry. Further, if a sustained or recurrent problem is diagnosed, educational intervention

> should be applied in the form of language stimulation programs and/or low level amplification in addition to ongoing medical or surgical treatment.

These guidelines, while developed for the very young, apply also to the older patient with otomastoiditis. The primary medical consideration is eradication of the disease; the secondary goal is restoration of hearing. Clearly, eradication of a disease process which threatens audition is itself a means to restore hearing.

Howie (1975) has collected incidence data concerning otomastoiditis in children. The data suggest that otitis media in children tends to be self-propagating. That is, if a child had a first bout of otitis media before the age of 18 months, it is likely that there will be several successive bouts over the years. In fact, having had the disease once, it seems to predispose the child to having it a second time, while the second bout predisposes to the third, etc.

Drug therapy is indicated for acute or subacute otomastoiditis. Purulence exists more often than not; hence, antibiotic therapy is indicated. Amoxycillin is probably the most frequent prescription, although ampicillin is also widely used *(Eichenwald, 1979)*. Whether or not the disease is purulent, it is often desirable to attack the accrued secretion with chemical decongestants, such as Actifed. At least one-third of acute and/or subacute otic infections demonstrate no purulence as causation. However, the incidence of secondary bacterial contamination is so high that current otological management includes antibiotic treatment in essentially 100% of cases *(see Newman, 1975)*. In cases of tubotympanitis and/or secretory otitis media, it is usual to apply various combinations of antibiotics, decongestants (which may or may not be antihistamines), and mechanical intervention. Newman claims that prolonged use of decongestants is not wise because "their drying effects may impede recovery . . ."

The mechanical intervention just mentioned takes several forms. One of the simplest and most direct is a procedure known as Politzerization. This is a simple technique whereby air is forced up the Eustachian tube by insufflation through the nose (figure 3-2). The purpose of such a procedure is to ventilate the middle ear. Middle ear ventilation is expected to inhibit the accumulation of fluid and also to relieve atelectasis, a condition of airlessness which appears as a chronic retraction of the tympanic membrane. Jaffe (1979) has shown that atelectasis may persist long after the incidence of otitis media has diminished in children with cleft palates, a population especially prone to otomastoiditis (figure 3-3).

If drug therapy fails, certain forms of surgical treatments may be required. For example, in a case of a very painful acute tubotympanitis which is not resolving, or in a case of long standing chronic otomastoiditis which is not resolving, it is frequently the otologist's decision to perform a myringotomy. The prefix *myringo-* refers to the tympanic membrane. The suffix *-otomy* refers to the "cutting of." A myringotomy is usually an office procedure whereby a very tiny incision (2 or 3 mm.) is made in the tympanic membrane and the fluid withdrawn by vacuum. In the case of acute tubotympanitis, this is done primarily for the relief of the pain produced by the rather considerable intratympanic pressure associated with the disease process and its resultant fluid-based distention of the tympanic membrane. According to Shambaugh (1967), a myringotomy *should* be done if the drum membrane is thickened and bulging.

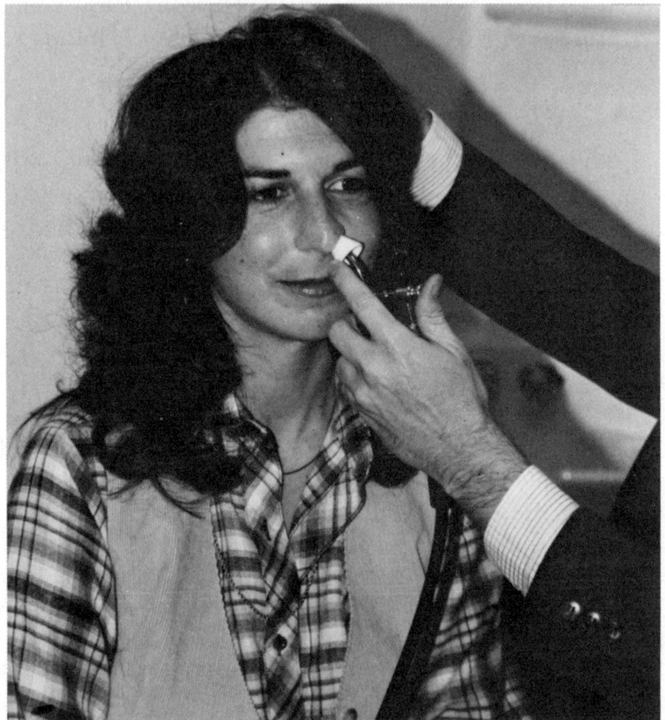

Figure 3-2. Politzerization.

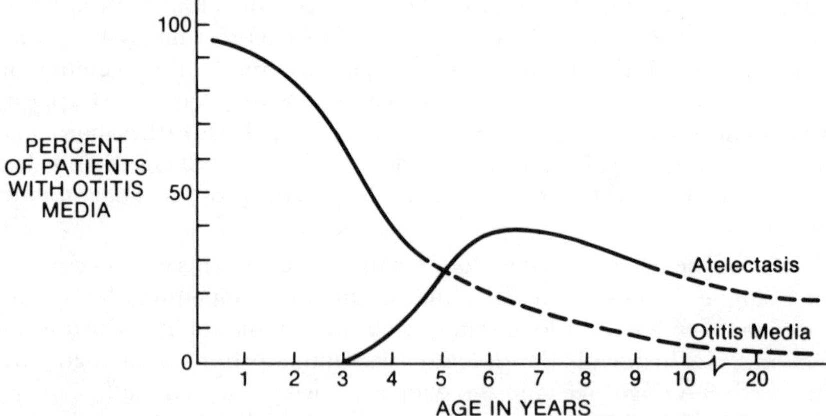

Figure 3-3. Retraction of the drum membrane (atelectasis) may continue and even increase at ages beyond which otitis media occurs frequently. *(Courtesy of Burton F. Jaffe, M.D.)*

40

For patients who have chronic otomastoiditis and/or recurrent subacute tubotympanitis — and these occur frequently in children — it is important that the myringotomy incision be kept open. It is desirable that an air passage be maintained to help air-dry the middle ear, to promote oxygenation of the tubotympanum and the mastoid air spaces, and to serve as a drain. All of these desiderata are intended to prevent the formation of a vacuum which could arise in the middle ear space if the Eustachian tube were closed or blocked, the middle ear cavity drained, and there would be no compensatory movement of air into the cavity from the outside. Normally, however, because a myringotomy usually involves a very tiny opening in the drumhead, it would heal in an hour or two. In order to keep the hole in the membrane open, a very tiny grommet (figure 3-4) is inserted into the myringotomy incision. This is usually done toward the inferior edge of the tympanic membrane to permit fluid to drain out but, primarily, for the purpose of permitting air to get in. If the middle ear cavity can be kept aerated, there is some decrease in the swelling of the cavity and of the mucosa of the Eustachian tube. As a result, no new vacuum is created in the middle ear and, of course, there is no additional exudate. The use of grommets has been wide-spread, and tends to be quite effective indeed.

The otological (i.e., surgical) treatment of glue ear is more complex than the treatment of other forms of otitis media. This highly viscid fluid usually resists break-up during a decongestant drug regime. It is just too thick for that. It is also too thick to be sucked out by a vacuum introduced through a tiny myringotomy incision, and it is so heavy that the placement of an aeration tube is of little benefit.

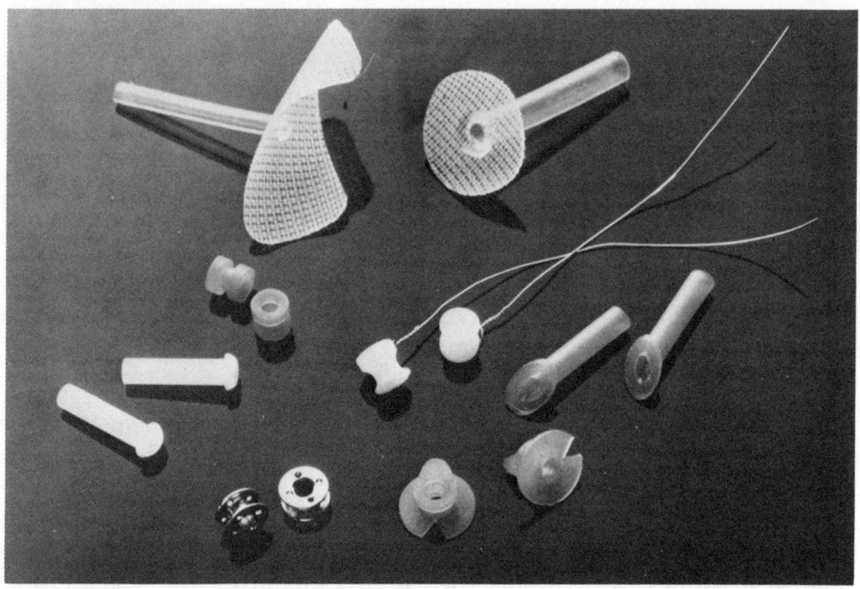

Figure 3-4. Myringotomy grommets. *(Courtesy of McGhan Medical Corp.)*

In such a case, the surgical procedure may require brief hospitalization and perhaps the use of a general anesthetic. The technique involves raising the tympanic membrane by making an incision in the skin of the ear canal, lifting the membrane with it, and then mechanically removing the adhesive glue-like substance. The fluid is often so heavy that it is common to require a surgical tweezer to remove it. Following removal, the ear canal needs to be sutured and to be packed with antibiotic-soaked gauze to prevent infection and to encourage healing. Glue ear is a serious matter, indeed, which may result in a maximum, or nearly maximum, conductive hearing impairment of 50 to 60dB.

A keratoma appears as a smooth white mass by otoscopic examination, and as it gets larger, of course, it becomes easier to see. Getting larger, it does damage to the middle ear, both to function and structure, in a variety of ways. Since it is a neoplasm — that is, a new tissue — it occupies space. And, since it occupies space in the middle ear, it alters the mass characteristics of the transmission system, thereby resulting in some amount of hearing impairment. Starting as a retraction pocket in Prussac's space or as a marginal perforation, as a keratoma becomes larger, it may also actually displace the ossicles and/or the stapedius muscle. It then alters the stiffness of the middle ear transmission system, in addition to interfering because of its very mass. Furthermore, a keratoma can become infected with bacteria, creating a secondary problem. The combination of infection and keratoma can virtually destroy the bony tissues of the middle ear. At a later stage of the disease, the tympanic membrane may be breached and a thick, green-colored, and foul smelling liquid may run from the ear (otorrhea) and everyone knows that treatment is essential. Drug therapy may resolve the secondary suppurative otitis media, but it will not affect the mass of the keratoma.

It is clear that the proper course of treatment for keratoma is surgical. The procedure is to remove the keratoma under the operating microscope (figure 3-5). The surgeon, of course, must assure that the entire neoplastic development is removed or it will continue to grow. A principal otological concern is that the keratoma is discovered and removed before it has done significant damage to the contents of the middle ear. On the other hand, if the keratoma has done a fair amount of damage, then tympanoplasty (middle ear reconstructive surgery) may be indicated. Furthermore, to assure that the keratoma is entirely removed, some form of mastoidectomy is necessary.

It is common for a surgeon to find it necessary to reconstruct the ossicular chain if the ossicles have been captured by the keratoma. Sometimes that is not required, nor is it required to remove part of the wall of the bony canal. On the other hand, it may be necessary to approach the middle ear space via the mastoid, and deal with the disease with a classic radical mastoidectomy. In any case, it is common for the ossicles to be damaged and, hence, reconstructive tympanoplasty must be done.

There are five types of tympanoplasty, but we need not detail them here. They range from repair of the drumhead (myringoplasty) and canal (Type I) through stapedectomy or fenestration (Type V). More typically, a Type IV tympanoplasty is done with mastoidectomy for the removal of keratoma, preparation of the oval window, and placement of a graft.

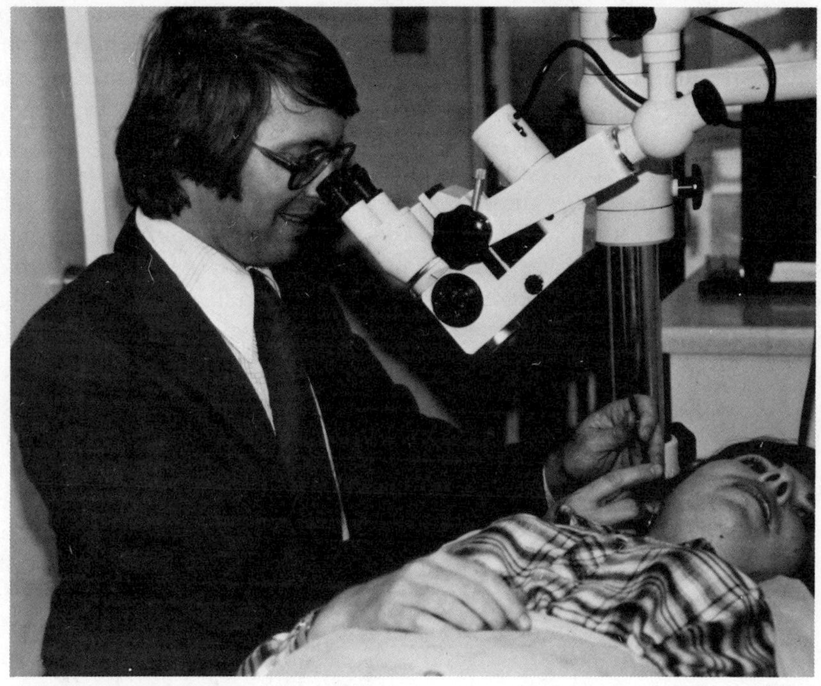

Figure 3-5. The operating microscope being used for an ear examination.

AUDIOLOGICAL CONSIDERATIONS

In the early stages of otomastoiditis there may be no measurable hearing loss for pure tones and no accompanying loss of sensitivity for speech, although tympanometry may be abnormal. In other words, the patient may not complain of an inability to hear. Instead, the complaint may center on pain or a sensation of fullness, and the underlying illness which has produced the condition. As the disease progresses, of course, there are obvious audiometric signs. As with most conductive hearing impairments, the audiogram is expected to be flat or rising. That is, the amount of loss of auditory sensitivity should be about the same for all frequencies or a little greater for lower frequencies than it is for higher frequencies.

AUDIOMETRY

One of the outstanding characteristics of any conductive hearing impairment — and one which necessarily appears with otomastoiditis — is the air-bone gap (figure 3-6). Since otomastoiditis is a condition of the middle ear, and the inner ear is unaffected, there is no loss of sensitivity at the level of the cochlea. Hence, if a signal were delivered directly to the inner ear so that it would bypass the middle ear conductive mechanism, an audiogram taken in this way would be normal. That type of measurement is accomplished, of course, by applying a bone conduction vibrator to the mastoid. As a result, the middle ear conducting mechanism is removed from the test situation and the cochlea is assessed directly. In a patient with otitis media, an audiogram obtained through bone conduction will be normal, illustrating that there is normal cochlear function. If the test is via air conduction — that is, by placing an earphone over the external ear and passing the signal through the affected middle ear cavity — the result will indicate a hearing loss. The difference between the air conduction audiogram and the bone conduction audiogram is called the air-bone gap, and its extent is a measure of conductive hearing impairment. Usually in cases with otomastoiditis — because there is normal cochlear reserve, and therefore no loss upon bone conduction testing — the air-bone gap is identical in size to the loss of sensitivity revealed by the air conduction audiogram.

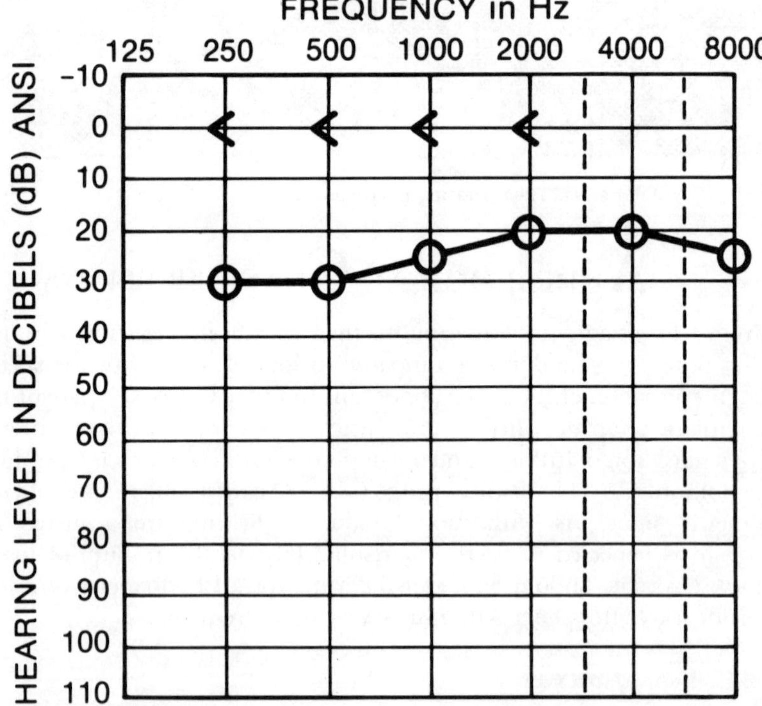

Figure 3-6. The air-bone gap.

TYMPANOMETRY

Tympanometry is a term which describes a procedure for measuring middle ear pressure and the compliance of the ear drum. A tympanogram may be considered in terms of the location of the peak pressure of the curve (positive, negative, or normal), the amplitude of the curve (high, low, or normal), and the shape of the curve (sloped, rounded, or peaked).

Changes as described above are produced by alterations of the stiffness and/or the mass of the middle ear transduction system. Figure 3-7, for example, is a tympanogram of a child with chronic otomastoiditis; the presence of fluid in the middle ear cavity has increased both the mass and the stiffness. The result is a tympanogram showing negative pressures in the ear canal as indicated by the peak of the curves being below zero. Similarly, the amplitude of the tympanogram is reduced. Figure 3-8 shows a tympanogram of a keratoma of the ear with ossicular destruction. Most midle ear pathologies have their own peculiar effects upon the tympanogram. Table 3-2 is a summary of those effects as specified by Feldman (1978).

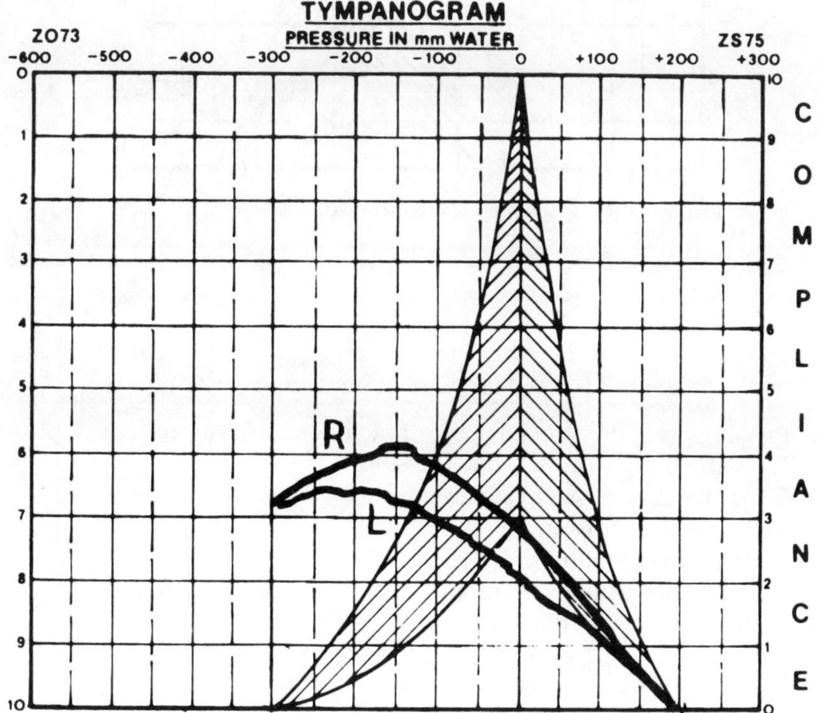

Figure 3-7. Tympanogram of a child with chronic bilateral otomastoiditis.

While the Feldman classification is both descriptive and helpful, it should be appreciated that individual patients with individual pathologies may display individual variations of the expected patterns. This is obvious when considering the number of different categories under which some pathologies appear. Tympanometry is an essential diagnostic tool, but it should be used in conjunction with other audiological procedures such as acoustic reflex measurements and, of course, along with otoscopic examination. The acoustic reflex may be absent in such patients; in any case, it will be shifted by the amount of the conductive loss.

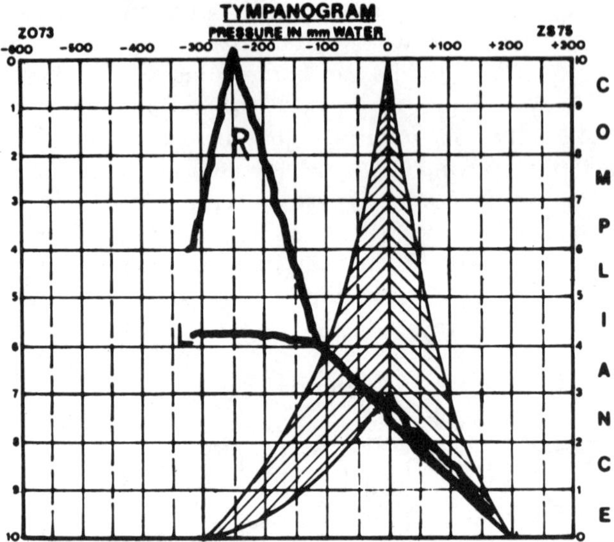

Figure 3-8. Tympanogram of a patient with a keratoma.

Table 3-2.
Feldman's (1978) Summary of Tympanometric Effects.

A. Pressure peak. Pressure related pathologies may be categorized as follows:
  1. Pathologies with negative pressure
    a) Blocked Eustachian tube
    b) Serous otitis media
  2. Pathologies with normal pressure
    a) Ossicular bony fixation
    b) Adhesive fixation
    c) Ossicular discontinuity
    d) Middle ear tumor
    e) Eardrum abnormality
  3. Pathologies with positive pressure
    a) Early acute otitis media
  4. Absence of pressure peak
    a) Middle ear effusion
    b) Open tympanic membrane
    c) Artifact.

B. Amplitude. Pathologies as they influence amplitude may be categorized as follows:
1. Pathologies with increased tympanogram amplitude
    a) Eardrum abnormality
    b) Ossicular discontinuity
2. Pathologies with decreased tympanogram amplitude
    a) Ossicular fixation bony or adhesive
    b) Serous otitis media
    c) Cholesteatoma, polyps, granuloma
    d) Glomus tumors
3. Pathologies not influencing tympanogram amplitude
    a) Blocked Eustachian tube
    b) Early acute otitis media.
C. Shape. Pathologies altering tympanogram shape may be categorized as follows:
1. Slope
    a) Pathologies which flatten or decrease tympanogram slope
        1) Serous otitis
        2) Ossicular fixation
        3) Tumors of the middle ear
    b) Pathologies which increase slope
        1) Eardrum abnormality
        2) Ossicular discontinuity
2. Smoothness
    a) Pathologies altering tympanogram smoothness
        1) Eardrum abnormality
        2) Ossicular discontinuity
        3) Vascular tumors
        4) Patulous Eustachian tube

SPEECH AUDIOMETRY

The patient with otitis media will have no difficulty understanding speech if it is sufficiently audible. That is to say, conductive hearing losses result in the same perceptual effect as a loss of loudness. Consequently, the patient with otitis media will display a loss of sensitivity for normal speech (i.e., depressed speech reception threshold) equal to his loss of sensitivity for air conducted tones. Speech discrimination scores will be close to 100% because they are measured at an intensity (30 or 40dB) which is well above the speech reception threshold. The patient will have no difficulty understanding speech if it is of sufficient intensity to overcome any loss of hearing by air conduction.

The amount of auditory handicap is related to the size and position of a keratoma and whether it has become secondarily infected. If the keratoma does not impede movement of the ossicular chain, there should be no hearing loss. If the ossicles are involved — erosion of the incus is common — as with other conditions which interfere with the sound transducing properties of the middle ear conducting mechanism, a keratoma should be expected to produce

PURE TONE AUDIOGRAM

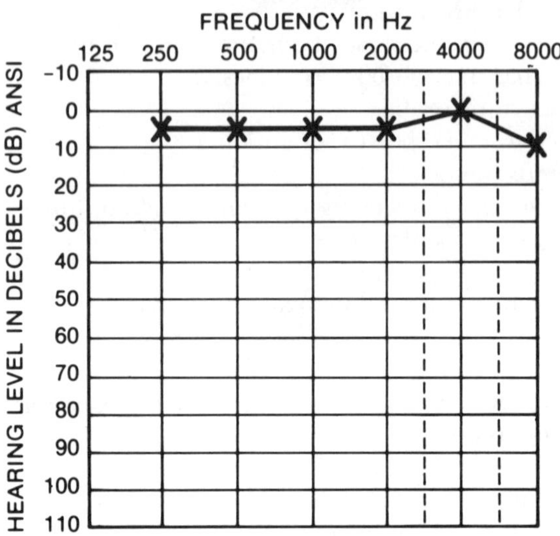

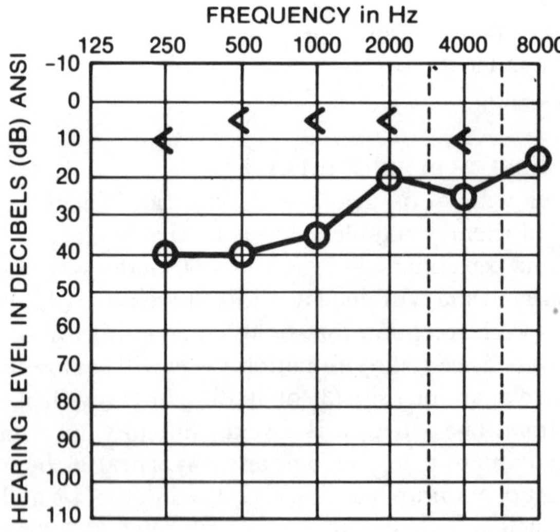

Figure 3-9. Audiogram of patient with a keratoma of the right ear.

a flat audiogram with accompanying hearing loss ranging anywhere from 35dB to 55dB (figure 3-9). The speech reception threshold should be congruous with the pure tone audiogram; and, given adequate loudness, the speech discrimination scores should be essentially normal.

It should be noted that the amount of hearing loss accompanying a keratoma may not be a true indicator of the actual damage to the middle ear resulting from the presence of the neoplasm. In other words, audiometry may not accurately reflect the pathology. In fact, sometimes a keratoma will conduct sound.

A long-standing keratoma may result in damage such that hearing cannot be completely restored except by surgical means. In the event surgery is not possible — Shambaugh (1967) reminds us that tympanoplasty is contraindicated if there is no air-bone gap — or fails to completely restore hearing, rehabilitative audiology assumes the primary responsibility. The hearing loss may be alleviated by amplification, sometimes via a bone conduction aid, and sometimes by more conventional models. Auditory training and speech reading instruction may also be desirable. Even so, continuous monitoring for recurrence of middle ear pathology is essential.

EDUCATIONAL SCREENING

Children with chronic or recurrent ear disease appear to have somewhat lower I.Q.s than matched controls as measured by standard tests *(Howie, 1978)*. That is not to say that ear disease itself lowers one's intelligence. What it suggests is that frequent or chronic ear disease may deprive a developing child of information essential for successful learning and for the development of normal spoken language. It appears, in fact, from the work of both Howie (1978) and Kramer (1978) that early and repeated ear disease may constitute the basis of a child's later behavioral and educational problems. As Katz (1978) indicated, "Disruption in auditory perception and language . . . are associated with fluctuating hearing impairment." A persistent hearing impairment may interfere with a child's ability to learn, due perhaps only to an inability to attend and to know what is going on all of the time *(Downs, 1978)*. Battin (1979), on the other hand, has cautioned that these mild conductive problems may constitute "additive stress factors" for children otherwise at risk, but that the same conductive problem in a non-risk child will not result in behavioral and educational problems.

Hence, recurrent otomastoiditis could be a problem for some children. Potsic (1978) has noted motor and affective changes in children with chronic otomastoiditis. Downs has proposed the fitting of very low-powered hearing aids for children with mild, conductive, long-standing hearing losses. It remains, of course, a debatable approach to management, but one which certainly merits serious consideration in view of the potentially marked educational implications for the very young child.

The early detection of all forms of otomastoiditis is essential. Audiologists must assume major responsibility as advocates and supervisors of audiometric screening programs at all levels from infancy to industry. The establishment of adequate standards for detection and the development of new procedures and instrumentation are constantly required. Methods must be tightened so that screening can be done more often, more effectively, and more cheaply than at present.

CASE STUDY 3-1:

RECURRENT OTOMASTOIDITIS WITH CLEFT PALATE

MP was referred for a complete audiological evaluation when she did not respond within normal limits on an audiometric screen at school. In the past, she had bilateral otomastoiditis, and five months before this evaluation Dr. D placed polyethylene tubes in both tympanic membranes. These tubes were still in place, but MP's father observed that she listened to the television at quite high levels and that she did not seem to hear quiet conversation.

Pure tone air and masked bone conduction thresholds revealed a mild, bilateral conductive loss, slightly worse in the right ear at low frequencies. Speech reception thresholds (27dB on the right and 25dB on the left) were consistent with the pure tone average, and word discrimination scores were normal bilaterally. Tympanometry was not attempted due to the presence of the tubes. MP's father was urged to have her reexamined by Dr. D.

Case Study 3-1: Recurrent Otomastoiditis with Cleft Palate

PURE TONE AUDIOGRAM

RIGHT EAR

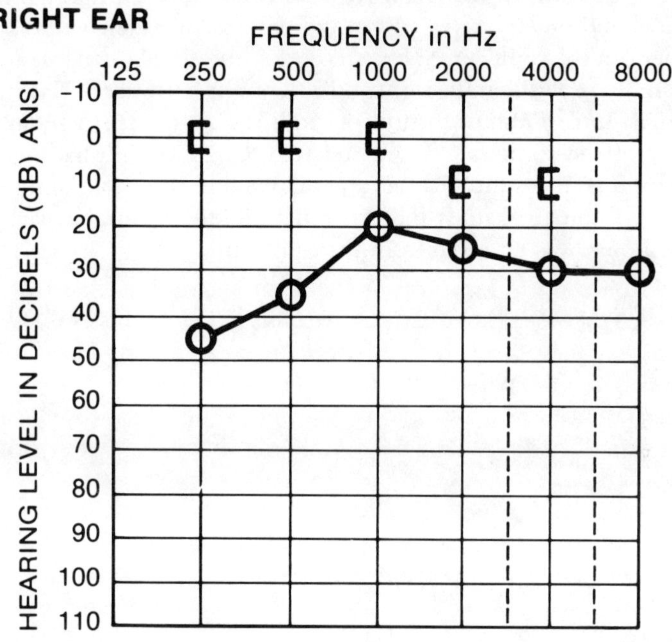

LEFT EAR

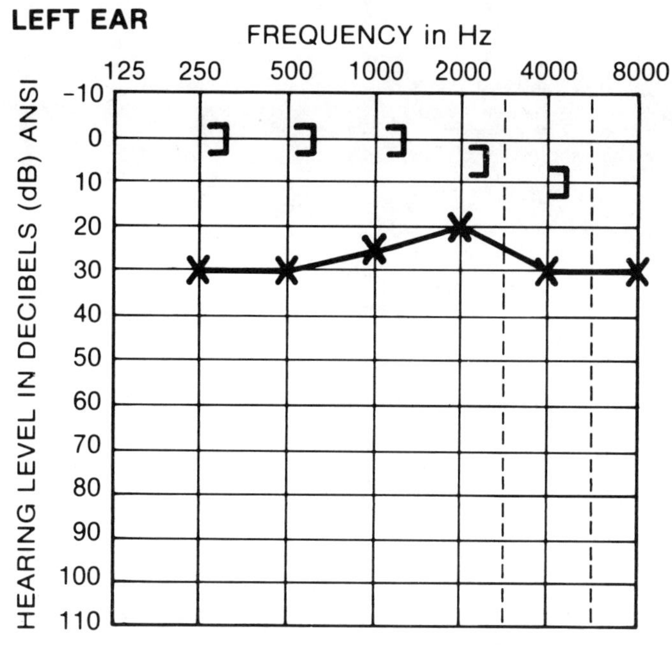

CASE STUDY 3-2: KERATOMA

TM, aged 18 years, was brought to the Speech and Hearing Center by his mother. Although he has a history of ear disease, he did not report any difficulty at the time of this visit. However, pure tone air and masked bone conduction audiometry revealed an audiogram consistent with conductive impairment in the right ear. Speech reception thresholds, consistent with the audiogram, were 32dB on the right and 5dB on the left. Speech discrimination was normal. Since TM has a history of ear disease, and since these data suggest pathology of the right ear, he was referred to Dr. D who had treated him previously. These results showed an unfavorable threshold shift from his earlier tests. Otological study indicated that middle ear surgery was in order, and a keratoma was removed from his right ear.

CASE STUDY 3-2: KERATOMA
PURE TONE AUDIOGRAM

LEFT EAR
FREQUENCY in Hz

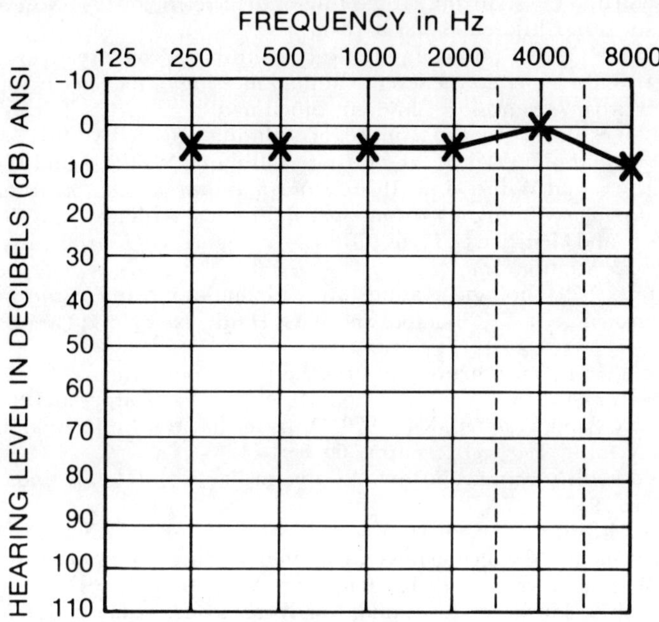

RIGHT EAR
FREQUENCY in Hz

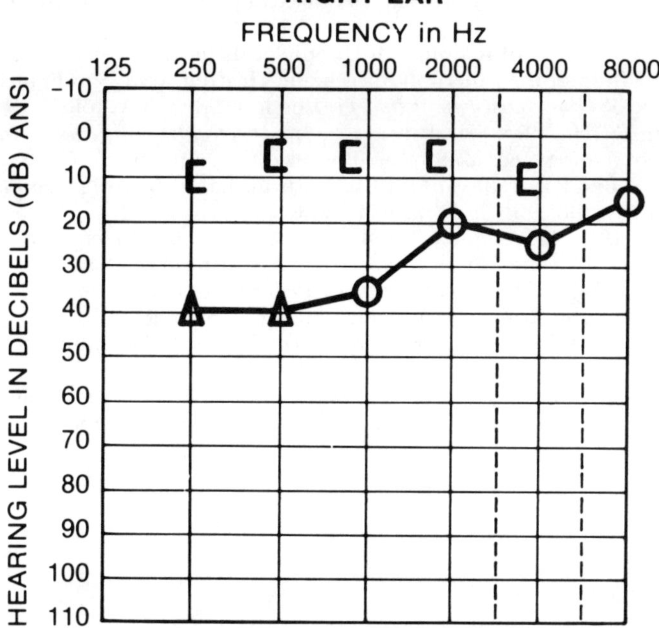

REFERENCES

Battin, R.R. 1979. The effects of early middle ear problems on later learning development revisited. *Corti's Organ* 4:4.

Downs, M.P. 1978. The interaction of critical periods with conductive losses. Presented to the sixth annual meeting of the Society for Ear, Nose and Throat Advances in Children. Santa Barbara.

Eichenwald, H. 1979. Rationale and efficacy of antibiotics use in ear, nose and throat practice. Presented to the seventh annual meeting of the Society for Ear, Nose and Throat Advances in Children. Cincinnati.

Feldman, A.S. 1978. Acoustic impedance-admittance battery. In *Handbook of clinical audiology*, 2d ed., ed. J. Katz. Baltimore: Williams and Wilkins Co.

Feldman, A.S. and Wilber, L.A. 1976. *Acoustic impedance and admittance — the measurement of middle ear function.* Baltimore: Williams and Wilkins Co.

Gerber, S.E. and Mencher, G.T. eds. 1978. *Early diagnosis of hearing loss.* New York: Grune & Stratton, Inc.

Goodhill, V. 1979. Otologic relationships with audiology. In *Hearing and hearing impairment,* eds. L.J. Bradford and W.G. Hardy. New York: Grune & Stratton, Inc.

Goodhill, V. and Brockman, S.J. 1979. Secretory otitis media. In *Ear diseases, deafness and dizziness,* ed. V. Goodhill. New York: Harper and Row, Inc.

Hanson, D.G. and Ulvestad, R.F. 1979. Otitis media and child development. *Ann. Otol. Rhinol. Laryngol.* Suppl. 60, 88:1-112.

Howie, V.M. 1975. Natural history of otitis media. *Ann. Otol. Rhinol. Laryngol.* Suppl. 19, 85:67-72.

Howie, V.M. 1978. The effect of early onset of otitis media on educational achievement. Presented to the sixth annual meeting of the Society for Ear, Nose and Throat Advances in Children. Santa Barbara.

Jaffe, B.F. 1979. The life cycle of middle ear disease in cleft palate children. Presented to the seventh annual meeting of the Society for Ear, Nose and Throat Advances in Children. Cincinnati.

Katz, J. 1978. The effects of conductive hearing loss on auditory function. *Asha* 20:879-886.

Kramer, R.I. 1978. Miniseminar on chronic otitis media. Presented to the annual convention of the American Speech and Hearing Assn. San Francisco.

Mawson, S.R. 1967. *Diseases of the ear.* London: Edward Arnold.

Newman, M.H. 1975. Hearing loss. In *Differential diagnosis in pediatric otolaryngology,* ed. M. Strome. Boston: Little, Brown and Co.

Payne, E.E. and Paparella, M.M. 1976. Otitis media. In *Hearing disorders,* ed. J.L. Northern. Boston: Little, Brown and Co.

Potsic, W. 1978. Miniseminar on chronic otitis media. Presented to the annual convention of the American Speech and Hearing Assn. San Francisco.

Ruben, R.J. 1972. The external ear. In *Pediatric otolaryngology,* vol. 2, eds. C. Ferguson and E. Kendig. Philadelphia: W.B. Saunders Co.

Shambaugh, G.E., Jr. 1967. *Surgery of the ear.* 2d ed. Philadelphia: W.B. Saunders Co.

Simons, M.R. 1979. Acoustic impedance tests. In *Ear diseases, deafness, and dizziness,* ed. V. Goodhill. New York: Harper and Row, Inc.

CHAPTER 4

Bony Abnormalities of the Middle Ear

Among other things, normal hearing depends upon the normal mechanical properties of the middle ear system. The middle ear is a kind of mechanical pump which takes the very tiny displacements of the tympanic membrane and expands them twenty-two fold in displacement of the membrane of the oval window. This results from two mechanical factors, the lever ratio and the areal ratio.

The lever ratio is a mechanical advantage resulting from movement of the ossicular chain (figure 4-1). Figure 4-2 illustrates the normal middle ear. Observe that the ossicular chain is not a piston; it does not go in a straight line from the tympanic membrane to the oval window. Rather, it rises into the attic of the middle ear and falls again across the relatively massive incus, thereby providing considerable increase of force at the incudo-stapedial joint. This increase of force — about eighteen times — is the lever ratio of the middle ear system.

The area of the tympanic membrane is substantially larger than the area of the oval window. Consequently, the effect of the larger membrane acting upon a small membrane is that of an.amplifier; that is called the areal ratio. It has been estimated that the ratio between the two areas ranges from 14:1 to 21:1 *(Kirikae, 1973)* in different individuals. In any case, the general effect is the same, that of increasing the force of the signal presented at the oval window, thus facilitating the initiation of the movement of the fluids within the cochlea.

Middle ear bony abnormalities may be of two distinct types: congenital malformations or the result of a disease process. Congenital malformations, although distinct from one another, may be considered as a group primarily because the medical/otological and audiological considerations are so similar. Disease processes might also be considered as a cluster. However, because one of them, otosclerosis, is so common and offers such a classical

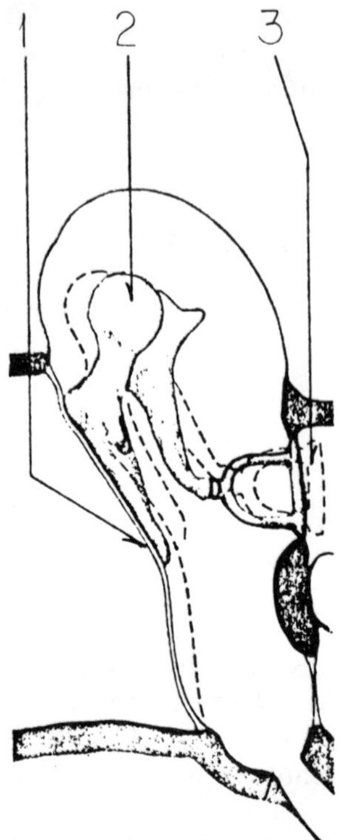

Figure 4-1. The areal ratio is produced by the fact that the area of the drum membrane (1) is much greater than the area of the oval window membrane (3), while the lever ratio is created by the rising of the ossicular lever (2) and then its fall.

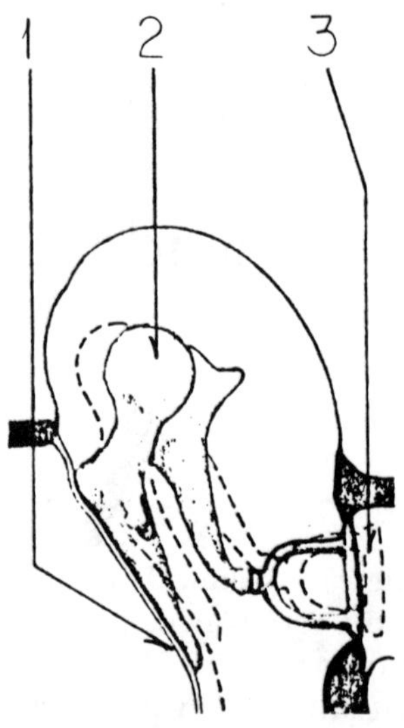

Figure 4-2. The middle ear: (1) tympanic membrane; (2) ossicular chain; and (3) oval window.

example of the effects and treatment of all forms of bony middle ear disorders, it has been singled out for discussion and presentation.

Congenital Malformations of the Middle Ear

Pathology and Etiology

There are well over fifty different syndromes which have an associated middle ear bony anomaly. There is no single etiology. The malformation may be genetic in origin, due to prenatal disease, the result of a toxin, the end product of a developmental interruption related to a regional defect, or simply a slight variant on a normal theme.

The various conditions described in chapter 2 (Anomalies of the External Ear) may be expected to have concommitant middle ear anomalies. Embryological development is such that anomalies of the external ear should cause the diagnostician to expect anomalies of at least part of the middle ear as well. The pinna need not be severely anomalous in this respect; if a pinna is too low, or is in the wrong position, or is at the wrong angle, or if the two pinnae do not match perfectly, then there is reason to suspect a middle ear anomaly. Jaffe (1978) has reported large numbers of surgically confirmed middle ear anomalies in which the first sign was the unusual position or appearance of one or both auricles.

What form may an anomaly take? One of the possibilities is a simple malformation of the malleus or incus as illustrated in figure 4-3. Another possibility is a fusion of the malleus and the incus so that they form one large ossicle rather than two. In such a case, of course, the advantage of the lever ratio which normally accrues from the joint action of the malleus and the incus is diminished or lost. In extreme cases, the middle ear cavity is absent or may be slitlike *(Nager, 1973)*. Most often, middle ear anomalies are limited to malformed or fused ossicles.

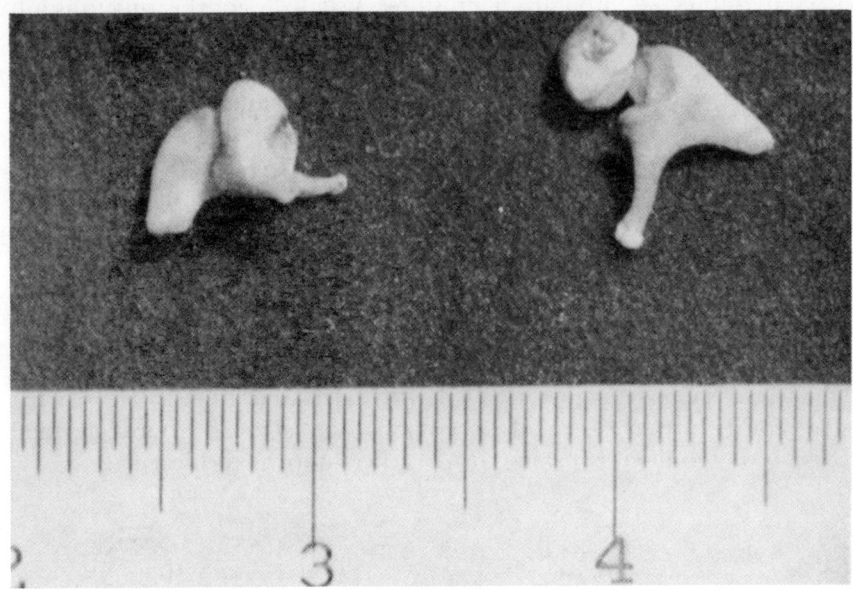

Figure 4-3. Deformed and fused incus and malleus on the left compared to normal on the right. *(Reproduced with permission of the W.B. Saunders Co.)*

MEDICAL CONSIDERATIONS

If the middle ear is anomalous, surgical intervention is usually preferred. At one extreme would be the peculiar case where the middle ear cavity is absent. In that situation, the only solution may be a complete middle ear construction or, in a severe dysplasia, use of a bone conduction hearing aid. At the opposite extreme would be an ear with moderately malformed ossicles which can be removed, reshaped, and replaced. In between these extremes is a broad range of combinations of anomalous or fused ossicles, and just as many solutions.

One major surgical alternative is replacement of the ossicles with ossicular homografts. In such cases, ossicles are removed from a cadaver and preserved for that purpose. This type of surgery is occurring with increasing frequency as the cadaveric material becomes more readily available. The subject of tympanic homografts has been described in considerable detail by Perkins (1975).

On occasion, an autograft may be a better solution. This means literally to use the same tissue. An example would be a case in which a malformed incus was removed, reshaped, and resituated. There is something surgically aesthetic, and perhaps psychologically preferable, about the use of an autograft over a homograft, but it is not necessarily preferable audiologically.

In some instances, an artificial prosthesis is a better choice. Such a device may be a piston attached at one end to the tympanic membrane and at the other end to the neck of the stapes; or, variously, a piston which attaches the tympanic membrane directly to the oval window. Examples of these are shown in figures 4-4 through 4-6. Prostheses usually restore hearing to as full an extent as homografts or autografts. Figures 4-7 and 4-8 present the audiograms of two patients, one with a homograft implant and one with a piston-type prosthesis in place. It is evident that the differences are not great.

AUDIOLOGICAL CONSIDERATIONS

If the middle ear system is not intact, the normal mechanical advantages of the ossicular chain obviously are not obtained. The associated hearing loss may be as high as 55dB by air conduction. As the audiometric configuration will be normal, bone conduction testing will usually reveal that a normal cochlea is present. A significant air-bone gap will be present. Results of speech testing will be similar to those seen in patients with middle ear disease. That is, if the sound is loud enough, the patient will understand virtually 100% of what is presented. In essence, because the middle ear serves as a transducer and mechanical amplifier, bypassing it will reflect normal cochlear reserve.

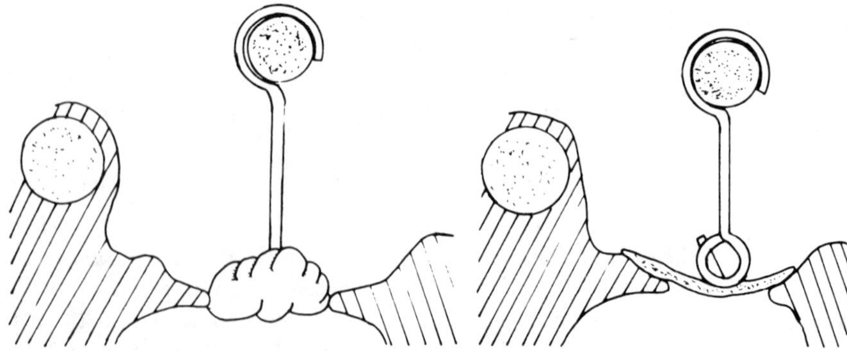

Figure 4-4. Wire prostheses for stapedectomy.

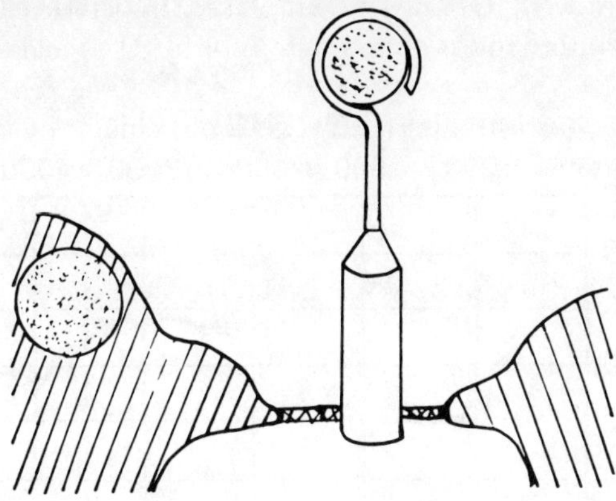

Figure 4-5. Wire teflon piston prosthesis for stapedectomy.

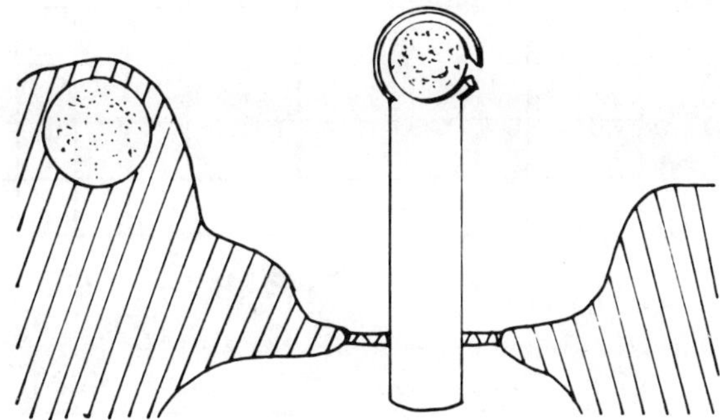

Figure 4-6. Shea teflon prosthesis for stapedectomy.

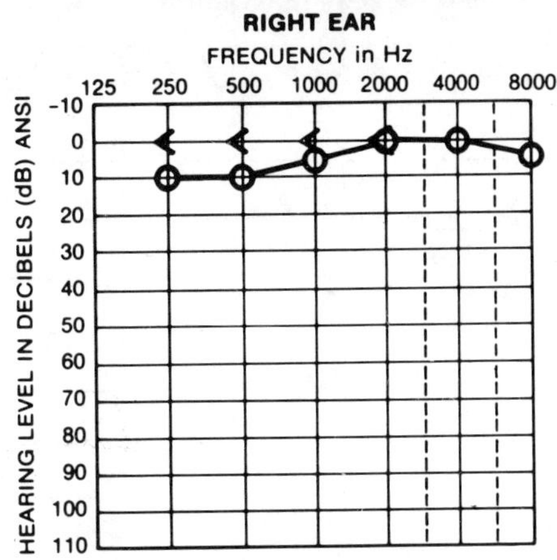

Figure 4-7. Audiogram of an ear with a homograft.

PURE TONE AUDIOGRAM

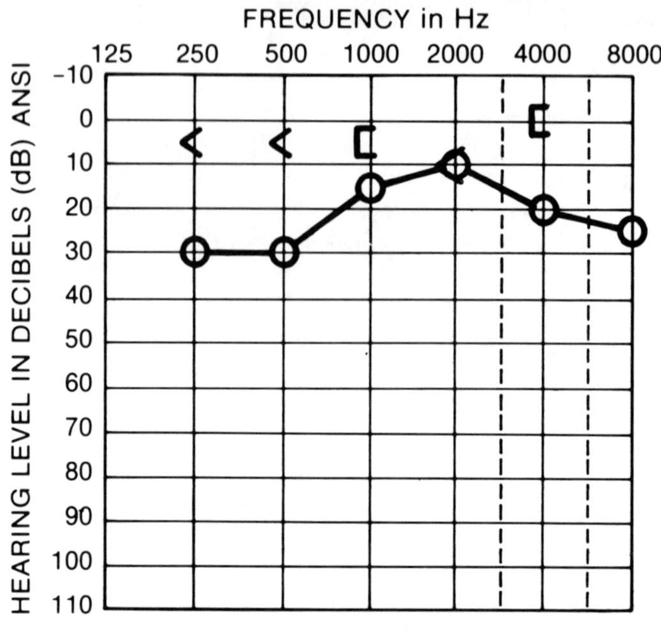

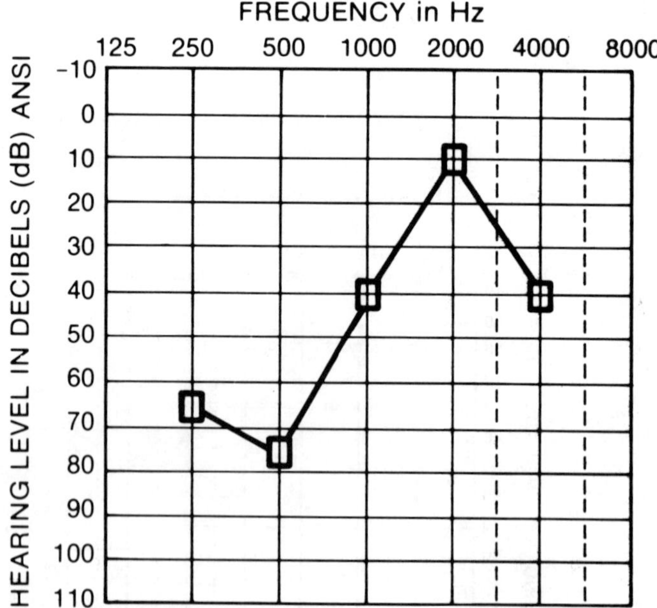

Figure 4-8. Audiogram displaying the benefit of a prosthesis placed in the middle ear on the right side.

Occasionally, a patient will be seen for audiological assessment who previously had normal hearing, but having suffered a blow to the head or trauma to the mastoid or temporal bone, has suddenly lost hearing. Tympanometry may reveal an extremely flaccid drum membrane. An air-bone gap of 50dB or more may be present, and otoscopically the ear may look normal. If the test is presented at a comfortable loudness level, the problem may be further compounded by an elevated speech reception threshold but normal speech discrimination. A disarticulation of the ossicular chain — a break in the physical continuity of the ossicles — may be responsible. The total audiometric picture, except for the case history, may be the same as that seen in a patient with a bony malformation of the middle ear. Figure 4-9 illustrates the similarity in the audiometric picture seen in patients with a disarticulation of the ossicular chain and those with congenital malformations of the middle ear. Clearly, the audiogram does not provide sufficient information to make an audiological diagnostic judgment. Tympanometry will provide the information that stiffness is markedly reduced (figure 4-10).

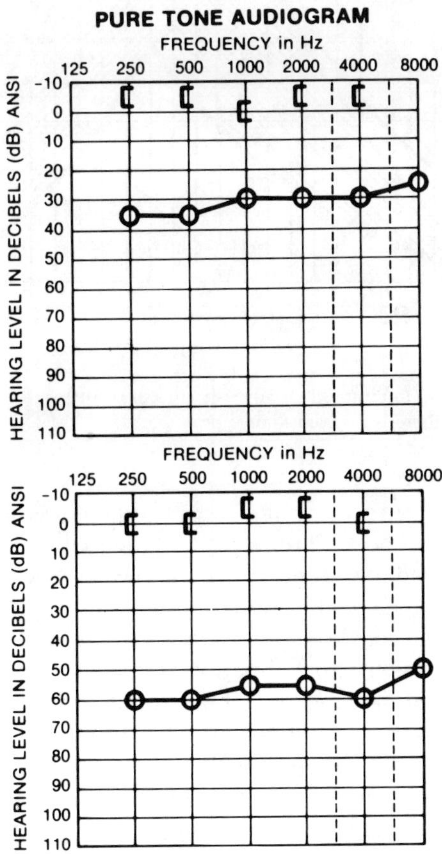

Figure 4-9. An ear having ossicular discontinuity (above) and another having an anomaly of the middle ear (below) displaying similar audiometric contours.

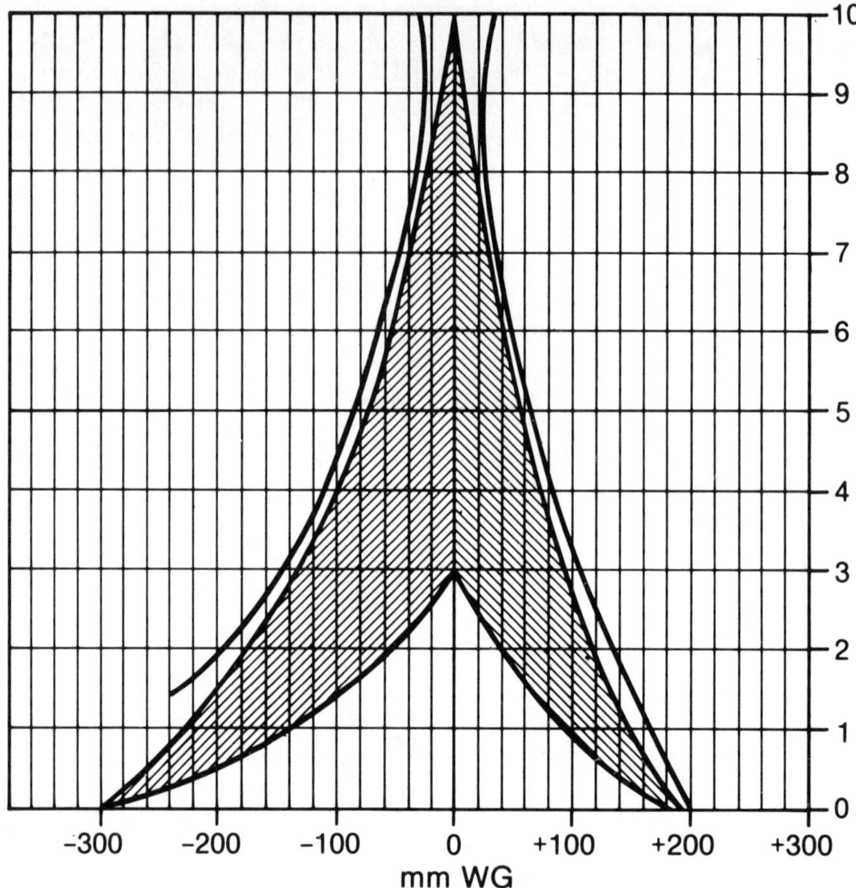

Figure 4-10. A tympanogram of an ear with a discontinuity of the ossicular chain. Note that there is no compliance peak.

Sometimes surgery is not the treatment of choice for a congenital malformation; or, because these types of anomalies are congenital, surgery is usually postponed until head growth has nearly reached maximum. In such a case, just as in bone conduction audiometric testing, the middle ear can be bypassed and the cochlea stimulated directly by applying a vibratory type of hearing aid to the mastoid (figure 4-11). Such a solution is called simply a "bone conduction hearing aid". The procedure is frequently satisfactory, but it is certainly less than perfect. Held on by a headband which is easily stretched, the vibrator may become so loosely held to the head that its effectiveness is diminished. Cosmetically, this type of hearing aid is marginally successful. The headband may disturb the hair or make the user self-conscious. Sometimes a regular air conduction hearing aid is a better choice, even though a bone conduction aid may offer better amplification. It is important that these issues be discussed thoroughly with the patient or patient's parents.

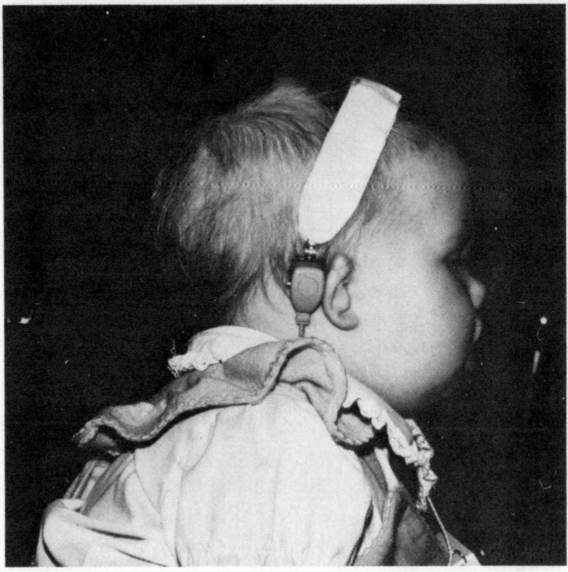

Figure 4-11. Bone conduction hearing aid.

OTOSCLEROSIS

Otosclerosis literally means "hard ears." Simply, *oto-* refers to an ear, while *sclerosis* is a hardening (e.g., arteriosclerosis: hardening of the arteries). At present, it is preferably called otospongiosis *(Goin, 1976)*.

First described by Valsalva in 1735, otosclerosis is characterized by a growth of new bone (figure 4-12) most often developing anterior to the oval window *(Lindsay, 1973)* and growing into the cavity of the middle ear. As the disease progresses, it will incorporate more and more of the stapes, inhibiting its movement. In many cases, the new bone also grows medial to the oval window reaching into the cochlear vestibule. This leads to a condition which has sometimes been described as "inner ear conductive impairment" *(Derlacki, 1976)*. This far more debilitating form of otosclerosis may be complicated by other symptoms, primarily vertigo and nausea.

A disease more prevalent in Caucasian women than in any other group, it has been estimated to occur in one of every five to ten *(Goin, 1976)*. It occurs half as often in white males as in white females, but it occurs only in about one in 100 black people, and virtually not at all in other races. Fortunately, the disease is quite minor in most patients. Only about 10% of persons with otosclerosis complain of hearing impairment; nevertheless, otosclerosis is the single most common cause of serious hearing loss in adulthood.

PATHOLOGY AND ETIOLOGY

Otosclerosis has been shown to be a hereditary, degenerative disorder, apparently produced by a dominant gene *(Konigsmark, 1972)*. Otosclerosis,

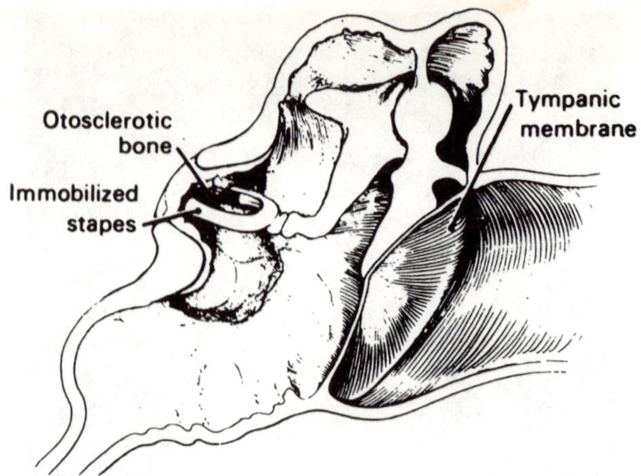

Figure 4-12. Bony growth in otosclerosis. *(Reproduced with permission of Williams & Wilkins.)*

because it is genetic and not congenital, is an example of those kinds of diseases which have been called familial degenerative or latent onset.

Because otosclerosis is dominantly inherited—hence, it runs in families—and, because it occurs more frequently in women than in men, the probability of the disease appearing in the daughter of a woman who has had it is fairly high. A logical question often heard, then, is "If it is not a sex-linked trait, how does it happen that the disease occurs more frequently in females than males?" The question is properly raised. The answer seems to be that, while the disease may be present in equal numbers in both sexes, it is aggravated and activated by certain metabolic and chemical changes that accompany pregnancy or menstruation. The disease rarely manifests itself before the third decade of life (although it has occasionally been reported in children), and it is in that decade (20-30 years of age) that most women bear children and undergo the associated biochemical changes. No special mechanism for this change has been isolated.

An otosclerotic lesion is characterized by an irregular growth of new bone which is interspersed with numerous vascular spaces. It sometimes replaces the dense bone of the labyrinth. When it is active and growing, the new bone is spongy and loose. When the growth stops, the new bone appears as a dense, mature, recalcified focus. The margins of this focus tend to be rather sharply defined. It is usually (but by no means always) confined to the place where the anterior crus of the stapes attaches to the footplate.

Medical Considerations

The patient will present with a conductive hearing loss and, as indicated earlier, may also complain of vertigo and nausea. Specific details regarding the audiometric findings are reviewed below under audiological considerations. In about 10% of cases, the otoscopic examination will reveal that the tympanic membrane exhibits a pinkish or rosy tint or even a reddish hue. This is called

Schwartze's sign, and is a positive diagnostic indicator of otosclerosis. Apparently, this tint is imparted to the tympanic membrane from dilated blood vessels in the mucosa of the promontory.

Some other pathologies affecting the middle ear may imitate otosclerosis. One is syphilis—sometimes called "the great imitator"—which, at least in its early stages, produces audiometric effects which can be confused with those of otosclerosis. Another is osteogenesis imperfecta which, although its external signs are usually obvious, also displays audiograms like those of otosclerosis.

After determination that the hearing difficulty is the result of otosclerosis, surgical intervention is almost always the treatment of choice. Otosclerosis presents one of the most dramatic and appealing examples of successful surgical intervention in that the diseased bony growth can be removed by surgery almost to the point of restoration of normal hearing. Medical (non-surgical) treatment has been attempted, but success has been minimal. Shambaugh (1966) attempted to treat otosclerosis with large doses of sodium fluoride. The majority of his patients showed no change, although a few displayed a return to normal on radiologic examination.

Historically, there have been three different surgeries employed for the correction of otosclerosis. These are called *fenestration, stapedolysis,* and *stapedectomy.* Only one of them, the stapedectomy, is truly successful and is utilized extensively today. However, a review of the development of all of the surgical procedures provides an interesting insight into the treatment of conductive hearing loss. Further, an audiologist may occasionally encounter a patient who has undergone one of the earlier surgeries, and the clinician must be aware of what has happened to that patient and what to expect from him.

FENESTRATION. Over 40 years ago, Lempert (1938) developed the procedure known as fenestration. While conceptually a simple procedure, surgically it is not. The concept of the operation is that, since the oval window is obliterated by bony growth, a new window (fenestra) needs to be made. Usually this window is drilled into the lateral semi-circular canal at the level of the promontory.

A successful fenestration operation cannot lead to a complete restoration of normal hearing. Figure 4-13 illustrates the state of the middle ear following fenestration. It can be seen that there is a new window, the ossicles are missing, the tympanic membrane has its medial attachment at the promontory between the oval and round windows, and the new oval window is exposed to the outside air. Fenestration fails more often than it succeeds, and thus is rarely done today.

STAPEDOLYSIS. In 1953, Rosen rediscovered a procedure called stapes mobilization or stapedolysis. Actually, that procedure had been done first by Kessel in 1878, but had fallen into disuse. As with the fenestration, the concept of the surgery is quite simple: if the stapes is stuck, free it. The procedure involves raising the tympanic membrane, exposing the contents of the middle ear, attaching a hook-like instrument to a crus of the stapes, and by jerking it, freeing the footplate from the otosclerotic growth. Frequently, the results of

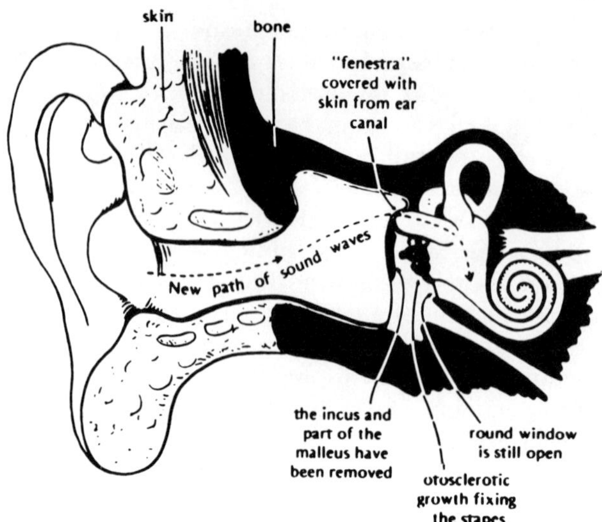

Figure 4-13. Fenestrated ear. *(Reproduced with permission of Holt, Rinehart, & Winston.)*

this procedure can be quite dramatic and the patient on the operating table can hear suddenly.

Rosen's rediscovery of stapedolysis reestablished otology as a surgical specialty. However, it was eventually determined that the long term effects of stapedolysis were not successful. The disease process which captured the stapes in the first place, and which was not removed by the surgical procedure, often seemed to continue. Consequently, far too many stapes became involved a second time and had to be operated on again.

STAPEDECTOMY. Eventually, stapedolysis fell into disuse in favor of going immediately to stapedectomy. An "-ectomy" is a removal. Stapedectomy, then, means to remove the stapes. Contrary to tonsillectomy and/or appendectomy, however, where something is removed without replacement, a stapedectomy includes the replacement of the stapes with some kind of prosthesis. Although a homograft has been used, a typical prosthetic device is not a simulation or a copy of the normal stapes; it is usually a simple wire crimped around the lenticular process of the incus and inserted into the oval window (figures 4-4 through 4-6). The point inserted into the oval window is packed with a material (such as gel-foam) which retains it in place while normal tissue growth occurs. Eventually, the packing is absorbed into the surrounding mucosa. There is a 97-99% success rate for this procedure in expert hands *(Paparella, 1973)*. A failure rate of only 3% for stapedectomy is excellent, especially when compared to the much larger percentages of failures associated with the stapedolysis and fenestration procedures.

The procedure is enhanced by other recent developments as well. Signal among them has been the development of the operating microscope. The ability to perform otic microsurgery with the great success now achieved in stapedectomy is primarily due to the use of the operating microscope (figure 4-

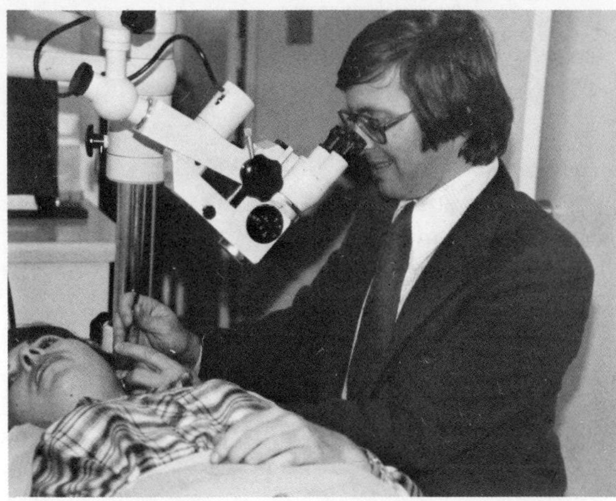

Figure 4-14. The operating microscope being used for an ear examination.

14). In addition, improvements in pharmaceuticals, as well as the development of new drugs, has significantly diminished the incidence of post-operative infection. Ampicillin and tetracycline are most commonly used as prophylactic antibiotics, and they have been most successful against the threat of labyrinthitis.

Nevertheless, there are instances of stapedectomy leading to an inner ear infection (endolabyrinthitis) which eventually lead to destruction of the cochlear end organ and a resultant dead ear. Fortunately, that situation is extremely rare. More often, but still rarely, the otosclerotic growth continues and the neoplastic bone eventually captures the prosthesis. In such a situation, many surgeons would prefer not to attempt to operate a second time on the same ear or on the other ear. For these types of patients, amplification usually offers an adequate solution.

As indicated above, otosclerosis very rarely re-occurs in the same ear. Thus, most surgeons will operate on only one ear at a time, the poorer one, as they are unwilling to assume even the 3% risk of failure and the consequent deafness suffered by the patient. If the operated ear is successful, and it will be most of the time, some patients will request that the other ear be operated on as well. Although two ears are not necessary for normal hearing in the customary acoustic environment to which we are all exposed, a unilateral hearing loss, however moderate, is a nuisance, and for some it is a handicap. Thus, the successful stapedectomy patient may often have the second ear done.

The value of stapedectomy cannot be overstated. Remember that otosclerosis is a disease which affects vast numbers of people. About 97% of those people can have their hearing restored to normal by a rather simple surgical procedure utilizing a local anesthetic and requiring only one or two night's sleep in a hospital. Consequently, literally hundreds of stapedectomies are performed daily. Hence, although otosclerosis is a very common disease, its resultant hearing loss is relatively easily corrected with dramatic effects. The development of both the stapedectomy procedure and the simple prosthesis to restore hearing have combined to form one of the major landmarks in otological science and one of the great achievements of the surgeon's art.

AUDIOLOGICAL CONSIDERATIONS

As with other diseases and disorders which primarily involve the middle ear, the handicap which accompanies otosclerosis is conductive in nature, and therefore, not likely to exceed 50 to 55dB HL. That is to say, no one will become "deaf" from this disease unless advanced otosclerosis reaches into the cochlear vestibule and produces a hearing loss as great as 90dB or more.

Otosclerosis has a characteristic audiometric configuration. Generally, in early otosclerosis, there will be a normal bone conduction audiogram and a mild hearing loss by air conduction, limited primarily to the lower frequencies. In other words, the loss tends to have a rising audiometric contour (figure 4-15). As the disease progresses, the contour of the air conduction audiogram will become flatter as the hearing loss for the higher frequencies becomes as great as the hearing loss at lower frequencies (figure 4-15). Furthermore, the air-bone gap is increased at most frequencies.

There is an audiometric peculiarity to otosclerosis, however, which sets it apart from other conductive hearing problems. In most patients, the air-bone gap is diminished at 2000Hz. That is, there is a "notch" or apparent sensory-neural hearing loss reflected in the bone conduction audiogram at 2000Hz *(Carhart, 1950)*. This pattern, called Carhart's Notch, rarely occurs at frequencies other than 2000Hz, and is unique to otosclerosis (figure 4-15). Its presence is one of those rare diagnostic signs which is clearly indicative of a particular disorder. The clinician should know, however, that its absence does not rule out otosclerosis as the disease process. Unfortunately, not all otosclerotic patients display it. Furthermore, it is important that Carhart's Notch not be confused with notches occurring in the audiogram for other reasons (e.g., acoustic trauma). Carhart's Notch is limited to the bone conduction audiogram; it does not appear in the air conduction audiogram.

Results of speech audiometric tests vary with the stage of the disease and the exact site of the conductive mechanism that is involved. Generally, a patient with an early, uncomplicated otosclerosis will demonstrate an elevated speech reception threshold in direct accord with the pure tone audiogram. Speech discrimination will be excellent, usually normal, if the signal is presented at a comfortable loudness level.

Patients with advanced otosclerosis that has entered the cochlear vestibule and beyond do not fare so well. As the audiogram reflects a decreased air-bone gap and an increasing sensory-neural hearing loss, the results of speech reception threshold tests and speech discrimination testing will mirror a corresponding difference in understanding. In severe cases, speech discrimination scores may drop below 70%. As long as it is only the conductive mechanism that is involved, speech tests are affected only by loudness changes. As soon as there is a concurrent cochlear involvement, the value of increased loudness is markedly decreased.

PURE TONE AUDIOGRAM

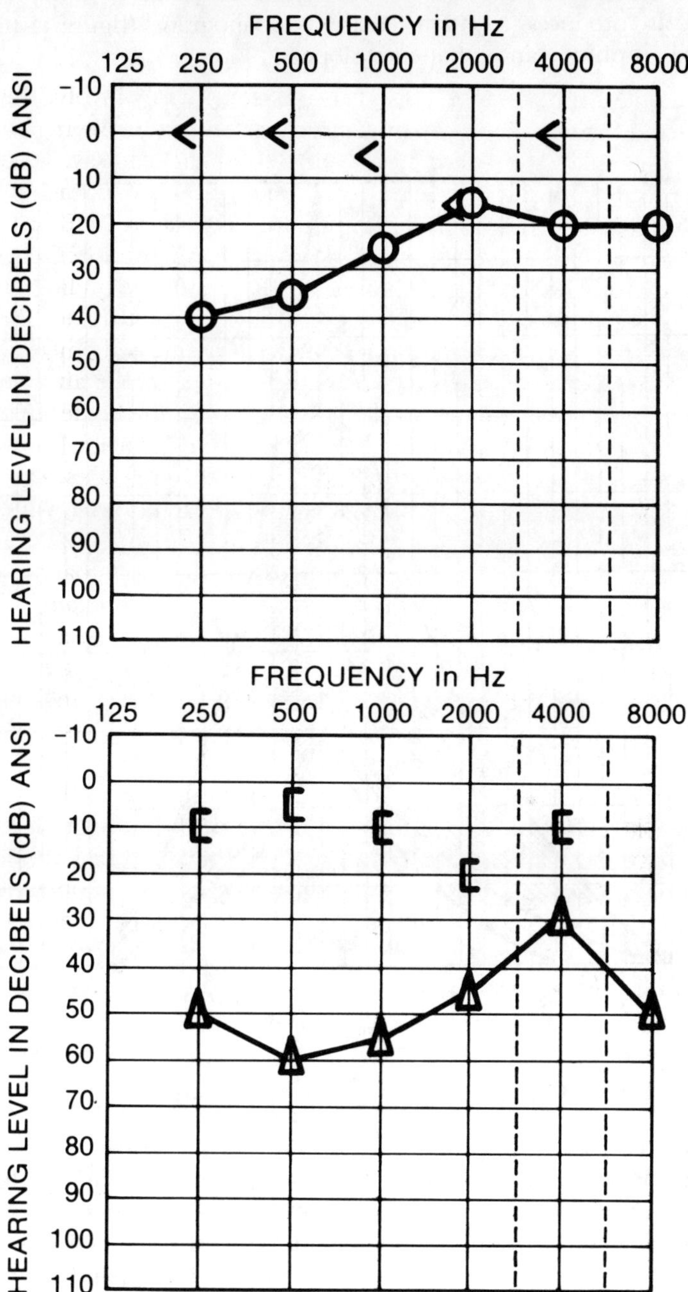

Figure 4-15. Early otosclerosis (above) compared to later otosclerosis (below). Note that both audiograms display Carhart's Notch.

TYMPANOMETRY. Otosclerosis may be the best example of increased resistance due to increases of stiffness. Clearly, if the movement of the stapes is limited, then the entire ossicular chain is restricted in its range of motion. Hence, otosclerosis produces a characteristic tympanogram (figure 4-16) with decreased amplitude and a flattened slope.

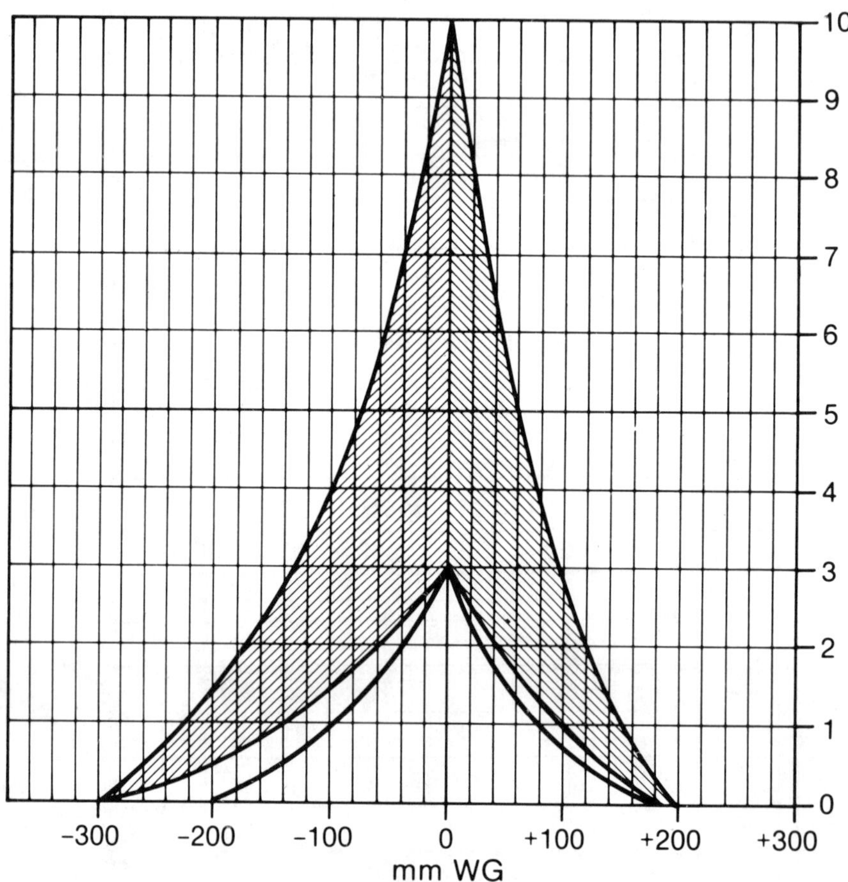

Figure 4-16. Tympanogram of an ear with advanced otosclerosis.

In summary, the audiologist's role is limited mainly to support diagnosis with most otosclerosis patients. A pre-surgical audiogram to assist in the diagnosis and a post-surgical audiogram to confirm the success of the operation may be all that is necessary. If, however, the patient has a problem which is inoperable or the surgery fails, the audiologist must assume the primary auditory rehabilitative responsibility for amplification, training, and counseling.

CASE STUDY 4-1:

SUCCESSFUL TYMPANOPLASTY

LR, a 27-year-old female, has a long history of chronic otomastoiditis. At this time, she presented with a non-healing perforation on the left side and has had several episodes of draining from the ear. She had a myringoplasty some years ago when she was 10 years old. Otologic examination by Dr. K revealed a 30% perforation of the left tympanic membrane, and he recommended tympanoplasty.

At surgery, a piece of temporalis fascia was taken for a graft. A tympanomeatal flap was created, the perforation rimmed, and the layers separated. Elevating the annulus revealed normal ossicles, but many middle ear adhesions. The adhesions were dissected free as much as possible, and the fascial graft was placed under the tympanic membrane and the mucosa of the middle ear. LR tolerated the surgery very well and was discharged from the hospital on the next postoperative day.

Pre- and post-surgical audiograms show that the surgery reduced a 20 to 25dB air-bone gap to about 5dB. Furthermore, the mild chronic conductive impairment present before surgical intervention was eliminated.

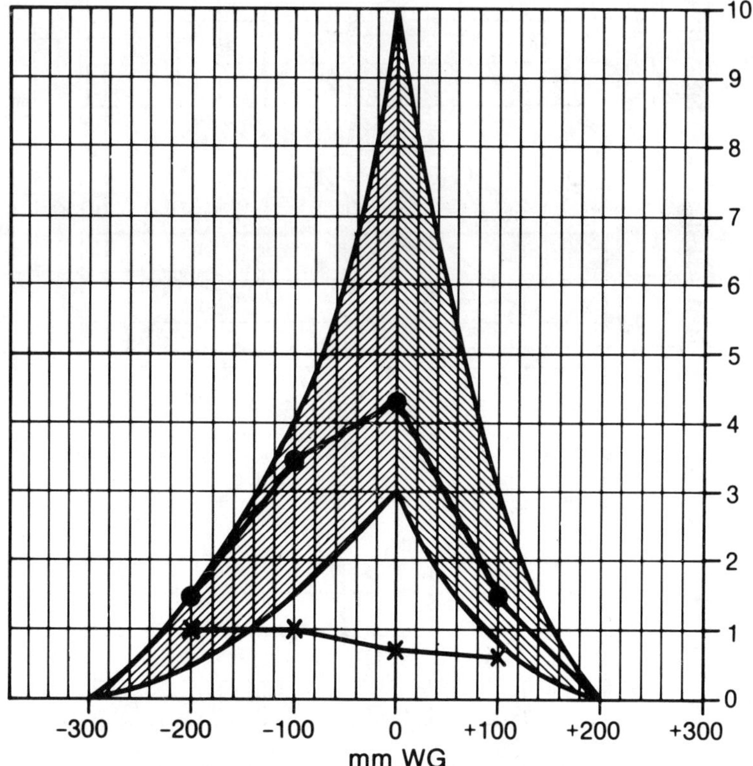

Case Study 4-1: Successful Tympanoplasty

PURE TONE AUDIOGRAM

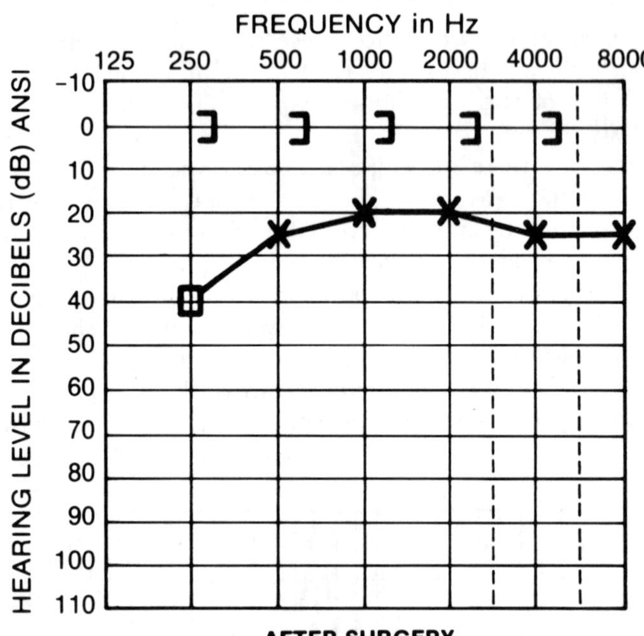

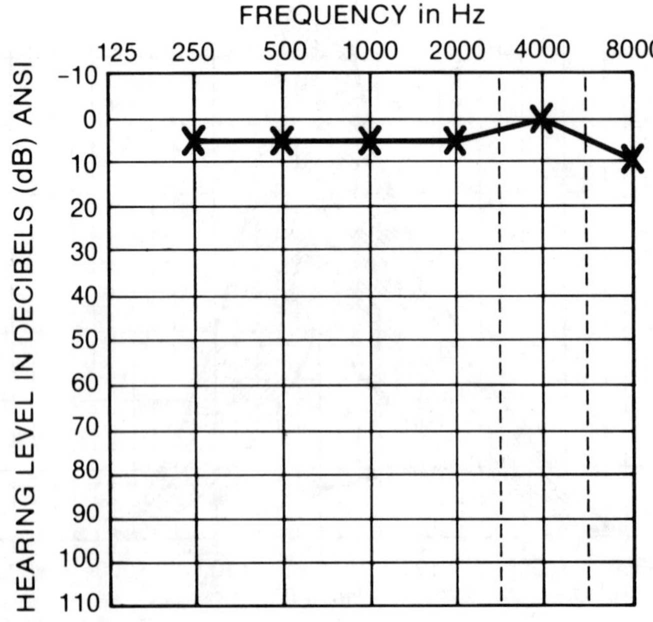

CASE STUDY 4-2:

SUCCESSFUL PROSTHESIS

JM is a 24-year-old female who has had a progressive hearing loss over the past three years. Otologic examination by Dr. S was unrevealing. Audiologic examination displayed an air-bone gap, Carhart's Notch, and a type C tympanogram. Dr. S decided to proceed with surgery, and indeed otosclerosis was present. A stapedectomy was performed and a wire prosthesis placed. JM recovered well and has had no further difficulty.

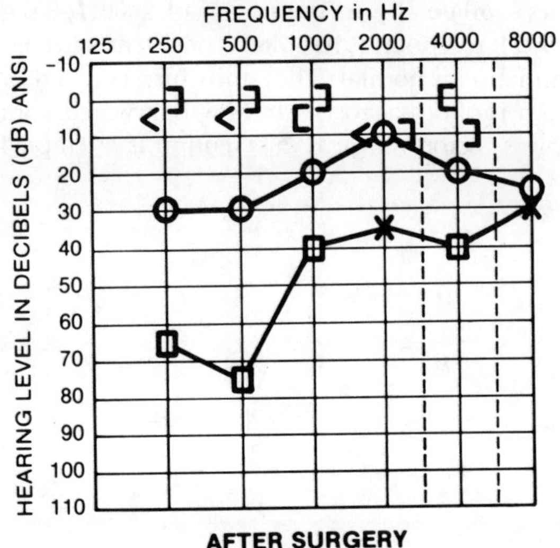

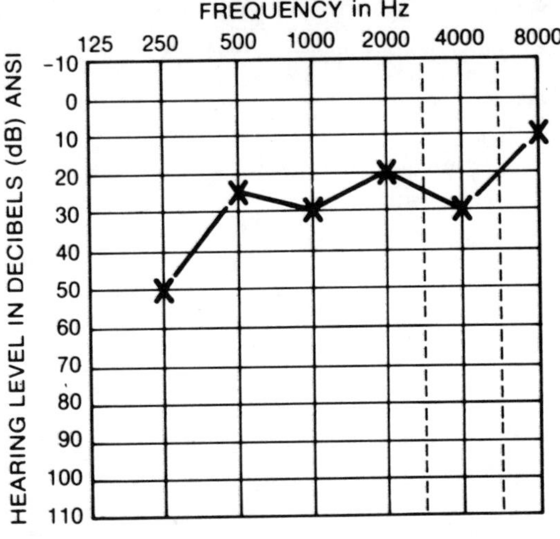

CASE STUDY 4-3:

EARLY OTOSCLEROSIS

DM, a 34-year-old male, has noticed some difficulty in hearing, a difficulty which has progressed over the past two years. He is a teacher, and now reports having trouble hearing in class. While he reports no history of ear disease or hearing loss, he states that his mother has a relatively severe hearing impairment of unknown origin. Otoscopic findings upon examination by Dr. B revealed normal tympanic membranes bilaterally, but the Rinne tuning fork test indicates a mild conductive loss.

Pure tone audiometry reveals an average loss of 35dB in the right ear and somewhat more than 25dB in the left. The contour of the bone conduction audiogram drops bilaterally in the region of 2000Hz suggesting Carhart's Notch. The speech reception threshold is consistent with the audiogram, and speech discrimination is normal. The family history and the audiometric data suggest a diagnosis of otosclerosis. Mr. M will be watched for the progression of the hearing loss before surgical intervention is attempted.

Case Study 4-3: Early Otosclerosis

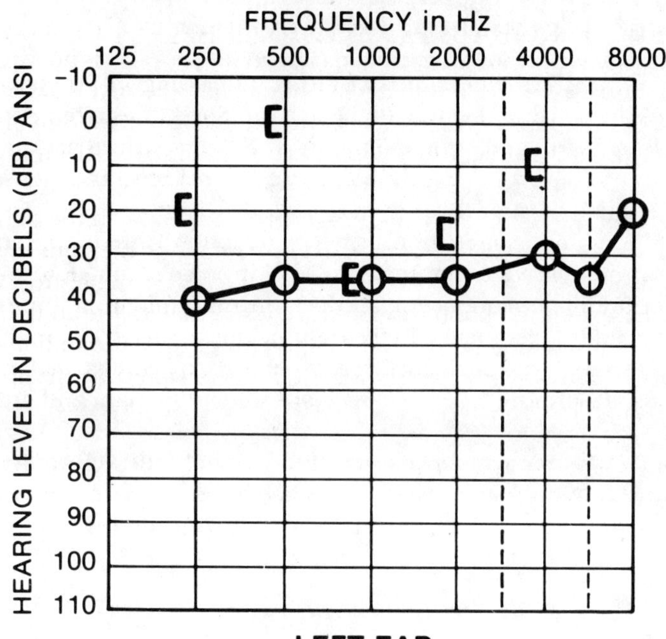

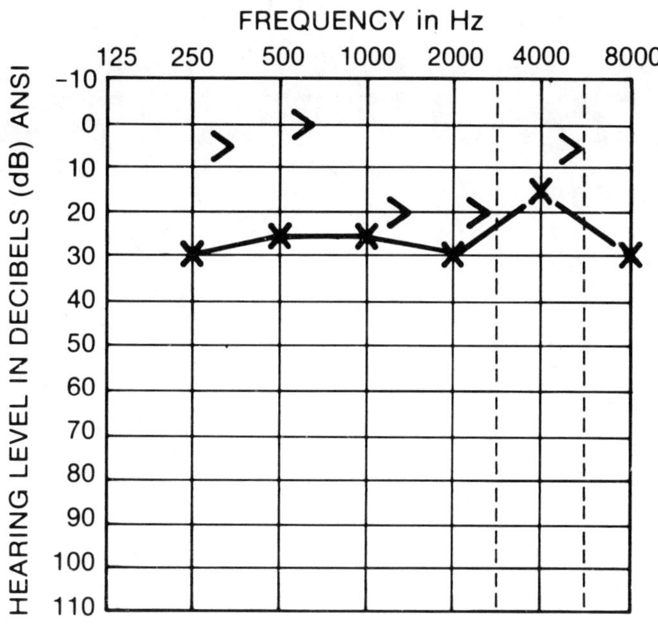

Case Study 4-4:

Advanced Otosclerosis with Probable Presbycusis

Mrs. G, age 72, complained of difficulty hearing in a noisy room; in particular, she noted problems with her left ear. She was seen by a "specialist" several years ago, and, apparently, it was suggested that she have a stapedectomy. She has a family history of otosclerosis, and her sister has undergone bilateral stapedectomy.

Pure tone air conduction, speech reception threshold, and word discrimination tests were administered. Masking was required during testing of the left ear for bone conduction and for word discrimination. Pure tone tests indicated a sensory-neural loss in the right ear, and a mixed loss in the left ear; moderate to severe on each side. Speech audiometry results were consistent with the results of pure tone tests: SRT of 45dB on the right and 75dB on the left.

Mrs. G. has been using her sister's hearing aid in her left ear for the past few months. It seems to be satisfactory for her; hence, it was recommended that she have her own ear mold made and continue wearing the aid.

CASE STUDY 4-4: ADVANCED OTOSCLEROSIS WITH PROBABLE PRESBYCUSIS

PURE TONE AUDIOGRAM

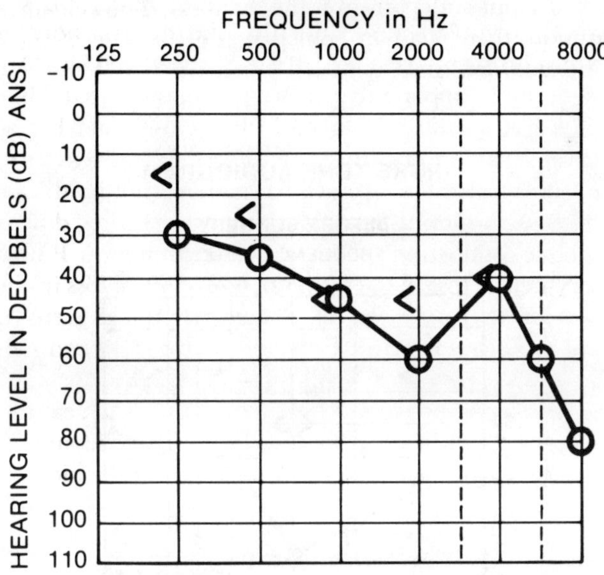

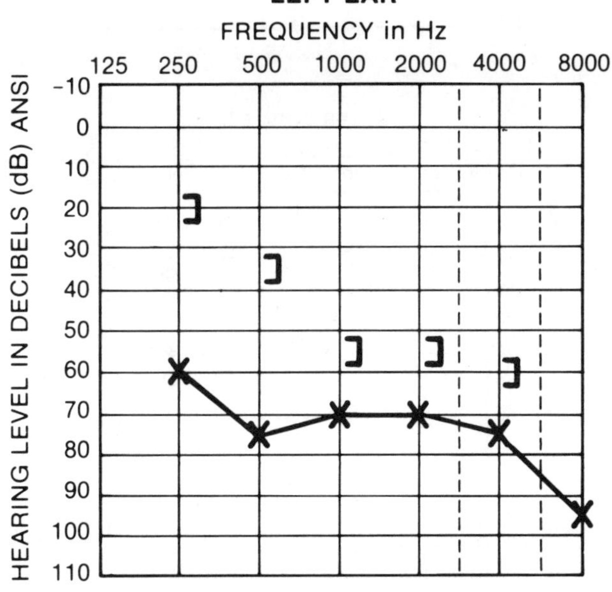

Case Study 4-5:

Post-surgical Otosclerosis

EP has had a progressive loss of hearing in the right ear. He has been seen previously and diagnosed as having otosclerosis. Post-surgically, he says that he hears 100% better but suffers from some dizziness. The evidence does not support his opinion: there is an air-bone gap as great as 20dB and a PTA of 25dB in the (operated) left ear.

PURE TONE AUDIOGRAM

BEFORE SURGERY

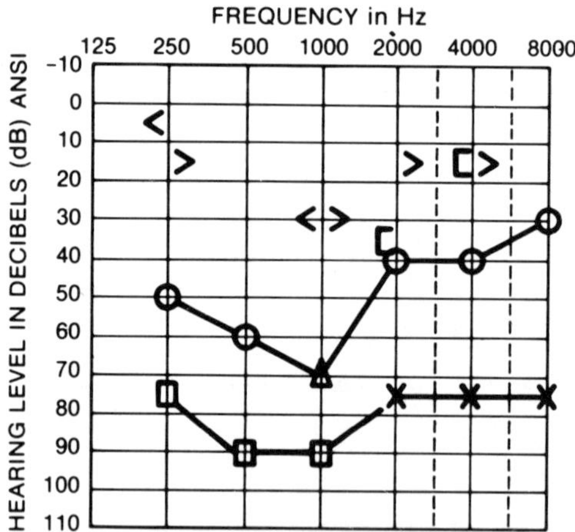

AFTER SURGERY

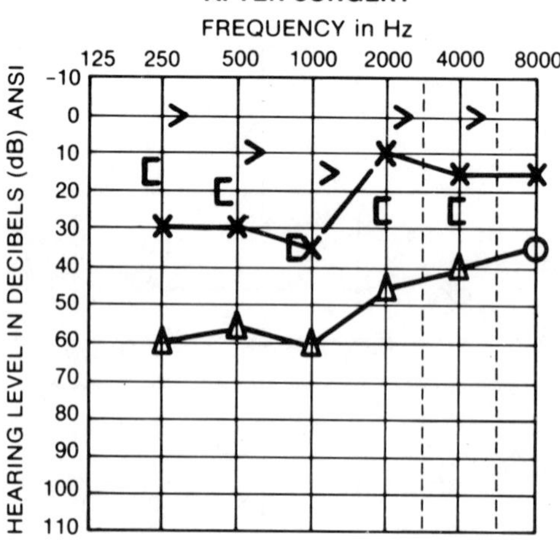

REFERENCES

Carhart, R. 1950. The clinical application of bone conduction audiometry. *Arch. Otolaryngol.* 51:789-807.

Derlacki, E. 1976. Otosclerosis. In *Hearing disorders,* ed. J.L. Northern. Boston: Little, Brown and Co.

Goin, D.W. 1976. Otospongiosis. In *Otolaryngology: A Textbook,* ed. G. English. New York: Harper & Row, Inc.

Jaffe, B.F. 1978. Topographical signs associated with congenital hearing loss. In *Early diagnosis of hearing loss,* ed. S.E. Gerber and G.T. Mencher. New York: Grune & Stratton, Inc.

Kirikae, I. 1973. Physiology of the middle ear including eustachian tube. In *Otolaryngology,* vol. 1, eds. M.M. Paparella and D.A. Schumrick. Philadelphia: W.B. Saunders Co.

Konigsmark, B.W. 1972. Genetic hearing loss with no associated abnormalities: A review. Part II. *J. Speech. Hear. Dis.* 37:89-99.

Lempert, J. 1938. Improvement of hearing in cases of otosclerosis: A new one-stage surgical technic. *Arch. Otolaryngol.* 28:42-97.

Lindsay, J.R. 1973. Otosclerosis. In *Otolaryngology,* vol. 2, eds. M.M. Paparella and D.A. Shumrick. Philadelphia: W.B. Saunders Co.

Nager, G.T. 1973. Congenital aural atresia: anatomy and surgical management. In *Otolaryngology,* vol. 2, eds. M.M. Paparella and D.A. Shumrick. Philadelphia: W.B. Saunders Co.

Paparella, M.M. 1973. Surgery of the middle ear, eustachian tube and mastoid. In *Otolaryngology,* vol. 2, eds. M.M. Paparella and D.A. Shumrick. Philadelphia: W.B. Saunders Co.

Perkins, R. 1975. Ear bank of project HEAR. *Trans. Amer. Acad. of Ophthalmol. and Otolaryngol.* 80:23-29.

Rosen, S. 1953. Mobilization of the stapes to restore hearing in otosclerosis. *New York State J. Med.* 53:2650-2653.

Shambaugh, G.E. 1966. Therapy of cochlear otology. *Ann. Otol. Rhin. Laryng.* 75:579.

PART **2**

Sensory

Hearing

Impairment

When speaking of sensory hearing impairment, in the strict sense in which the term is utilized here, concern is limited to those conditions where the pathology is restricted to the cochlea, that is, the auditory end organ. Throughout most of the literature, the terms sensory-neural, sensori-neural, and sensorineural are employed. While a histopathologist (one who studies pathological conditions of tissue) may be unable to totally discern sensory (cochlear) from neural (retrocochlear) pathology, there are situations in which the distinction is audiologically useful. For example, the distinction may be potentially life-saving in a differential diagnosis between cochlear and retrocochlear pathology, as some brain stem lesions could be lethal. Consequently, the term *sensory-neural*—where the hyphen should be read as "and/or"—is utilized in this text. That is to say, our discussion is about those disorders which are sensory and/or neural.

Part Two deals specifically with sensory disorders. That is not to say that such disorders do not also involve neural components or even conductive components in some instances. But, audiometrically and rehabilitatively, the distinction between sensory and neural impairment is important, even critical; thus the division in this book.

CHAPTER 5

Congenital

Hearing

Impairment

The word *congenital* means present at birth. It does not imply any particular cause, meaning only that the patient was born with the disorder. The term *genetic* refers to those disorders, whether or not congenital, that are carried by the genes, Since approximately half of all congenital hearing impairments are genetic, and half are not, it is easy for there to be confusion. Fraser (1976) summarized the problem succinctly when he said:

> It is a paradox which underlies the distinction between congenital and genetically determined disease that genetic types of childhood deafness may frequently not be congenital, whereas acquired types due to causes acting in the prenatal period may often be truly congenital. This is one of the reasons why diagnostic confusion may occur between these two types of deafness, in that congenital hearing losses which are acquired in fetal life due to infection or other causes may be falsely attributed to genetic determination.

There is a certain amount of difficulty in addressing an issue as ultimately complex as congenital deafness. Consideration must be given, for example, to how great a loss is required for it to be considered "deafness." If discussion is limited to that small portion of the hearing-impaired population which suffers from a truly profound (by anyone's definition) hearing loss at birth, then the best available statistics indicate that about 1 child among 1000 born in the United States or Canada today will be in that category *(Mencher, 1976)*. Roughly the same proportion is evident in other western countries, although Barr (1965) reported only 1 profoundly hearing-impaired child in 2000 births in Sweden. In other parts of the world, the incidence is substantially greater. In the middle east, for example, it is about double the incidence rate in the U.S. *(Feinmesser and Tell, 1976)*, while in some parts of Latin America it is even greater *(WHO, 1967)*.

When attempting to determine the incidence of congenital deafness, the problem is knowing that the impairment was, in fact, present at birth. There are at least two very good reasons why this is a problem:

1. Most children who are born in hospitals are not screened for hearing loss until they are 9 to 12 months of age or even older. This is a particular tragedy since accurate screening methods do exist, methods which are not being utilized. As a result, and aside from the eductional/moral issues of not screening in the nursery, no one knows which children have hearing impairment at birth;

2. Large numbers of children are not born in hospitals.

In the United States today only about 75% of all births occur in hospitals. It has been suggested by Gerber (1977) that the incidence of birth defects, including hearing impairment, is likely to be greater in the unexamined 25% than in the 75% available for an examination. This is because the non-hospital population is likely to have a larger proportion of children born in remote areas, or born to families of considerable ignorance or poverty to whom the kinds of medical and hospital services that the middle class is accustomed to are not available or else are not utilized.

In summary, if there is to be universal agreement as to what "profound" hearing loss means and how many cases there are in any given community, there needs to be a clear definition of the term. Furthermore, there needs to be a comprehensive analysis of the incidence of hearing loss at birth. Since neither of these is a reality, a clear and accurate reporting of the incidence of congenital deafness is a very difficult thing to do.

PATHOLOGY and ETIOLOGY

The etiology of congenital deafness may be considered in terms of two main categories: genetic and non-genetic. Some forms of genetic deafness have associated abnormalities; most do not *(Konigsmark, 1971)*. Those deafnesses which are non-genetic in origin may be due to infection, trauma, maldevelopment, and metabolic or toxic disorders.

CONGENITAL GENETIC DEAFNESS

FORMS OF TRANSMISSION. About half of all cases of congenital deafness are inherited *(Fraser, 1971)*. The form of genetic inheritance may be autosomal recessive, autosomal dominant, or X-linked recessive. The vast majority (approximately 2/3) of congenital deafness which is genetic in basis arises from an autosomal recessive gene.

Autosomal Recessive. According to Carrel (1977) there are at least five abnormal genes in each person that do not appear as distinct entities. When one of these genes is located on a non-sex chromosome (i.e., autosomal) and is matched with another autosomal recessive abnormal gene mate, the risk for producing a deaf child is one in four. Since the risk is but one in four, there are three chances in four that a normal hearing child would be produced by such a mating. If no hearing-impaired child has been produced for several generations, it is likely that the carrier of such a gene structure would be unaware of the potential of its presence. Consequently, there are many cases where normally hearing parents produce a hearing-impaired child and honestly deny knowledge of any family history of deafness. Furthermore, if the baby was a first child, it would not have been automatically considered at risk, and therefore it would most likely not have been evaluated by a neonatal hearing screening program which was based solely on the high risk register.

Bergstrom (1976) studied 427 patients who were known to be hearing-impaired at a very early age. She found that somewhat more than 40% of the patients could ascribe their hearing impairments to heredity, while slightly more than 31% related causation to factors other than those which are inherited. Furthermore, and perhaps most interestingly, Bergstrom found that 28% of the patients did not know the cause of their hearing losses. It is probable that a significant proportion of that 28% whose etiology was unknown were first born to normal hearing parents who were carrying matched autosomal recessive genes. In fact, Konigsmark (1971) estimated that this phenomenon could account for as many as 35% of those who are congenitally deaf.

If such a set of parents had had the same autosomal recessive genes, rather than any other one of the available five or ten, then their risk for producing deaf children would be 100% *(Carrel, 1977)*. Such a family is one in which a normally hearing couple has produced three severely hearing-impaired children. There is no evidence that anything could have occurred within that family other than that "throw of the dice" which results in a matching of the same autosomal recessive genes for deafness.

Autosomal Dominant. In the case of the dominantly inherited deafness, the genetic programming from only one parent is sufficient to produce the disorder. The risk of having a hearing-impaired child due to an autosomal dominant condition is 50%. In other words, if one parent carries the gene, each child has a 50% risk of being hearing-impaired. If both parents carry the same autosomal dominant disorder, the risk is 75%.

In some autosomal dominant conditions, the hearing disorder may not manifest itself, even though the child may receive the abnormal gene. An outstanding example of such a variable expression is Waardenburg's Syndrome (figure 5-1). Some proportion of people born with Waardenburg's Syndrome have no hearing impairment, some have a moderate hearing impairment, and some have a unilateral hearing impairment. Yet, all of the people in each group carry the gene for the syndrome. Figure 5-2 displays a pedigree for recessive deafness, while figure 5-3 displays one for dominant deafness.

X-Linked Recessive. In slightly more than 3% of the cases of congenital deafness there is a form of inheritance which is called X-linked recessive. This means that the gene locus which determines the condition is on the X chromosome, one of the sex chromosomes. Females have two X chromosomes and males have one X and one Y. Since the male has only one Y chromosome, if he carries the deafness gene on that chromosome it is necessary for him to

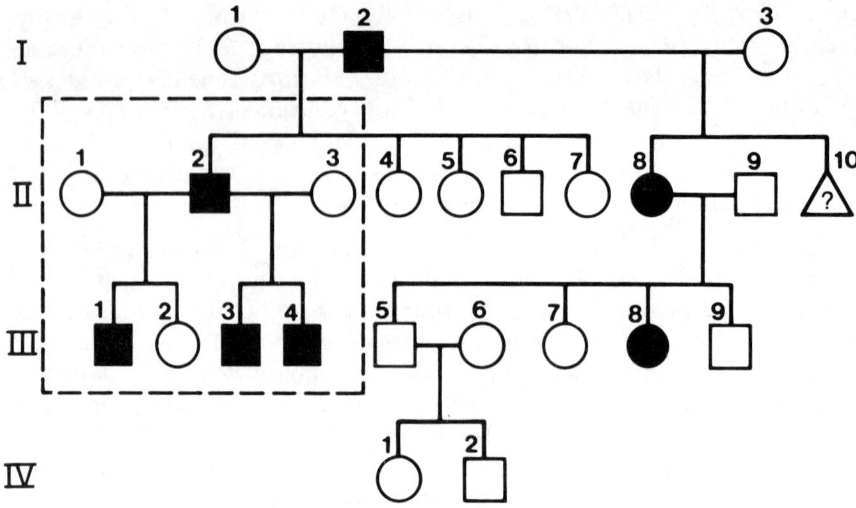

Figure 5-1. Pedigree of a family with Waardenburg's Disease. □normal male ■affected male ○normal female ●affected female

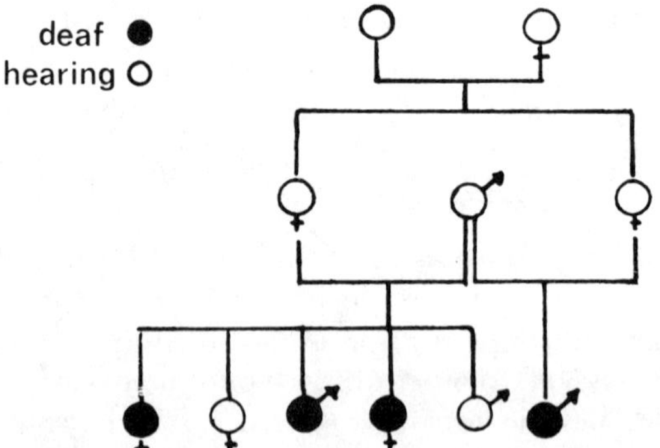

Figure 5-2. Pedigree of a family displaying a recessive mode of inheritance of deafness.

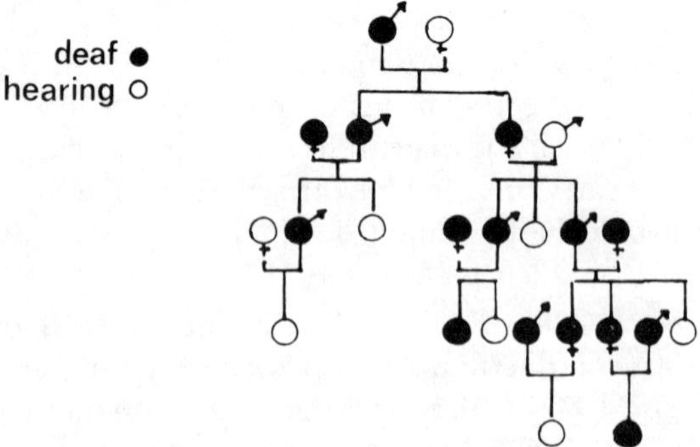

Figure 5-3. Pedigree of a family displaying a dominant mode of inheritance of deafness.

mate with a female who also carries the gene on only one of her two X chromosomes in order for them to produce an affected child. In such a case, there is a 50% chance of producing a son with a hearing loss or a daughter who will be a carrier of the trait, but without a hearing loss herself. Transmission is always from mother to son as shown in figure 5-4.

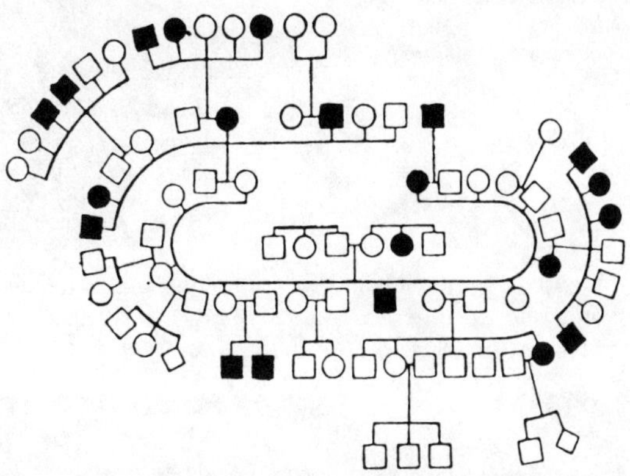

Figure 5-4. Pedigree of a family displaying the X-linked mode of inheritance of deafness. ☐normal male ■affected male ○normal female ●affected female

FORMS OF PATHOLOGY. All of the modes of transmission discussed above produce deafness with or without associated abnormalities. Most often they do not. Anomalies of the external and middle ear are not considered here because they have been reviewed in chapters 1 and 2. Nevertheless, it should be noted that they could quite properly fit into this discussion as well. Inner ear anomalies have not been considered earlier, and although they are generally rare, they certainly deserve mention.

The most extreme and rare form of an inner ear anomaly is called the Michel Anomaly (figure 5-5). In such a case there is no inner ear and, in fact, in some cases the entire auditory nerve may be absent. The disorder occurs in only about 1% of the profoundly deaf population. By contrast, according to Bergstrom (1976), about 70% of the congenital inner ear anomalies are of the Scheibe type (figure 5-6). These usually are seen with the bony labyrinth intact, but with the loss of some of the vestibular and metabolic organs of the inner ear, along with an atrophy of the organ of Corti. The third major type of inner ear anomaly is called the Mondini Anomaly (figure 5-7). In the Mondini, there is an alteration of the tissue of the cochlear duct and its contents. For example, the first one and one-half turns of the cochlea may be normal, but the remaining turn absent or markedly malformed. There are other anomalies of the inner ear (i.e., Alexander and Bing-Siebenmann), but they occur rarely. All are congenital anomalies which are usually genetic in origin.

ASSOCIATED ANOMALIES. Those congenital or genetic disorders which have associated anomalies are usually called "syndromes"; that is, a collection of

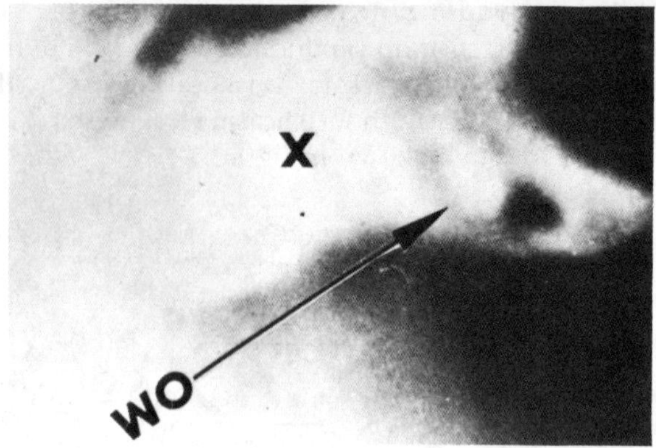

Figure 5-5. Michel anomaly showing an ossicular mass (OM) and an undeveloped inner ear (X). *(From F.O. Black et al., Congenital Deafness. Colorado Associated University Press, 1971.)*

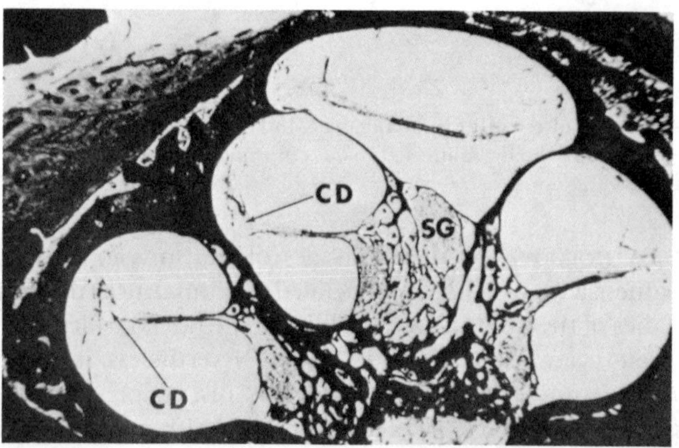

Figure 5-6. A Scheibe anomaly showing a poorly developed cochlear duct (CD) but a normal spiral ganglion (SG). *(From Schuknecht, H., in F. McConnell and P.H. Ward, eds., Deafness in Childhood, Vanderbilt University Press, 1967.)*

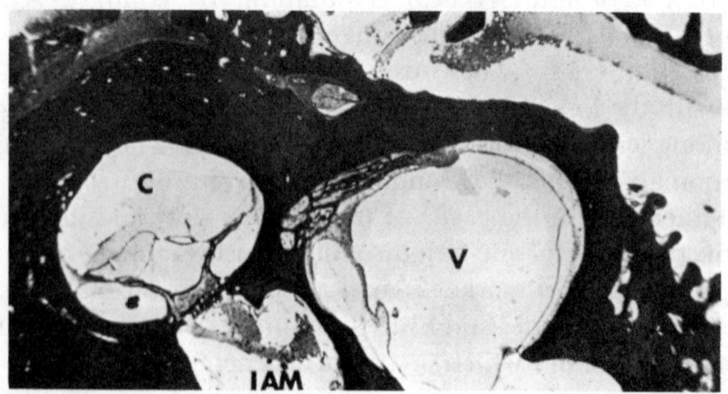

Figure 5-7. The Mondini anomaly. Notice that the cochlea has only 1-1/2 turns.*(Ibid.)*

associated abnormalities and symptoms. For purposes of convenience, the associated anomalies are classed as:

1. Integumentary (pertaining to the skin)
2. Skeletal
3. Eye
4. Other

Perhaps the most inclusive example of a congenital familial disorder with overt abnormalities of the type discussed is Waardenburg's Syndrome. This is because it characterizes many of the inheritable abnormalities which may occur. It is a dominant genetic disorder with variable expression. Since it is dominant, it will be passed to the offspring in the manner described earlier; but it is characterized, as are many dominant disorders, by the variable expressivity of its stigmata. This means that the collection of symptoms which constitute the syndrome described by Waardenburg (1951) appears with all degrees of severity, including not appearing, from one patient to another.

Waardenburg's Syndrome (figure 5-1) is classified by the Konigsmark (1971) nosology as congenital deafness with integumentary system disease. Its signs are all in the realm of pigmentary disorders. For example, a patient may present with an alteration of eye color, heterochromia iridis, in which the eyes are of different colors and/or more than one color may appear in the iris of each eye. Patients often have an alteration of hair color which is revealed by an unpigmented streak. The medial canthi of the eyes may be widely separated. The separation may be exaggerated by a characteristic flattening of the bridge of the nose. In some patients there is a typical "heart shaped" mouth. Due to the variable expression of symptoms, some of these signs may not appear at all. Similarly, hearing loss may not appear, or it may present from mild to profound in one or both ears.

Integumentary Anomalies. A number of syndromes count congenital sensory-neural hearing loss and skin abnormality among their chief sequelae. Best known is albinism. Tietz (1963) reported an extended family in which fourteen members demonstrated the disorder. The hearing loss was severe. In addition to albinism, or absence of the coloring pigmentation to the skin, integumentary anomalies may involve abnormal patterns of pigmentation. For example, hereditary piebaldness (strips of hyper- and hypo-pigmentation) and Lentigines (leopard-like spots) may accompany severe congenital sensory-neural hearing loss. These disorders tend to favor males, although not exclusively.

Skeletal Anomalies. Perhaps the most frequently seen example of a genetic congenital hearing loss with associated skeletal defect is Klippel-Feil Syndrome (figure 5-8). Called an "otocervical" disorder, it involves the ear and the cervical vertebrae. The patient seems to have a shortness or absence of neck. In conjunction with that, there is limited mobility of the head and what appears to be a lowered hair line in the back.

The syndrome does tend to run in families, but, because its appearance is not so frequent or easily predicted, the disorder is said to be of "autosomal dominance with poor penetrance." As with Waardenburg's Syndrome, the

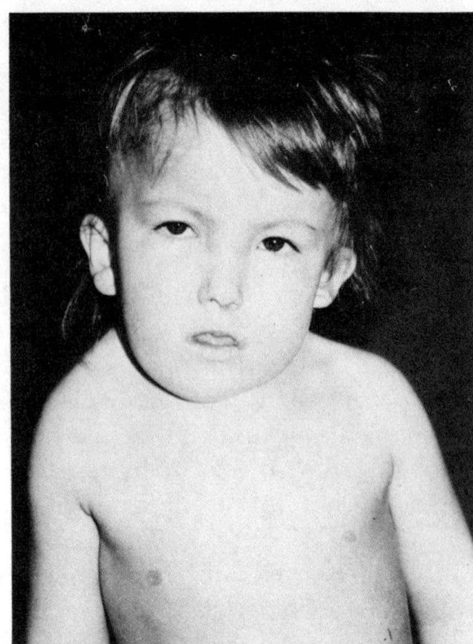

Figure 5-8. Klippel-Feil Syndrome.

disorder, and most of the others like it, have variable expressivity. That is, there is no consistent audiological pattern associated with it. Again, as with most other disorders in this category, it does usually involve some middle ear malformation (i.e., misshapen stapes, absence of oval window, etc.), and thus, conductive losses occur often. However, sensory-neural hearing losses occur more often, while mixed losses occur most often.

Ocular Anomalies. Usher's Syndrome, which appears in 3% to 10% of profoundly deaf children, offers the best example of a recessive genetic condition with hearing loss and associated ocular abnormalities. The first signs the patient notices are a narrowing field of vision and defective night vision. This usually occurs in early adulthood. The syndrome is specifically characterized by retinitis pigmentosa, a slowly progressive, bilateral, tapeto-retinal degeneration. Eventually, total blindness occurs. The disorder may also be accompanied by mental retardation, epilepsy, psychological abnormalities, physical anomalies, and vertigo. The hearing loss is usually in the moderate to severe range, sensory-neural, and frequently involves the high frequencies *(Northern and Downs, 1978)*. Because the visual problem is progressive, the earlier the diagnosis, the more intensive the audiological counseling can be, and thus, the more effective it will be. Family members should also receive genetic counseling.

Other eye anomalies, extending as far as total absence of eyes *(anophthalmos)* occur with hearing disorders. In fact, Rapin and Ruben (1979) reported eye anomalies in twelve of sixteen children with ear anomalies. Markedly bulging eyes, *exophthalmos,* is characteristic of Crouzon's Disease;

and widely separated eyes, *hypertelorism,* accompanies several of the congenital deafness syndromes.

Other Anomalies. There are two excellent examples of congenital genetic syndromes with hearing loss and other associated anomalies which could loosely be called "other," but which are of such significance that they should not be treated so off-handedly. The first of these is called Mucopolysaccharidosis (Hurler Syndrome and Hunter Syndrome). The second is called Down's Syndrome (Trisomy 21 Syndrome; Mongolism).

a) *Mucopolysaccharidosis (M.P.S.).* There are actually seven disorders in this group, all of which are characterized by increased urinary mucopolysaccharide excretion. While all may present with hearing loss, only M.P.S. I (Hurler Syndrome) and M.P.S. II (Hunter Syndrome) count hearing impairment among their major stigmata. Hurler Syndrome is often reflected in mental deficiency and a specific constellation of deformities including reduced stature, osseous and articular (bone and joint) deficits, large heads, widely spaced eyes, and flattened nasal bridges (figure 5-9). In contrast, Hunter Syndrome is less severe (figure 5-10). They are considered to be an inborn error of metabolism *(Northern and Downs, 1978).* Most patients appear normal at birth, features gradually becoming coarse as the degeneration proceeds. These disorders are also typified by failure to grow, chronic nasal problems, mental retardation, and stiffness of the joints. Patients with Hurler Syndrome usually die by the age of 10 years. Hunter Syndrome patients usually live longer, but an early death is expected.

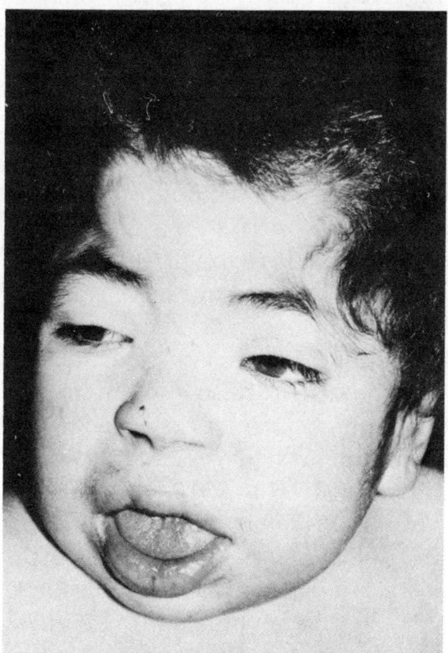

Figure 5-9. Hurler's Syndrome. Note coarseness of features, large head, and flattened bridge of nose.

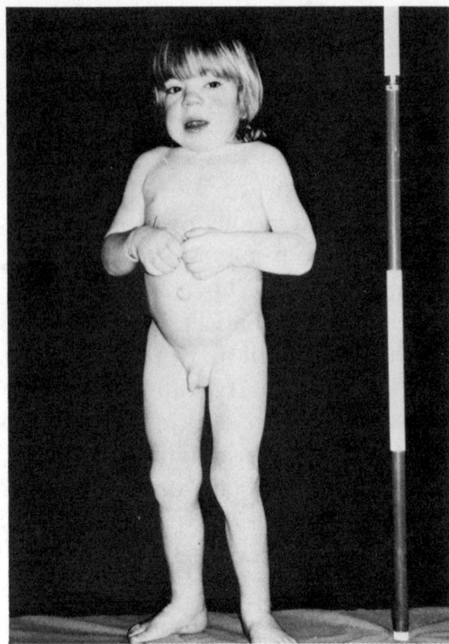

Figure 5-10. Hunter's Syndrome. Child aged 5-8 with history of ear disease. Note reduced growth, joint abnormalities, and enlarged and malproportioned head.

Patients with Hurler Syndrome usually have some progressive hearing loss. Similarly, about half of the Hunter Syndrome patients have a moderate hearing loss, primarily sensory-neural. Because these disorders are also characterized by bone and joint malformations, middle ear and cochlear anomalies are common. A mixed conductive and sensory-neural hearing loss may be present as a result of ossicular chain malformation and an inner ear anomaly (*Leroy and Crocker, 1966; Konigsmark and Gorlin, 1976; Kelemen, 1977*).

b) Down's Syndrome. Perhaps the best known congenital disorder is Down's Syndrome, once known as Mongolism. Recently, the discovery that this disorder is the result of an extra chromosome has led to it also being called the Trisomy 21 Syndrome. Incidentally, other major chromosomal disorders (Trisomy 13-15 and Trisomy 18) also result in severely involved children with marked degeneration of the organ of Corti, and most die in the first year of life.

Estimates of occurrences suggest that Trisomy 21 (Down's Syndrome) children appear in 1 in 600 to 1 in 770 live births *(Northern and Downs, 1978)*. The children may exhibit any combination of over 50 different anomalies. Mental retardation, short fingers (especially the fifth), simian folds across the palm of the hands, and a flattened facial expression with a characteristic anti-mongoloid slant of the eyes are present in virtually all patients (figure 5-11).

Audiograms obtained from Down's Syndrome patients vary dramatically from person to person. Generally, because of the frequent physical anomalies of the pinnae and ear canals, it is reasonable to expect, at worst, middle ear

92

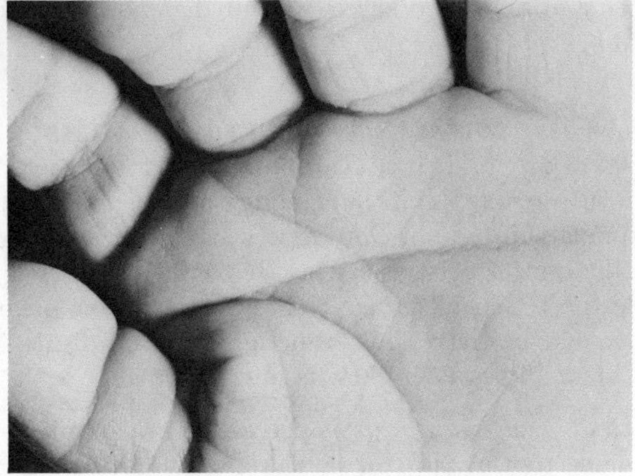

Figure 5-11a. Down's Syndrome.

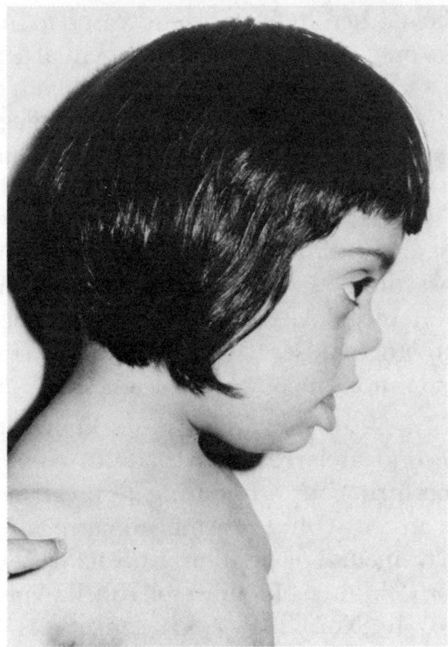

Figure 5-11b. Down's Syndrome.

anomalies, and at best, a long series of middle ear infections. Most studies report the presence of middle ear problems in 50% to 80% of the cases. Gerber (1977) has indicated that deafness is rare in this group. On the other hand, most authors agree that mild to moderate sensory-neural hearing loss is present in a large percentage of the cases, with mixed sensory-neural/conductive hearing loss present most often. It should be noted that the degree of mental retardation may influence the audiometric results obtained, and sensory-neural hearing loss may appear far more severe than it really is.

Play audiometry is usually very successful with these patients even at full adult chronological age.

Congenital Non-Genetic Deafness

While 50% of the children who are born deaf have a genetic etiology, it is apparent that 50% do not. Significant among causes of non-genetic congenital deafness are prenatal infections. Any viral, bacterial, protozoal, etc., infection can damage the central nervous system prenatally and, therefore, can cause congenital deafness. Generally, bacterial infections during pregnancy do not cross the placental barrier. Thus, although bacterial disease may cause a hearing loss in a child, it is unlikely to affect a fetus.

VIRAL DEAFNESS. The word *virus* is derived from a Latin word meaning poison, the same root as *virulent,* and implies a potent, destructive agent *(Bergstrom, 1977).* Some viruses may cause devastating effects on the fetal ear when they produce intrauterine infections which may be innocuous or even asymptomatic in the mother. In fact, there is reason to suppose that any viral disease which occurs prenatally may lead to congenital deafness. For example, one center reported a severely hearing-impaired girl born to a mother who had contracted viral influenza in the seventh month of her pregnancy. Granted, the cause-effect relationship is based on supposition; but, nevertheless, the principle is correct and cannot be ignored. Viral disease may also result in severe inner ear or systemic effects when contracted in postnatal life. Notable among these diseases are measles, mumps, and meningitis (see chapter 6).

Two of the most common viruses associated with congenital hearing loss are rubella and cytomegalovirus. With the exception of rubella and cytomegalovirus, no other viruses have been clearly documented as playing a major role in the causation of congenital deafness.

Rubella. Historically, of all the viral diseases known to cause congenital hearing loss, the world at large has been most concerned about rubella (German measles) occurring any time during the pregnancy and leading to the development of an infant with a hearing impairment, visual impairment, cardiac defect, and/or mental retardation. Rubella has been one of the worst cripplers of newborn children. In times of rubella epidemics, such as the epidemic of 1964-65 in North America, as many as 25% of births with congenital hearing impairment can trace their deafness to this disease. It is a myth that rubella is dangerous only during the first trimester of pregnancy. In fact, according to the longitudinal studies of Bordley, Brookhauser, et al. (1967) and Baldursson, Bjarason, et al. (1972), over 23% of the children with a hearing loss were born to mothers who contracted rubella during the second or third trimesters of the pregnancy.

The causal relationship between maternal rubella in pregnancy and congenital defects was first recognized by Sir Norman Gregg in 1941 *(Brookhauser and Bordley, 1973; Hardy, 1973; Monif and Jordon, 1977; Hanshaw and Dudgeon, 1978).* It was nearly 20 years following Gregg's discovery before progress was made either in an understanding of the pathogenesis of rubella, including the mechanisms of fetal damage, or in the development of a means of prevention. Before the isolation of the rubella virus, it was necessary to depend on clinical symptoms as the criteria for the diagnosis of the viral infection. Even now, the diagnosis of rubella is very often difficult and must be based on virological confirmation.

Fetal infection by the rubella virus generally occurs by one of the following routes: 1) the transplacental passage of virus, 2) spreading up the birth canal with infection of the membranes, or 3) as a result of direct contact or contamination during the birth process. Neonatal infection may be acquired from the mother or the nursery attendants *(Hardy, 1973; Bergstrom, 1977)*.

Prenatal rubella infection differs in several important aspects from postnatally acquired rubella. Rather than being a mild, self-limiting disease, intrauterine rubella is often associated with a severe disseminated infection and a chronic infectious state which persists throughout fetal life. In some cases, infection may be incompatible with life and fetal death ensues; the symptoms in those who survive depends on the organs involved and the degree of the damage to them.

Maternal rubella acquired in the first trimester of pregnancy usually results in fetal malformations: congenital cataracts, congenital heart disease, microcephaly, and/or mental retardation *(Top and Wehrle, 1976)*. Hanshaw and Dudgeon (1978) indicated that, in all of the prospective studies that have been reported, the risk to the fetus is greater in the first eight weeks of pregnancy than in the second. Although the first trimester is the major "at risk" period, there is no distinct dividing line for risk at the thirteenth week of gestation. Hanshaw and Dudgeon (1978) reported that malformations of the heart and eye are uncommon after the twelfth week, but a large number of cases of hearing loss, delayed development, and neurological deficits are noted by the fourth month, but less frequently thereafter.

Information on the risk of fetal damage from maternal rubella after the fourth month of gestation is sparse. Hardy, Sever, and Gilkeson (1969) reported that 15 of 22 infants born to mothers who had clinical rubella sometime between the thirteenth and thirty-first weeks of gestation had evidence of fetal damage. The defects noted consisted mainly of poor or delayed development and speech disorders *(Bordley et al., 1967)*.

Kohji et al. (1979) conducted a correlational study of the relationship between gestational age at the time of prenatal rubella and the type of congenital anomaly. They analyzed instances of congenital rubella syndrome for which the last menstrual period and the date of appearance of rubella rash were known. The history of prenatal rubella in these cases was from 16-131 days (approximately 2 to 19 weeks) of gestation. Kohji et al. found 46 cases of deafness out of 55 such patients. They also found that there was no special relationship between the time of prenatal rubella and the degree of hearing loss. Thus, despite the paucity of documented evidence on the incidence of defects associated with rubella contracted beyond the twentieth week of pregnancy, it can be concluded that the risk of incurring hearing loss diminishes after the twentieth week.

One aspect affecting the reported incidence of defects due to prenatal rubella is the age at which the children are assessed for evidence of damage. Hanshaw and Dudgeon (1978) cite several studies which indicate the progressive nature of hearing loss as a result of prenatal rubella. Studies reported by Manson, Logan, and Loy (1960) of children born in England and Wales (1950-51) following prenatal rubella indicated that the incidence of sensory hearing loss detected at age two years was 2% and that of suspected sensory hearing loss was 6%. When the same group of children was reassessed at 4 to 5 years of age, 12.8% were found to have sensory deafness. A third follow-up of this same group of children at age 8 to 11 years showed that the incidence of sensory deafness was 16%. Bearing in mind that as children get older they respond better to audiometric testing and further that the incidence of sensory hearing loss in a population of normal 8-11 year olds is markedly less than 16%, this information suggests that there is progressive hearing loss due to prenatal rubella. This observation stresses the importance of continued assessment of children known to or thought to have been exposed prenatally to rubella.

The histopathology of prenatal viral disease is often identical to that of an acquired endolabyrinthitis and is structurally the same as some of the congenital anomalies of the inner ear. In fact, Bordley et al. (1967) described the pathology as that of the Scheibe type. A most interesting observation was reported by Lindsay and Matz (1966). They had acquired the temporal bones of a child who had a well-documented congenital hearing impairment, and who subsequently had mumps which caused an additional hearing loss. Studies of the temporal bones revealed that the cochleae were abnormal, indeed, but there was no way to tell which abnormality was congenital and which was acquired.

Temporal bone studies of children congenitally deafened by rubella have revealed localized lesions in the inner ear. These are mainly confined to the stria vascularis, Reissner's membrane, and the tectorial membrane *(Bergstrom, 1977; Hanshaw and Dudgeon, 1978)*. Necrosis of the epithelium of the cochlea with damage resulting from small hemorrhages and inflammatory cells in the stria vascularis are common findings. The main histopathological changes observed by Friedman and Prier (1973) consisted of inflammation and necrosis, with adhesions between Reissner's membrane and the tectorial membrane. The latter may be found retracted away from the organ of Corti and covered by inflamed cells. The degenerative and inflammatory processes are often ongoing, leading to profound deafness in the child, and offering an explanation for the late onset of hearing loss in some children. Another problem encountered in congenital rubella is related to a lesion in the brain which results in a form of central auditory imperception (see chapter 11).

In some cases hearing loss is the only defect associated with congenital rubella. Severe deafness was a prominent feature following a rubella epidemic in Iceland in 1963-64 *(Baldursson et al., 1972)*. Thirty-seven children with rubella syndrome were detected, none had cardiac or ocular defects, but there were varying degrees of hearing loss among them. Many of the children had behavioral disorders but normal intelligence. Another similar type of epidemic was seen in Trinidad between 1960-61 *(Karmody, 1969)*. Serological tests for rubella on children with deafness of unknown etiology indicated that maternal rubella in subclinical form was probably the cause of a high proportion of such cases.

The pattern of hearing loss associated with maternal rubella was reported in a study by Brookhauser and Bordley (1973). They found that the hearing loss was sensory in character with a mild conductive component present in a few cases. Severity of the loss varied from patient to patient and between the ears of the same patient. Audiometric patterns varied among individual patients and between the ears of the same patient. Some patients showed no response at any frequency in either ear, while others responded to most frequencies but with a distinct asymmetry between ears. Audiograms most frequently associated with rubella showed a curve with greatest loss in the middle frequencies between 500 and 2,000Hz. Poor speech discrimination was seen in many cases. A subsequent follow-up study of rubella infants reported a decrease in auditory acuity from the initial hearing tests in about 25% of the cases. This has been observed also by Downs (1976), Tell (1976), and Mencher (1976).

Recent studies suggest that there is a high coincidence of conductive hearing loss related to otitis media in children with rubella associated hearing losses *(Bordley et al., 1967; Sellars, 1969)*. Hardy and Bordley (1973) reported that although the primary hearing loss is sensorineural, all rubella children may have concurrent middle ear difficulty, suggesting that the host for the rubella virus in cases of progressive hearing loss may lie in the middle ear disease.

Mencher et al. (1978) noted several cases of progressive sensory hearing loss in rubella children with a full history of middle ear disease, and a contrasting absence of sensory hearing loss in children from the same epidemic with a negative history of middle ear disease. It appears, therefore, that the rubella virus survives in the diseased middle ear tissue and reenters the inner ear, producing additional sensory hearing loss.

Anderson, Barr, and Wedenberg (1970), in reviewing 20 children with hearing loss due to prenatal rubella, found that 13 of 19 parental pairs had hereditary abnormalities in hearing. From this, Proctor (1977), like Anderson, Barr, and Wedenberg, concluded that genetic disposition to hearing impairment appears to be a prerequisite for rubella deafness. This seems to be a fairly broad generalization, especially in consideration of the other defects resulting from rubella in the first trimester of pregnancy. Probably, there are cases in which there is no genetic predisposition to rubella hearing loss. Clearly this hypothesis needs further investigation.

The problem is further compounded by the fact that the virus has a very long life. Bordley et al. (1967) reported two hearing-impaired children born to mothers who had contracted rubella prior to conception, and they also reported one hearing-impaired child in whom they could culture a live rubella virus at a post-partum age of 15 months. The disease is insidious, and caution is required as infants may be severely damaged due to prenatal rubella in cases where the mother has been relatively free of symptoms.

Fortunately, rubella is on the wane. Immunization has rendered it a preventable disease, and its incidence is markedly decreasing. However, we must not become sanguine about this fact. Carrel (1977) expressed his concern that our decreasing attention to prenatal rubella may lead to increasing numbers of children who are not immunized against this potentially devastating disease.

Rapid progress has occurred in the development and testing of rubella virus vaccines *(Sever and Bethesda, 1973)*. The criteria for an ideal vaccine include: safety and no untoward reactions; no adverse effects on the fetus; not transmissable from vaccinees to women of childbearing age; and finally, long-lasting immunity. Several strains of rubella vaccine have been tested and results indicate that not all are satisfactory for mass immunization programs. Local health departments can provide more specific information.

Rubella embryopathy is numerically the most important known prenatally acquired cause of congenital childhood deafness, and the highlighting of such an avoidable cause of deafness clearly shows the urgent need for an effective immunization program. The total number of cases of rubella deafness is substantial in any year and in epidemic years can rise to catastrophic figures.

If the vaccines used to prevent rubella are effective there should be a gradual decline in the incidence of rubella. This would not only prevent unnecessary suffering for individual children and their families, but it would also reduce the number of children requiring special education for the deaf and partially hearing. The resultant economic saving would be remarkable.

Cytomegalovirus. Concern cannot, and should not, be limited to rubella. Cytomegalovirus (CMV) is far more common today than prenatal rubella. It is estimated that 2%-3% of pregnant women excrete this virus, and that it may be found in 1% to 1.5% of all newborns. The disease resulting from cytomegalovirus is "silent" (that is, asymptomatic) in 98% of the infants who have it *(Marx, 1977)*. Furthermore, Marx estimated that by the age of 30 years, fully 80% of the population of the United States at some time will have carried a live cytomegalovirus. So the disease is extremely common and apparently easily transmitted.

In the 1960's, scattered reports of congenital deafness resulting from cytomegalovirus (CMV) infection began to appear *(Gerber, Mendel, and Goller, 1979)*. CMV was first isolated in 1956, although it had been suspected as a cause of cytomegalic inclusion disease for the greater part of this century *(Amstey, 1977)*. Ten times as many infants are infected by cytomegalovirus at birth as by rubella. The infection is asymptomatic in the mother, who may shed organisms for weeks or months in saliva, urine, breast milk, feces, or tears *(Bergstrom, 1977)*. Transmission may occur during pregnancy by the transplacental route. Intra-partum infection is possible during the passage of the fetus through the birth canal in women with cervical CMV but this is usually not associated with disease, and the infant who may be ill one month later, is asymptomatic otherwise. In postnatal life, CMV is transmitted only by intimate contact in adults, frequently by sexual contact and by fresh blood transfusion. Although, theoretically, babies with congenital CMV may be infectious, there is little evidence that CMV is readily disseminated to other patients or personnel in a hospital setting *(Affias and Embil, 1978)*.

When CMV comes in contact with the unborn infant, the infection may be contained by the several host defense mechanisms of the fetus, or there may be disease ranging from subtle abnormalities not detectable at birth to severe generalized disease in the newborn period. The latter, more recognizable form of the disease has been far better documented than the milder manifestations. Classically, cytomegalic inclusion disease is characterized by enlarged liver and spleen (hepatosplenomegaly), jaundice (hyperbilirubinemia), blood and skin abnormalities (thrombocytopenia with petechiae or purpura), and variable involvement of the central nervous system, including cerebral calcifications, microcephaly, chorioretinitis, deafness, and psychomotor retardation *(Weller and Hanshaw, 1962)*. There are several variations and combinations of these findings. Overt congenital CMV, which occurs in only 2% of the cases, is usually fatal *(Aballi and Korones, 1963)*.

Hyperbilirubinemia is a common manifestation of congenital CMV infection occurring in more than half of symptomatic infants in the first week of life. Hyperbilirubinemia is one of the high risk factors for sensory-neural hearing loss. Since it is a common symptom of congenital CMV, monitoring the bilirubin level is one way to be alert to the hearing status of newborns who might develop a hearing loss associated with CMV.

There is growing evidence that most infants with congenital CMV infection have little or no clinical manifestations of the disease but develop subtle neurological deformities that become apparent in the late preschool and early school years.

Hanshaw et al. (1976) sought to determine if CMV-infected, asymptomatic children were developmentally different from uninfected controls as they approached the demands of elementary school education. Of the 53 children who were found to be seropositive for CMV at birth, 44 had psychometric and pediatric evaluations at 3.5-7.0 years of age. The group's mean I.Q. was nine points below that of a group of matched controls and bilateral hearing loss was present in 5 of 40 children with antibody against CMV and only in 1 of 44 matched controls without antibody. The predicted school failure rate, based on I.Q., behavioral, neurological, and auditory test data was 2.7 times that of matched socio-economic controls and eight times that of randomly selected controls. In one particularly severe case, the child did not have symptoms of CMV in the newborn period, and the possibility of congenital infection was not considered by his physicians. He was microcephalic, hypotonic, and had a profound bilateral, sensory hearing loss. His I.Q. was below 30 at 7 years of age and he continued to excrete CMV in his urine. Hanshaw et al. (1976) concluded, on the basis of their study, that clinically inapparent congenital CMV infection definitely could have an adverse effect on CNS development.

In 1968, the first CMV case involving pathology of the cochlear end-organ was described by Myers and Stool. The infant died in the first month of life and hearing had not been evaluated. Cytomegalic inclusion-bearing cells were found in epithelial cells of the saccule, utricle, and semicircular canals and also on the epithelial cell layer (endolymphatic side) of Reissner's membrane and the stria vascularis. Hydrops of the saccule of both ears, of one utricle, and of the scala media of both ears was present. The stria vascularis was degenerated and contained a cystic structure in one ear.

According to Dahle et al. (1974), a severe-profound, high frequency, progressive sensory hearing loss is often associated with congenital CMV infection. The hearing sensitivity of 18 children with subclinical cyto-megalovirus infection was studied. Nine of the 18 children had some hearing loss ranging from slight high frequency impairment to a severe-profound unilateral loss. Indirect evidence for a progressive disease process was discovered by analyzing the number of cases with a hearing loss in relation to the age at time of testing. It was found that only 2 of 18 children under 30 months had a hearing loss, whereas 7 of 18 children over 30 months had a hearing loss. The most severe hearing losses were seen in children over 40 months.

Dahle et al. (1979) presented four case studies in which CMV may have been the cause of progressive hearing loss. The four subjects were part of a longitudinal study involving 182 children seen for audiological evaluation and serological studies. All four of the cases had progressive hearing loss and a history of chronic middle ear disease since early infancy. This suggests that, as with rubella, there is a need for close monitoring for progressive hearing loss.

Gerber, Mendel, and Goller (1979) reported a case study of a child with congenital CMV whom they monitored audiometrically over a long period of time. The child's examination at birth was unremarkable. It was reported that at the age of 4 weeks she apparently was not responding to events occurring in her acoustic environment. At the age of 2 months, an audiological diagnosis revealed no responses to speech or narrow band noise at 90dB HL in the sound field. At that time tympanometric measures appeared normal. At 10 weeks she was seen for electric response audiometry and responses were obtained at levels indicating a moderate flat hearing loss in the left ear and an upward sloping audiogram for the right ear. Impedance testing again revealed normal compliance and a pediatric examination revealed a positive titer for cytomegalovirus. At 22 weeks, electric response audiometry revealed responses at 95 and 103dB HL. On her last visit at the age of 31 weeks, auditory brainstem responses were obtained at the limits of the system, 103dB bilaterally. Thus, in this case, it appears that CMV led to degenerative sensory hearing impairment and it is therefore possible that this is a natural sequela of CMV infection.

Recently, attention has been turned to the possible development of a vaccine to prevent CMV. If 1% of delivered infants excrete CMV at birth, then out of 3,000,000 infants in the United States, 30,000 were born with this infection in 1975 *(Amstey, 1977)*. This is an extremely large number of children and should encourage the development of some type of preventive measure.

At the present time, there is no therapy for congenital CMV infection. Severe congenital anomalies are not usually produced by CMV; however, intrauterine infection produces an inflammatory reaction in the fetal tissues that leads to the observed changes at birth. It is the child with mild disease or the asymptomatic virus excretor who may benefit from therapy. It is hoped that this therapy may prevent subclinical disease, mild handicaps, mental retardation, or deafness. According to Hanshaw (1979), a number of antiviral agents has been used in the treatment of congenital and acquired cytomegalovirus infections. Although virus excretion has been temporarily halted in some instances, no role in the treatment of these infections has been established for these agents. Further, Hanshaw states that the use of these agents is potentially toxic and has not been adequately studied.

Protozoal Infections. The most dramatic example of congenital non-genetic deafness caused by protozoal infection is toxoplasmosis. It has been said that 10% to 20% of all profound childhood deafness is caused by this infection *(Theissing and Kittel, 1962)*. Children affected by *toxoplasma gondii,* which is acquired transplacentally, usually are multiply involved. Hydrocephalus, seizures, mental retardation, visual impairment, and neuromuscular deficit are frequent sequelae in addition to the hearing loss. The disease apparently develops as calcium deposits on the stria vascularis and the spiral ligament. The resultant hearing loss is therefore slowly progressive. The hearing impairment may begin in early childhood as a mild loss and will advance toward profound deafness with time. The disease does not respond well to drug therapy, and, because of the multiple involvements, prognosis is poor. Audiological differential diagnosis is extremely difficult; nevertheless, habilitative efforts can be quite rewarding.

Congenital syphilis also leads to severe sensory hearing impairment. However, the hearing loss which results from this protozoa rarely is manifest before the second decade of life. It is discussed further in the next chapter.

MEDICAL CONSIDERATIONS

In order to provide the maximum in educational and audiological programming, and thus, presumably, the maximum opportunity for normal development, the congenitally deaf or hard-of-hearing child must be identified at the earliest possible time in life. The recommended procedures for screening newborns are in print and are presumably well known to physicians and others engaged in early identification efforts *(Mencher, 1976; Northern and Downs, 1978)*. Predicated on longitudinal research data, the recommendations were refined at the 1974 Nova Scotia Conference on Early Identification of Hearing Loss and adopted by the United States Joint

Committee on Infant Hearing. They have also been adopted by the Canadian Advisory Coalition on Childhood Hearing Impairment (CACCHI), the Canadian equivalent organization.

The procedures focus on the use of a high-risk register in the newborn nursery called the A B C D's of Hearing Loss *(Downs and Silver, 1972)*. Table 5-1 reflects the register as originally proposed and a recent addition adopted at the Saskatoon Conference on the Early Diagnosis of Hearing Loss *(Gerber and Mencher, 1978)*.

Children falling in the high-risk register may be behaviorally screened in the nursery by use of commercially available calibrated sound generators, by use of automated devices such as the crib-o-gram *(Simmons and Russ, 1974)* or by electrophysiological approaches such as electric response audiometry. Those children failing the screening examination and/or those referred directly to diagnostic centers are to be evaluated by both audiological and medical techniques which follow a specific sequential procedure. The audiological techniques are discussed later (see Audiological Considerations).

TABLE 5-1.

The criteria for identifying a newborn at risk for hearing impairment is the presence of one or more of the following:

A. Affected family: history of hereditary childhood impairment in the family, first cousins or closer.

B. Breathing difficulty: significant asphyxia associated with acidosis (a pH level of greater than 7.3 with asphyxia has been associated with sensory-neural hearing loss).

C. Transplacental infection: rubella or other non-bacterial intrauterine fetal infection (e.g., cytomegalovirus, Herpes infections, syphilis).

D. Defects of Ear, Nose and Throat: malformed, low-set or absent pinnae; cleft lip or palate (including submucous cleft); any residual abnormality of the otorhinolaryngeal system. Any first arch syndrome.

E. Elevated Bilirubin Level: Serum bilirubin level judged by the primary care provider to be potentially toxic.

s. Small at Birth Weight: birthweight less than 1500 grams.

When a child has been identified as at risk for hearing loss, and has failed a preliminary hearing screening, procedures to confirm or deny the presence of hearing impairment should be implemented immediately and with the utmost care. Most family physicians or pediatricians will refer to otological centers when the investigation progresses to the stages outlined.

Medical approaches to the patient are aimed at two definitive purposes: 1) identification of a hearing loss, and 2) identification of the etiology of any hearing loss. It is significant, therefore, that each of the items seen in table 5-2 be considered in terms of the entire discussion as to causes and types of congenital hearing losses as presented in this chapter.

Table 5-2.

A comprehensive assessment of any child suspect for hearing loss should include these procedures:

A. Essential to the Assessment
1. Standard pediatric examination
2. Pneumatic otoscopy and/or otomicroscopy
3. Fundoscopic examination
4. Observations for specific physical abnormalities

B. Strongly Recommended in the Assessment
1. General laboratory examinations
2. Appropriate serology examinations for toxoplasmosis, rubella, cytomegalovirus, and herpes
3. Urinalysis
4. Family audiograms

C. Include When Indicated
1. Thryoid function
2. Polytomography of middle and inner ear
3. Electrocardiogram
4. Chromosomal study
5. Fluorescent trepanemal antibody (FTA) Absorption test for syphilis
6. Appropriate testing for mucopolysaccharidosis

Procedures such as pneumatic otoscopy are aimed at separating sensory-neural from conductive problems. Fundoscopic examination is germane to relating etiology to rubella or retinitis pigmentosa (although that is not likely to be spotted in a newborn). Urinalysis may identify kidney disease or one of the mucopolysaccharidoses. An examination of thyroid function may reveal Pendred's Disease, while chromosomal studies may specify a large number of different etiologies. Chromosomal examinations may also lead to genetic counseling and thus, possibly, to the prevention of future children with hearing loss.

It is important that all disciplines concerned with identification of deafness in children—specifically audiology, otology, and pediatrics—be familiar with and understand the procedures reviewed here, the limitations of their usage, and the rationale for the priorities specified. Only through a clear understanding by all involved of the what, why, and how of sister disciplines can the team approach be developed and the best interests of the patient be served.

Finally, the general otological considerations for a patient with a congenital sensory-neural hearing loss are no different than they would be for

103

any normally-hearing person, except perhaps, that greater caution is required. Identification of middle ear disease in a patient with a congenital sensory-neural hearing loss is far more difficult. That is, the sensory loss may hide any change in middle ear function which would normally have been reflected in a conductive hearing loss. Furthermore, when dealing with a patient having a unilateral hearing loss, the significance of the development of ear disease in the one good ear is doubled.

AUDIOLOGICAL CONSIDERATIONS

The handicapping effects of congenital hearing impairment are extensive and variable. The genetic deafnesses range from mild to profound with audiometric contours from flat through odd shaped, affecting one or both ears. Some genetically based hearing impairments are degenerative; some are not. Among those which are degenerative, some appear within the first weeks of life, and some not until much later. Some children with hereditary degenerative hearing losses appear, at first, to have no hearing loss, but become quite profoundly impaired.

Congenital hearing losses which are not genetically based are equally variable. Hearing impairment consequent to prenatal viral diseases is usually very severe. For example, audiograms associated with prenatal rubella have sometimes been called "corner audiograms" because the only responses are in the lowest frequencies and at the highest intensities. In comparison, hearing losses associated with some prenatal familial dispositions, such as diabetes or thyroid diseases, are not as severe.

The point is that it is not easy to predict the severity and/or extent of a congenital hearing loss. To every rule, there is an exception. The only constant is that genetically based hearing losses appear with equal severity in both children and adults.

Furthermore, in spite of, or perhaps because of, the variety of conditions, audiometric patterns, and causes for hearing losses within this group of disorders, there seems to be little, from an audiological point of view, to distinguish congenital from acquired hearing impairment.

There is a set of audiological diagnostic tests and procedures which, when utilized, should result in a comprehensive auditory assessment of a suspect infant. Procedures developed at the Saskatoon Conference *(Gerber and Mencher, 1978)* in conjunction with the development of the medical sequence considered earlier (table 5-2), include:

1. An extensive Behavioral History by parental report,
2. Observations of Behavioral Responses to appropriate auditory stimuli,
3. Visual Reinforcement Audiometry (where age appropriate),
4. Acoustic Immitance Measurements (including Tympanometry, Acoustic Reflex, and Static Compliance),
5. Electric Response Audiometry (as indicated).

Obviously, the age and physical condition of the patient, as well as the information available from and about the family, and the type and degree of any hearing loss will influence which procedures will yield which information, and under which conditions.

The results of the assorted special audiological tests ought to be consistent with each other and with the audiometric contour. As with other forms of cochlear pathology, a patient with a congenital hearing impairment may demonstrate the phenomenon known as recruitment (see chapter 8) or an abnormal sensitivity to changes in loudness. It is necessary that the audiologist be aware of the presence of recruitment during testing procedures, and, of course (re)habilitation, particularly if amplification is recommended.

For most profound losses, the expectation is that test procedures will be at the limits of the clinical audiometer. However, some caution should be exercised in this regard. When dealing with a patient who cannot respond to any of the sounds which an audiometer can generate, one cannot conclude that there are no sounds to which this patient responds. The only safe conclusion is that the equipment cannot generate sounds to which the patient can reply. Expectations regarding speech reception and speech discrimination scores being consistent with pure tone audiograms, to the same extent expected in an adult with an acquired hearing impairment, must be tempered with reality.

Audiometric data should not lead to the assumption that a profoundly hearing-impaired patient should not be provided with amplification. The fact that an audiogram is not acquired in the usual manner does not preclude a hearing aid evaluation. There is often great success in providing amplification to very, very young hearing-impaired infants who do not demonstrate auditory behavioral responses. Further, when examining *and* when providing rehabilitative programming, the audiologist must consider all the special problems of someone who has never had any hearing or never had sufficient hearing to communicate aurally.

Finally, when dealing with a child who is congenitally severely impaired, it is unfair and, perhaps, even unkind, to expect performance in a foreign language, that is, speech. Unquestionably, the language of signs is the native language of most congenitally deaf. It behooves the professional to deal with those patients in their native language, just as would be done for those who were native speakers of Spanish or French. This should not be construed as an argument for or against oral language, sign language, or total communication. It should serve only to remind the reader to start from the patient's perspective, skills, and experiences, not from his/her own.

CASE STUDY 5-1:

WAARDENBURG'S SYNDROME

LH, whom we have been following since birth, is now 13 years old. She exhibits all the stigmata of Waardenburg's Syndrome, as does her mother and several members of her mother's family. She is presently enrolled in a special class for the hearing impaired at a junior high school. She wears two post-auricular hearing aids.

She was referred for an annual evaluation by the school audiologist. The data reconfirmed that she has a profound bilateral sensory-neural hearing impairment. Air conducted signals elicit responses at only 250, 500, and 1000Hz. There are no responses at the limit of the audiometer for any higher frequency in either ear. Her hearing aids seem to be functioning adequately, providing her with an aided speech awareness threshold at 45dB in the sound field. Unaided, her speech awareness threshold is 85dB.

PURE TONE AUDIOGRAM

RIGHT EAR

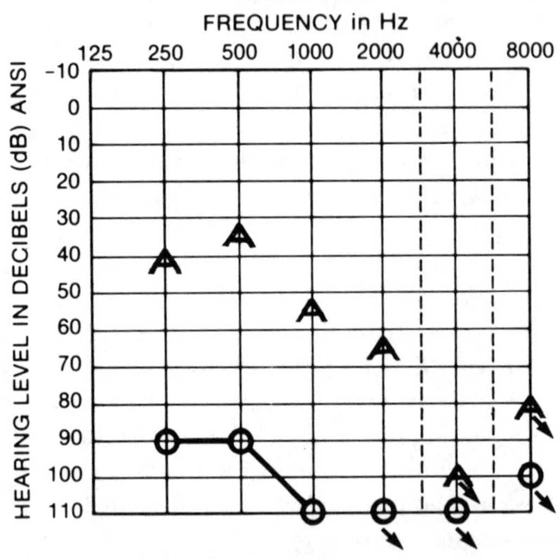

LEFT EAR

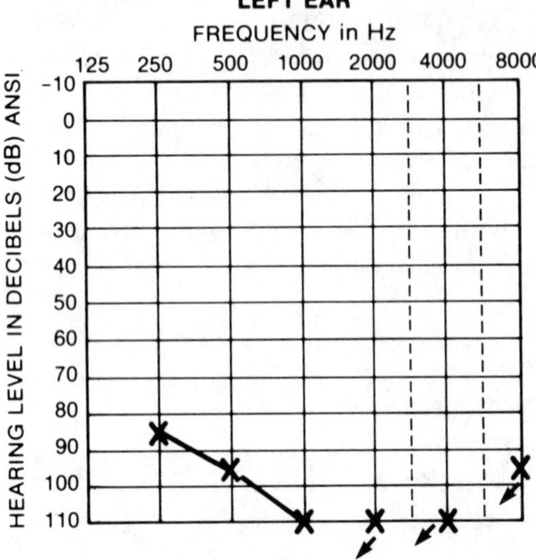

REFERENCES

Aballi, A.J. and Korones, S.B. 1963. The newborn infant. In *Synopsis of pediatrics,* ed. J.G. Hughes. St. Louis: The C.V. Mosby Co.

Affias, S. and Embil, J.A. 1978. Congenital infections and the TORCH syndrome. *The Nova Scotia Medical Bulletin* 57:43-47.

Amstey, M.S. 1977. Maternal viral infection with adverse results: cytomegalovirus and herpes virus. *Seminars in Perinatology* 1:1-10.

Anderson, H., Barr, B., and Wedenberg, E. 1970. Genetic disposition as a prerequisite for maternal rubella deafness. *Arch. Otolaryng.* 91:141-174.

Baldursson, G., Bjarnason, O., Halldorsson, S., Juliusdottir, E., and Kjeld, M. 1972. Maternal rubella in Iceland 1963-1964. *Scandinavian Audiol.* 1:3-10.

Barr, B. 1965. Early primary screening. In The young deaf child, ed. H. Davis. *Acta Otolaryngol.* Suppl. Stockholm, 206: 45-47.

Bergstrom, L. 1976. Congenital deafness. In *Hearing disorders,* ed. J.L. Northern. Boston: Little, Brown and Co.

Bergstrom, L. 1977. Viruses that deafen. In *Childhood deafness,* ed. F.H. Bess. New York: Grune and Stratton, Inc.

Bordley, J.E., Brookhouser P.E., Hardy, J., et al. 1967. Observations on the effect of prenatal rubella in hearing. In *Deafness in childhood,* eds. F. McConnell and P.H. Ward. Nashville: Vanderbilt Univ. Press.

Bordley, J.E., Brookhouser, P.E., and Worthington, E.L. 1971. Viral infections and hearing: a critical review of the literature. *Laryngoscope* 81:557-579.

Brookhouser, P.E. and Bordley, J.E. 1973. Congenital rubella deafness. *Arch. Otolaryngol.* 98:252-256.

Carrel, R.J. 1977. Epidemiology of hearing loss. In *Audiometry in infancy,* ed. S.E. Gerber. New York: Grune & Stratton, Inc.

Dahle, A. J., McCollister, F.P., Hamner, B.A., et al. 1974. Subclinical congenital cytomegalovirus infection and hearing impairment. *J. Speech Hear. Dis.* 39: 320-329.

Dahle, A.J., McCollister, F.P., Stagno, S., et al. 1979. Progressive hearing impairment in children with congenital cytomegalovirus infection. *J. Speech Hear. Dis.* 44:220-229.

Downs, M.P. and Silver, H.K. 1972. The A.B.C.D.'s to H.E.A.R.: Early identification in nursery, office and clinic of the infant who is deaf. *Clin. Pediatr.* 11:563-566.

Feinmesser, M. and Tell, L. 1976. Evaluation of methods for detecting hearing impairment in infancy and early childhood. In *Early identification of hearing loss,* ed. G.T. Mencher. Basel: Karger.

Fraser, G.R. 1971. The genetics of congenital deafness. *Otolaryngol. Clin. N. Amer.* 4:227-247.

Fraser, G.R. 1976. *The causes of profound deafness in childhood.* Baltimore: The Johns Hopkins Univ. Press.

Friedman, H. and Prier, J.E., eds. 1973. *Rubella.* First annual symposium of the eastern Pennsylvania branch, American Society for Microbiology. Springfield, IL: Chas. C. Thomas.

Gerber, S.E. 1977. High risk conditions. In *Audiometry in infancy,* ed. S.E. Gerber. New York: Grune & Stratton, Inc.

Gerber, S.E. and Mencher, G.T. eds. 1978. *Early diagnosis of hearing loss.* New York: Grune & Stratton, Inc.

Gerber, S.E., Mendel, M.I., and Goller, M. 1979. Progressive hearing loss subsequent to congenital cytomegalovirus infection. *Human Communication* 4:231-234.

Gregg, N.M. 1941. Congenital cataract following German measles in the mother. *Trans. Ophthal. Soc. Austr.* 3:35-46.

Hanshaw, J.B. 1979. Cytomegaloviral infection. In *Textbook of pediatrics,* eds. V.C. Vaughn, R.J. McKay, and R.E. Behrman. Philadelphia: W.B. Saunders Co.

Hanshaw, J.B. and Dudgeon, J.A. 1978. Viral diseases of the fetus and newborn. *Major problems in clin. pediatr.* 17:1-9.

Hanshaw, J.B., Scheiner, A.P., Moxley, A.W., et al. 1976. School failure and deafness after "silent" CMV infection. *New England J. Med.* 295:468-470.

Hardy, J.B. 1973. Fetal consequences of maternal virus infections in pregnancy. *Arch. Otolaryngol.* 98:218-227.

Hardy, J.B., Sever, J.L. and Gilkeson, M.R. 1969. Declining antibody titers in children with congenital rubella. *J. Pediatr.* 75:213-220.

Hardy, W.G. and Bordley, J.E. 1973. Problems in diagnosis and management of the multiply handicapped deaf child. *Arch. Otolaryngol.* 98:269-274.

Karmody, C.S. 1969. Asymptomatic maternal rubella and congenital deafness. *Arch. Otolaryngol.* 89:720.

Kelemen, G. 1977. Morquio's Disease and the hearing organ. *ORL* 39:233-240.

Kohji, U., Yukiaki, N., Kenji, O., et al. 1979. Congenital rubella syndrome: correlation of gestational age at time of maternal rubella with type of onset. *J. Pediatr.* 94:763-765.

Konigsmark, B.W. 1971. Hereditary and congenital factors affecting newborn sensorineural hearing. In *Conference on newborn hearing screening*, ed. G.C. Cunningham. Berkeley: California Department of Health.

Konigsmark, B.W. and Gorlin, R.J. 1976. *Genetic and metabolic deafness.* Philadelphia: W.B. Saunders Co.

Leroy, J.G. and Crocker, A.C. 1966. Clinical definition of Hunter-Hurler phenotypes. A review of 50 patients. *Amer. J. Dis. Child* 112:518-530.

Lindsay, J.R. and Matz, G. 1966. The differentiation of acquired congenital from genetically determined inner ear deafness. *Ann. Otol. Rhinol. Laryngol.* 75:830-843.

Manson, M.M., Logan, W.P.D. and Loy, R.M. 1960. *Rubella and other virus infections during pregnancy.* London: H.M. Stationery Office.

Marx, J.L. 1977. Cytomegalovirus: A major cause of birth defects. *Science* 190:1184-1186.

Mencher, G.T. ed. 1976. *Early identification of hearing loss.* Basel: S. Karger.

Mencher, G.T. 1976. Personal communication.

Mencher, G.T., Baldursson, M.S., Tell, L., and Levi, C. 1978. Mass behavioral screening and follow-up. Presented to the meeting of the National Research Council-National Academy of Sciences, Assembly of Behavioral and Social Sciences Meeting of the Committee on Hearing, Bioacoustics and Biomechanics, Omaha.

Monif, G. and Jordon, P.A. 1977. Rubella virus and rubella vaccine. *Seminars in Perinatology* 1:41-49.

Myers, E.N. and Stool, S. 1968. Cytomegalic inclusion disease of the inner ear. *Laryngoscope* 78:1904-1915.

Northern, J.L. and Downs, M.P. 1978. *Hearing in children.* 2d ed. Baltimore: Williams & Wilkins Co.

Proctor, C. 1977. Congenital rubella and sensorineural hearing loss. *Laryngoscope* Suppl. 7. 87:1-60.

Rapin, I. and Ruben, R.J. 1979. Clinical appraisal of auditory function. Presented to the symposium on Developmental Disabilities in the Preschool Child. Chicago.

Sever, J.L. and Bethesda, M.D. 1973. Present status of vaccines for rubella. *Arch. Otolaryngol.* 98:265-268.

Simmons, F.B. and Russ, F.N. 1974. Automated newborn hearing screening, the crib-o-gram. *Arch. Otolaryngol.* 100:1-7.

Tietz, W. 1963. A syndrome of deaf-mutism associated with albinism showing dominant autosomal inheritance. *Am. J. Hum. Genet.* 15:259-264.

Tell, L. 1976. Personal communication.

Theissing, G. and Kittel, G. 1962. Die Bedeutung der Toxoplasmose in der Atiologie der connatalen und fruh erworbenen Hörstorungen. *Arch. Ohr. - Nas. u. Kehlk - Heilk* 180:219.

Top, F.H. and Wehrle, P.E. 1976. *Communicable and infectious diseases*. 8th ed. St. Louis: C.V. Mosby Co.

Waardenburg, P.J. 1951. A new syndrome combining developmental anomalies of the eyelids, eyebrows, and nose root with pigmentary defects of the iris and head hair and with congenital deafness. *Amer. J. Human Genet.* 3:195-253.

Weller, T.H. and Hanshaw, J.B. 1962. Virologic and clinical observations on cytomegalic inclusion disease. *N. Engl. J. Med.* 266:1233-1244.

World Health Organization 1967. *The early detection and treatment of handicapping defects in young children.* Report on a working group convened by the Regional Office for Europe of the World Health Organization.

6

Adventitious Hearing Impairment

Consider again that one in 1000 births results in an infant with a profound hearing loss, and that about one in 400 or fewer infants is born with some lesser degree of hearing impairment *(Carrel, 1977)*. On the other hand, in the United States alone, there are about 10 million people of all ages with hearing impairment sufficient to cause some degree of handicap. Clearly, the vast majority of hearing-impaired people became that way post-natally; hence, their hearing loss is said to be *adventitious*. In fact, the rate of increase in the number of people with hearing loss throughout each decade of life is really rather astounding.

First is a group of children with a hearing loss which is apparently of latent onset, but which occurs so early in life that it has the same effect as deafness at birth. Second, at any given moment, as high as 5 or 6% of the school age population has a hearing impairment, although usually conductive, and therefore medically treatable. Third, and finally, is a vast group of people with handicapping hearing impairment acquired in childhood or in adulthood. Many of the impairments arise from some of the same kinds of things which cause congenital deafness.

Adventitious hearing impairments are related to systemic disturbances, diseases (viral, bacterial, or protozoal), or degenerative disorders. Some of the losses are *idiopathic;* that is, they are said to cause themselves. Usually that term is used because there is no clearly known or definitive cause for the problem. On the other hand, some of the hearing losses have rather obvious causes including drugs (ototoxicity), noise (trauma), and age (presbycusis). The overt results of systemic disturbances, diseases, and hereditary degenerative disorders are similar; therefore, they are considered together in this chapter. Because ototoxicity, noise trauma, and presbycusis have their own special effects on hearing, they are reviewed independently in chapters 7, 8, and 9.

PATHOLOGY and ETIOLOGY

SYSTEMIC DISORDERS

All of those diseases, conditions, and pathologies which effect the general metabolic system and/or chemical homeostatis have a potential for resulting in hearing impairment. Within this group are such diverse problems as thyroid disease, diabetes, kidney disease, and even perhaps Ménière's Disease, an idiopathic hearing impairment which may possibly be systemic in nature. The audiologist should be aware that hearing impairment may accompany such things as diabetes and thyroid disease; however, kidney diseases and Ménière's Disease are far more significant causes of hearing loss and therefore are discussed at length.

THYROID DISEASE. Thyroid disease offers one of the more interesting and peculiar examples of an adventitious disorder. One form of thyroid disease, called Pendred's Disease (figure 6-1), is genetic and usually appears with deafness at birth and with a goiter developing later in life. The peculiarity is that the deafness is present at birth, while the symptoms of the disease itself appear much later. Pendred's Disease produces 5% of all cases of deafness *(Fraser, 1976)*.

There is evidence of progressive hearing impairment in some cases of Pendred's Disease which may be abated by appropriate thyroid therapy. Cases of idiopathic hypothyroid disease with similar auditory symptoms and similar responses to thyroid therapy have also been reported *(Cotton, 1977)*.

In the majority of cases with Pendred's Disease the hearing loss is not adventitious, but rather it is the onset of the complete thyroid disease which is. In fact, it may be the hearing loss which provides the earliest possible sign of the presence of the disease. Pendred's Disease, a unique member of the family of thyroid diseases, has been the focal point of extensive research by Fraser (1976).

KIDNEY DISEASE. Kidney disease is a more typical cause of severe adventitious hearing loss. Since the kidneys are required to remove naturally occuring toxins from bodily systems, it follows that if they fail, those toxins will also not be removed from the endolymphatic and perilymphatic spaces. Due to the intimate association between kidney function and other bodily functions, it is not surprising to discover that fluctuations of auditory sensitivity frequently accompany kidney disorders.

A study by Visencio and Gerber (1979) reported unexpected and unpredictable variations in pure tone thresholds among patients undergoing dialysis treatment for kidney failure. This study correlated auditory function with dialysis treatment and thirty different blood tests. The expectation was that, as certain chemicals varied in levels present in the blood stream, so would auditory sensitivity. Sometimes it did, and sometimes it did not. The results suggested that the function of the kidneys

112

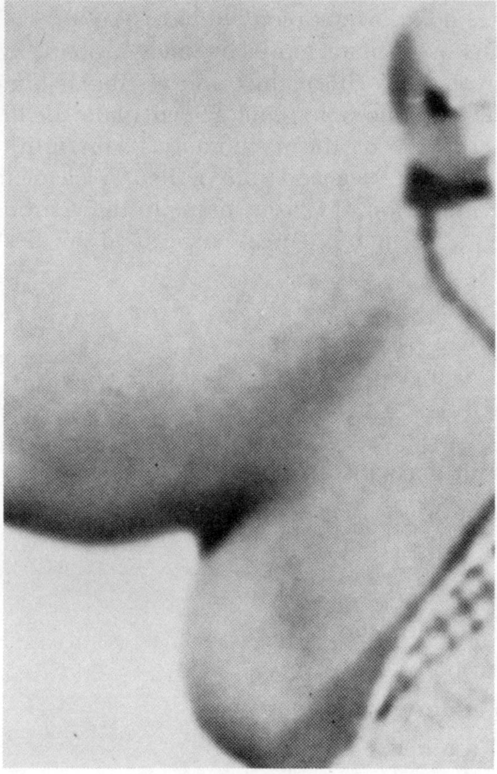

Figure 6-1. Pendred's Disease showing the goiterous enlargement of the thyroid gland in a deaf patient.

is so broad and so complex that no easy prediction can be made about the variability of auditory sensitivity. The only generalization which is possible is that hearing impairment should be expected to accompany kidney disease, but the severity of the impairment is not necessarily highly correlated with the severity of the disease, nor is recovery or relief from the disease necessarily highly correlated with recovery of hearing.

There is a congenital disorder known as Alport's Disease *(Alport, 1927)*, which is characterized by nephritis (i.e., infection of the kidneys) and congenital deafness. The hearing loss is progressive, males showing the degeneration faster and more frequently than females. The disease is often fatal. Nevertheless, amplification and rehabilitation techniques offer necessary support. Constant monitoring of hearing is required as the disease reaches various stages of progression and stabilization.

Meniere's Disease. Ménière's Disease is an outstanding example of an acquired idiopathic hearing impairment which is limited to the auditory system. Pulec (1976) claimed that the etiology of Ménière's Disease is allergic; but that other kinds of systemic deficiencies may also give rise to the disorder. Pulec also claimed that in 45% of his patients with Ménière's Disease there was no known etiology (table 6-1).

Ménière's Disease is characterized by endolymphatic hydrops which is a watery swelling of the cochlear duct and vestibular organs. Schuknecht (1975) lists a series of pathologies: enlargement of the cochlear duct, dilation of the saccule, rupture of the membranous labyrinth, collapse of the membranous labyrinth, degeneration of neural elements in the apical cochlea, and proliferation of fibrous tissue in the vestibule. In summary, Schuknecht says, "Ménière's Disease is caused by dysfunction of the endolymphatic sac."

Table 6-1. Causes of Ménière's Disease*

Allergy	14%
Adrenal-pituitary insufficiency	7
Congenital or acquired syphilis	6
Hypothyroidism	2
Vascular	3
Estrogen insufficiency	2
Combination of above	12
Internal auditory canal stenosis	3
Physical trauma	3
Acoustic trauma	2
Viral	1
Idiopathic	45%

First described in 1861 by Prosper Ménière, for whom it was named, it is characterized by a unique group of symptoms. There is hearing loss. There is tinnitus (noise in the ear). There is vertigo (a characteristic form of dizziness). All three of these symptoms must be present to enable a diagnosis of Ménière's Disease. If all three are not present simultaneously, then the disorder may be something else; although, of course, Menière's Disease cannot be completely ruled out. The disease may occur at any age but usually appears before age 50 *(Mawson, 1967)*; however, it has been known to be present in children. The disease is more likely to occur in a male than a female. It does not occur in black people. Over 85% of the cases are unilateral.

One of the most striking characteristics of Ménière's Disease is its cyclic nature. The report of a tendency to feel disoriented is often an early sign of

---

*From: Jack Pulec, "Ménière's Disease." In J. Northern (ed.), *Hearing Disorders*. Boston: Little, Brown and Co., 1976.

Ménière's Disease. Most patients who suffer from this disease are not affected all the time. They get "attacks" of hearing loss, tinnitus, and vertigo. The handicapping effects of Ménière's Disease vary with the severity of the symptoms. Some patients are severely handicapped, unable to walk, unable to hear, and suffer from frequent and violent attacks of nausea and vomiting. On the other hand, some patients have mild, rare attacks of fleeting dizziness, with some annoying tinnitus. Over a period of time, the hearing impairment and the tinnitus worsen, even though they may be relieved somewhat between attacks. Cody (1978) stated that perhaps the most characteristic thing of Ménière's Disease is a fluctuation of auditory acuity with a "tendency to progressive deterioration in the hearing ability . . ."

One patient had her first attack of Ménière's Disease in rather old age and was greatly surprised. She had had no earlier problems of the kind, and had no more hearing loss than one normally expects as a function of age. Suddenly, one day, she was rendered quite ill with nausea and vomiting and very distressing ringing in the ears. She had frequent attacks of Ménière's Disease for a period of several months. After that time, she had virtually no more attacks of vertigo and tinnitus, but her auditory sensitivity deteriorated rapidly. About five years after her first attack, she had regained her ability to walk steadily; but she heard very poorly, even with a properly fitted hearing aid.

HEARING LOSS OF SUDDEN ONSET. Hearing loss of sudden onset with no known etiology is another of the more dramatic and interesting problems encountered by the audiologist. Goodhill and Harris (1979) have described the problem as an "otologic emergency . . . which may occur as the result of lesions of the external, middle, or inner ear, or as the result of internal auditory meatus, cerebello-pontine angle, or CNS lesions." Because outer and middle ear obstruction or damage are usually amenable to medical and/or surgical treatment, most other authors do not include those lesions within the category. The discussion here focuses on sensory hearing loss of sudden onset (e.g., overnight or perhaps within a very few weeks) and of no known etiology.

The etiology of the problem has been variously attributed to viral disease, vascular insult, endocrine imbalance, and allergic reaction. No doubt, individual cases merit each of those etiologies. The most prevalently listed etiologies are viral and vascular. Mumps, discussed elsewhere in this chapter is certainly a major factor. In many histopathologic studies, the destruction within the cochlea is quite similar to that seen in mumps and/or meningitis. There may be such things as atrophy of the stria vascularis, displacement of the tectorial membrane and/or collapse of the cochlear duct *(Snow, 1973; Goodhill and Harris, 1979).*

Often the disorder is diagnosed as a vascular accident, and the patient is led to believe that there has been a small "stroke." Although an occlusion of a blood vessel of the inner ear by an embolus or thrombus has probably not occurred, the problem may be due to vascular spasm, capillary sludging, hyper-coagulation, or a host of other vascular system disorders.

There has been some recent evidence to suggest that severe hearing loss of a sudden nature may be due to a rupture of the membranes within the labyrinth or to a labyrinthine fistula. The reader is referred to Goodhill and Harris (1979) for an excellent discussion of this topic.

Rubin (1968) developed a classification system for categorizing the effects of the disorder based on severity of the hearing loss and audiometric configuration. These classifications range from Type I with a mild low frequency hearing loss, to Type II with a fairly flattened 60dB loss across all frequencies, to Type III which is typical of a severe hearing loss and markedly reduced speech discrimination. The tinnitus and vertigo which often accompany the onset of the disorder — and which frequently lead to a tentative diagnosis of Ménière's Disease — will usually disappear after a week or two. Furthermore, as the disease abates, the hearing will often return, sometimes to completely normal.

ACQUIRED DISEASE

VIRAL DISEASES. No matter which viral disease is the cause of deafness, the mechanism, the destructive pattern, and the auditory consequences are the same. In most cases the organ of Corti is affected primarily at the basal turn: individual hair cells are severely damaged or missing. The stria vascularis may become atrophied. The tectorial membrane appears shriveled or rolls up, while Reissner's membrane may completely collapse to the point that it attaches itself to the basilar membrane *(Berkow, 1977)*.

The relative significance and the danger to the hearing mechanism associated with the so-called "diseases of childhood" vary somewhat, and the effects of individual diseases may differ prenatally from postnatally. For example, rubella is less significant as a cause of acquired deafness postnatally than prenatally. On the other hand, measles (i.e., rubeola) has far more significance postnatally. McCabe (1963) determined that measles was the most common cause of acquired hearing loss among children in residential schools for the deaf. That is, of course, no longer true, primarily because of mass immunization programs against the viral diseases of childhood. Children are now innoculated against rubella, rubeola, pertussis, influenza, and poliomyelitis. Nevertheless, people still do develop these diseases and do suffer hearing losses subsequent to that illness. For example, the reader is reminded of the temporal bone study of Lindsay and Matz (1966) which described a child who had mumps with hearing impairment overlaid upon an existing congenital sensory-neural hearing loss.

Among the most significant diseases which result in acquired sensory hearing loss is meningitis; in fact, according to Catlin (1978), "it is the leading postnatal cause of hearing loss among school-age deaf children." The incidence of profound hearing impairment subsequent to viral or bacterial meningitis has increased in the past many years because of the increasing number of people surviving the disease. Sometimes, especially in

116

early infancy, the hearing impairment is accompanied by other neurological disorders which may also be severely debilitating *(Robertson, 1978).*

Vestibular difficulties and the severity of the hearing impairment are the most striking things about post-meningitic deafness. It is usually profound to the extreme. For example, the audiograms of 28 children in special classes for the hearing-impaired were examined in our center and grouped according to severity. The purpose was to illustrate to parents what an audiogram shows and what is meant by such terms as profound, severe, and moderate hearing loss. The profoundly hard-of-hearing group was entirely mutually inclusive of the post-meningitic children. That is, all of the children with profound hearing losses were those who had had meningitis, and all of the children who had had meningitis were in the profound hearing loss group.

BACTERIAL DISEASES. In chapter 3, purulent otomastoiditis, a bacterial disease, was discussed at length. It differs from secretory otitis media by the presence of bacteria in the fluid rendering it purulent. According to Eichenwald (1979) and Howie (1977), the most frequently found pathogen (35%) is pneumococcus (i.e., Streptococcus pneumoniae) followed in frequency by Hemophilus influenzae (29%). In addition to the risk to the middle ear, there is a risk of mastoiditis and bacterial meningitis. In fact, pneumococcus is the micro-organism which most often produces meningitis. Sometimes a purulent labyrinthitis is a consequence of bacterial meningitis; sometimes it is a precursor. It may be characterized by pain in the ear, high fever, headache, and even coma.

Clearly, bacterial meningitis is a dangerous disease, threatening to life itself, as well as a threat to produce nervous system disorders including deafness. In fact, a procedure as drastic as labyrinthectomy is sometimes required to prevent purulent labyrinthitis from reaching the brain by lymphatic drainage from the mastoid or by some other means.

PROTOZOAL DISEASES. Syphilis (Lues), a protozoal disease, provides a very good illustration of a condition which may produce sensory and/or neural hearing loss of delayed onset. If the disease is congenital, degeneration typically begins in the second decade of life, although 37% of the cases may have otologic signs before the age of 10 years *(Shulman, 1979).* There is also a form of congenital syphilis in which symptoms do not appear until late in life. If the disease is acquired, primarily through sexual contact, symptoms may appear at any time and their rate of progression and severity are highly variable.

Congenital syphilis may never result in a hearing impairment; but when it does, it is rapid in development, starting as a unilateral problem, and becoming symmetrical and profound rather quickly. Some individuals, particularly females and most particularly those who were pregnant, have reported fluctuation in the early stages of their hearing losses. Sometimes, loss of hearing and what appears to be VIIIth Nerve involvement are the first signs of the presence of the disease. The patients are almost always also troubled with vertigo and tinnitus. Therefore, all the signs of Ménière's Disease and/or VIIIth Nerve tumor are present. No wonder that this disease has been called "the great imitator." Diagnosis focuses on medical questions related to case history, physical examination, blood serology, and vestibular tests. Treatment is usually based on antibiotics or steroid therapy.

Hearing loss is much less frequent when the syphillis is acquired. If there is a hearing problem, it is often the product of an associated meningitis or secondary problem. In either case, though, the result is usually severe hearing impairment.

DEGENERATIVE DISORDERS

In the previous chapter it was noted that some genetic disorders are congenital, while some that appear later in life are not. The outstanding example is otosclerosis (chapter 4) which is dominantly inherited but does not usually appear until the third decade of life. Furthermore, as is discussed in chapter 9, some forms of so-called "early" presbycusis are likely to have a genetic component.

Some genetically based hearing disorders that are not present at birth appear early in life. These are collected under the general headings of early onset recessive deafness and early onset dominant deafness. There is some difficulty with the term "early" as it is used here, in that it is not really known at what age the hearing loss develops. Most authorities agree, however, that degeneration is well under way by the time the patient is three years of age, and frequently, even younger than that.

Some diseases discussed in this chapter also lead to degenerative hearing losses. For example, that pattern is well established for syphilis and, more recently, it has been established for cytomegalovirus. Cytomegalovirus, probably the most common of all viral diseases, has long been suspected of producing auditory degeneration, but it has only recently been documented as doing so *(Dahle et al, 1979; Gerber, Mendel, and Goller, 1979)*. Systemic disorders, such as idiopathic hypothyroidism and Cretinism, may also result in a degeneration of auditory function unless promptly and properly treated. Kidney disease also falls into this general category.

Diseases which lead to degenerative hearing loss may be associated with other degenerative disorders. Some are genetic and adventitious (chapter 5). Usher's Disease *(Vernon, 1969)* marries congenital deafness with progressive visual loss. Pendred's Disease *(Fraser, 1976)* combines hearing loss with progressive thyroid deficit. Hunter's Disease pairs hearing loss with progressive retardation, dwarfism, and hepatosplenomegaly (enlargement of the cells of the liver and spleen). Hunter's Disease is an example of a whole family of diseases collectively called mucopolysaccharidosis, all of which are genetically determined and which display degenerative hearing loss *(Konigsmark and Gorlin, 1976)*.

Multiple sclerosis is an excellent example of a group of demyelinating diseases which may affect the auditory and vestibular pathways. Known to cause visual disturbance, poor coordination and control of muscle groups, and vestibular difficulties, the disease is characterized by periods of remission and exacerbation. Sataloff (1966) and Strome (1977) suggested that hearing loss may be both profound and transient, with spontaneous remission accompanying a general improvement of the patient. Strome also reported that the cochlear and vestibular nuclei have been suggested as the site of the primary lesion; audiological studies indicate retrocochlear pathology. Speech discrimination scores are lower than would be predicted from pure tone thresholds, a phenomenon also seen in presbycusis (chapter 9), another disorder associated with disintegration of the central pathways. There has been no single consistent audiometric pattern associated with multiple sclerosis. However, Strome cautions"... fluctuating sensorineural hearing loss in a young adult with or without vertigo should suggest the possibility of multiple sclerosis . . ."

The significant factor in degenerative disorders is that some of the patients may very well be dying, and the hearing loss is clearly a secondary consideration. Nevertheless, the patient should receive appropriate amplification and rehabilitation for as long as possible. In fact, the audiologist's assistance may be the most critical and essential factor in helping the patient to adjust to the situation, in maintaining communication, and in dealing with an extremely difficult problem.

MEDICAL CONSIDERATIONS

Adventitious hearing impairments are as different otologically as they are etiologically. Usually, but not necessarily, postnatal viral or bacterial disease does not lead to as severe a hearing impairment as when the disease occurs prenatally, although there is a risk of necrotizing otitis media. The major exception, of course, is meningitis which does not occur prenatally at all, and which can result in the most severely handicapping hearing disorders. Many patients with acquired sensory hearing losses are truly profoundly hearing impaired; many are not. It is also important to note that hearing impairment subsequent to viral or bacterial disease is usually unchanging — the hearing loss should not get worse.

No discussion of acquired sensory hearing impairments would be complete without a consideration of *tinnitus*. Tinnitus, properly pronounced with the stress on the first syllable, is a term commonly used to describe noise in the ear. Different people describe the sound differently: ringing, buzzing, whistling, humming, running water, etc. It is a symptom which appears when internal sounds are subjectively louder than external or environmental noises *(Goodhill, 1979)*.

The physician, in this case usually an otologist, will consider the presence of tinnitus an important diagnostic clue to otologic or neurologic disease. It appears in both conductive and sensory disorders; in fact, it may be one of the first signs of otosclerosis, presbycusis, or VIIIth nerve tumor. It could, of course, simply be the ringing we all occasionally experience. When a physician examines a patient for auditory deficit, and tinnitus is a factor, the focus of the investigation will be on the location (inside the head or the image of sound in the room), pitch, loudness, and time alterations of the noise. There may be diagnostic clues associated with variations in each of those parameters.

The specific cause of tinnitus is unknown, but certain hypotheses are tenable under certain circumstances. For example, tinnitus following exposure to intense noise may be a sign of auditory fatigue, and tinnitus following a blow to the head may indicate compression of a blood vessel. If the tinnitus is the sign of a disease, it may disappear with cure or relief of the problem, although frequently it does not.

Recently, there have been attempts to fatigue the tinnitus with masking sounds *(Northern, 1979)*. These methods have been tried because there is no specific medical or surgical cure for the problem. Masking has been moderately successful, but continued research is necessary to further evaluate the large numbers of commercial "tinnitus maskers" which have suddenly appeared on the market.

SYSTEMIC DISEASES

It would be difficult to find a common medical or surgical treatment plan for systemic disorders, as each disease is unique. Diseases of the kidney would most certainly require different management from diseases of the thyroid or of the other organs. Therefore, any discussion of medical considerations pertaining to systemic diseases must consider each of the symptoms, and not as a cure for the disease. Goodhill and Harris (1979) have developed a model program for the patient with Ménière's Disease. They feel that *management* is a far better term than treatment for these patients. Their management plan is ". . . based on fluctuating physiologic changes in a dynamic organ, the endolymphatic labyrinth, with osmotic, vascular, and endocrine interrelationships." It is primarily a medical model, with care for other physical problems (e.g., diabetes) left to the family physician. The management schedule is presented as table 6-2. Goodhill and Harris report that most patients will respond, as far as vertigo is concerned, to the therapy plan outlined. They also suggest that surgical management may be indicated if the patient is nonresponsive to treatment.

Table 6-2. Management of Ménière's Disease*

Management of Mild Attack

1. Bed rest in position of greatest comfort
2. Bland, low-sodium diet with only moderate intake of fluids, and distilled water
3. Dimenhydrinate, 50 mg every 3 hours, or diazepam, 5 mg.
   If nausea is present, substitute promethazine

---

*From Goodhill & Harris, 1979.

hydrochloride, 50-mg suppository
4. No smoking, no coffee, no tea, no "Cokes," no alcohol

Management of Severe Attack

1. Bed rest
2. Dimenhydrinate, 50 mg IM, repeated every 3-4 hours as necessary
3. Prochlorperazine, 25-mg suppository, if severe nausea is present, accompanied by vomiting; or diazepam, 10 mg every 4 hours; or droperidol, 25 mg IM every 4 hours
4. If attack has been prolonged and the patient is dehydrated, I-V fluids may be necessary

Long-range Management Between Attacks

1. Complete review of detailed history of patient's way of life, contacts, stresses, etc., in an effort to find precipitating causes and possible allergies
2. Careful review of audiologic, vestibular, and radiographic findings to rule out possibility of a cerebellopontine angle tumor, other intracranial disease, FTA-abs serology, etc.
3. Eliminate smoking, coffee or tea, and stimulating drugs. Control habits and environmental factors which produce fatigue and stress
4. Low-sodium diet with use of distilled water rather than spring water or tapwater for all cooking and drinking purposes. Empirical hypoallergenic diet, eliminating milk, eggs, chocolate, shellfish, corn, pork, nuts, and their products
5. Periodic utilization of diuretics such as hydrochlorothiazide, 50 mg once or twice daily. Such therapy frequently will relieve the feeling of fullness in the ear, relieve the vertigo and the tinnitus, and will occasionally be accompanied by significant hearing improvement. Choice of diuretics will depend upon prudent evaluation of the general medical status of patient
6. Intermittent use of diazepam, phenergan, or dexedrine
7. Consultations with other physicians will be necessary if there are significant signs of special problems, such as allergy, emotional stress, and neurologic problems

There are two types of operative procedures: 1) drainage and 2) destructive. Drainage procedures are designed to preserve hearing and stop vertigo. Basically, they involve inserting a needle through the round window into the scala media and through to the saccule. This procedure ruptures the saccule and relieves the hydrops, but it may result in further hearing loss in 20% of the cases *(House, 1975)*.

Another surgical procedure for the patient disabled by Ménière's Disease is the endolymphatic-subarachnoid shunt. The purpose of the operation is to relieve the hydrops by opening the endolymphatic sac into the subarachnoid space (in the brain cavity) so that the fluid may drain.

There are procedures similar in purpose to drainage which may have the same effect. These involve ultrasound or cryosurgery. One such surgery is called labyrinthotomy. In that procedure, the cavity of the middle ear is opened and an ultrasonic probe is applied to the part of the lateral semi-circular canal which bulges into the middle ear cavity. This destroys a minimum amount of tissue in a very circumscribed area in the hope of reducing the vertigo to the point where the patient is no longer handicapped.

In a more extreme case, or a case of failure of a drainage operation, the surgeon must sometimes do a destructive procedure. This is devastating, literally involving a destruction of the entire inner ear and vestibular contents. The result, of course, is a dramatic loss of both vertigo and hearing. It results in an utterly "dead" ear with no hope of recovery. Consequently, these procedures are done only in the most extreme cases. House (1975) defined the candidate for destructive surgery as one whose hearing level is poorer than 50dB or 60dB and whose discrimination score is less than 50% in the offending ear, and one whose vertigo is totally incapacitating. When the patient has bilateral Ménière's Disease, about 10% to 20%   *(Goodhill and Harris, 1979),* surgery is done only if one ear is totally deaf.

The patient who has had a unilateral surgical procedure still has essentially normal hearing in the sound field, but has lost localization ability. One can adjust to the loss of that ability, and skillfully utilize the remaining ear. These patients have an excellent potential for normal living.

With the exception of Ménière's Disease, there is little that can be done surgically specifically for acquired sensory hearing impairments. They are not subject to surgical intervention, nor are they usually amenable to medical-otological treatment. Of course, the underlying disease is a medical problem which needs to be treated, and that treatment may have a beneficial effect vis-a-vis the hearing impairment (e.g., as in hypothyroidism). Cochlear implants, a subject to be discussed later, may offer some hope for the future.

ACQUIRED DISEASES

Any of the so-called diseases of childhood (which are not necessarily limited to children) may lead to a viral labyrinthitis. Chicken pox, mumps, the common cold, and such things as influenza and poliomyelitis are all produced by viruses that may attack the inner ear. Measles had been the most frequent cause of virally produced severe hearing impairment *(McCabe, 1963).* Antibiotic drugs, in general, are ineffective against viruses. Consequently, there is little that can be done during the acute stage of these diseases other than to minimize febrility and treat external symptoms. There is no way to cure the auditory deficit resulting from viral labyrinthitis *(Mawson, 1967)*.

Meningitis, whether acquired from a virus or a bacterium, demands heroic treatment. Mawson points out that the physician would normally immediately attack a suppurative otitis media and/or mastoiditis, but the meningitis must be treated first. Bacterial diseases usually respond to antibiotic treatment. However, if there is a risk of meningitis subsequent to mastoiditis, then surgical intervention in the form of mastoidectomy may be indicated.

Syphilis may manifest itself as a suppurative otitis media, but the syphilis spirochete may find its way to the inner ear. The otitis media associated with syphilis would be treated locally and as a purulent otomastoiditis, in addition to the general treatment for syphilis, usually penicillin. Syphilis also appears as a late onset sensory-neural hearing impairment. This syphilitic hearing loss is degenerative and treatment is limited at best.

The genetically based degenerative hearing losses also are not amenable to otological intervention. But the otologist has a central role in such cases. While he cannot treat the disorder, he must assume a role as advisor, genetic counselor, and referral source. In fact, in all those cases of adventitious hearing loss, when the treatment is done or not possible, the otologist has an absolute obligation to refer the patient to the audiologist who would assume case management *(Goodhill, 1979)*.

AUDIOLOGICAL CONSIDERATIONS

The audiometric configuration should be similar in all sensory hearing losses; that is, usually a greater loss for the higher frequencies than for the lower frequencies. Speech reception thresholds are usually consistent with the pure tone audiogram. Speech discrimination usually is as good as, or as poor as, the audiogram suggests.

In spite of these broad generalizations, it must be understood that each disease entity may have its own characteristic patterns. For example, hearing losses associated with thyroid diseases may be profound. On the other hand, those associated with kidney disease are as diverse as the patients; Visencio and Gerber (1979) found that pure tone thresholds on the same ear were sometimes improved by dialysis and sometimes not.

More often than thyroid or kidney disease, the most profound hearing impairments arise from viral or bacterial endolabyrinthitis. Sometimes it is impossible to get a response; sometimes only a "corner" audiogram may be obtained. In such a case, of course, speech audiometry is out of the question.

The phenomenon of severe to profound *unilateral* hearing loss is peculiar to mumps among all acquired hearing impairments associated with viral disease. It is known, of course, that mumps involves the parotid gland on either one side or both sides. But, mumps may lead to a unilateral profound hearing loss, whether the disease occurs on one side or both. A typical example is a case of a young teacher who contracted bilateral mumps, but the disease resulted in a permanent, profound unilateral hearing loss.

The audiologist should inquire about mumps in every patient who complains of a unilateral hearing loss. However, deafnesses of sudden onset due to vascular disease or accident also are typically unilateral. In addition, some of the degenerative genetic disorders sometimes appear unilaterally. Syphilis, too, may present with a unilateral impairment, but the loss soon becomes bilateral *(Paparella and Capps, 1973).*

Ménière's Disease has associated audiometric characteristics as well. Patients with Ménière's Disease usually have a rising audiogram, that is, one with a more severe hearing loss for lower frequencies than for higher frequencies (figure 6-2). In earlier discussions, it was indicated that a rising audiogram with an air-bone gap is a sign of middle ear disease. In patients with Ménière's Disease, the problem is cochlear (sensory); there is no air-bone gap. As the disease progresses, and the hearing deteriorates, the audiometric contour becomes flattened and then, eventually, falling with greater deficit in the high frequencies than in the lows. That is, after time the audiometric contour assumes the shape which we have come to customarily associate with sensory-neural hearing impairment. During the early stages of the disease, when the hearing loss is primarily limited to the lower frequencies, the patient has very little loss for speech discrimination. As both the magnitude and configuration of the hearing loss change, then so do the speech reception threshold and speech discrimination scores. Other audiological tests are usually consistent with the pure tone audiogram, and results of special tests (e.g., for recruitment) are characteristic of cochlear impairment.

Furthermore, remember that the presenting complaint of patients with Ménière's Disease is usually one of dizziness. In fact, the presence of vertigo is one of the distinguishing signs of this disorder; and if there is no vertigo, one should probably look elsewhere than the inner ear for the site of the pathology. If the patient does complain of vertigo, then the vestibular system needs to be examined, and it is frequently the audiologist in an otological practice who does the tests. While this is not a book on vestibular disorders or vestibular tests, the hearing clinician needs to be aware of them. The essential test is *electronystagmography* (ENG). Nystagmus is an oscillation of the eyes from side to side which occurs when a normal vestibular system is disturbed. Abnormalities of the vestibular system may be reflected in this oculomotor activity, and can be measured by electronystagmography. An electronystagmograph is a device which records even tiny nystagmic movements. The way an ENG is arranged is shown in figure 6-3. Many things influence ENG results; Glattke (1978) points out that the ENG ". . . results from a combination of labyrinthine and proprioceptive or exteroceptive cues." Hence, the diagnosis of Ménière's Disease — or, for that matter, any other isolated clinical entity — cannot

PURE TONE AUDIOGRAM

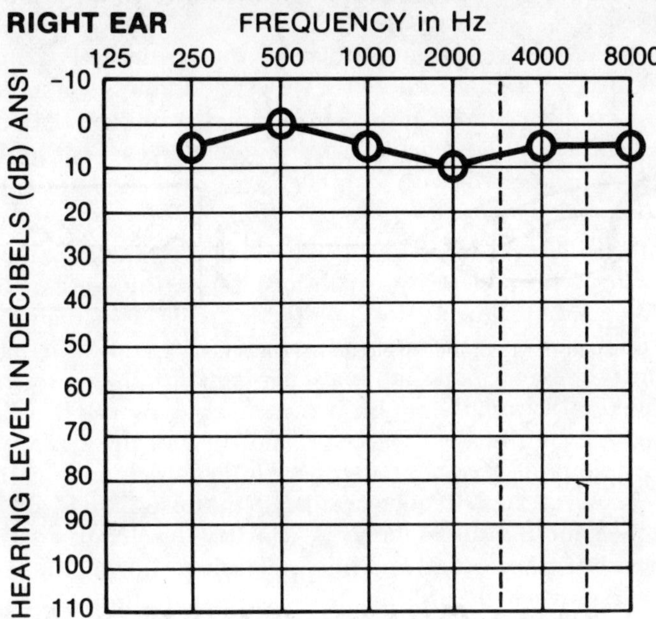

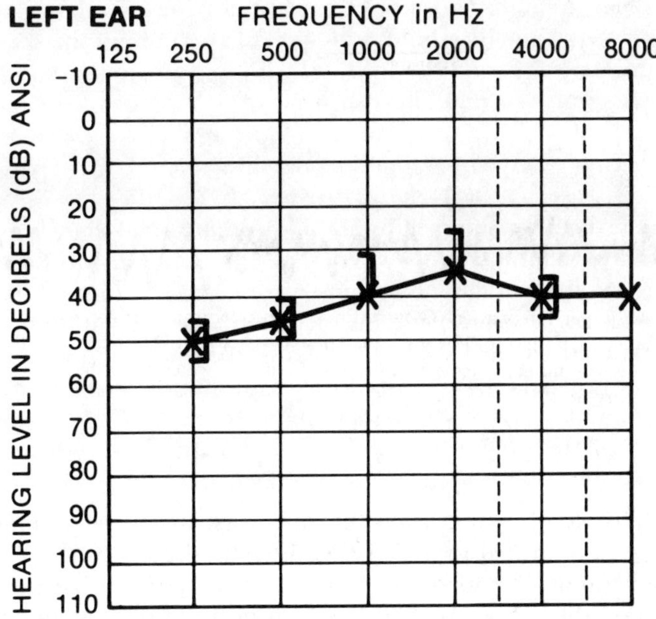

Figure 6-2. Audiogram of a patient with Ménière's Disease on the left ear. Note that the audiogram has a rising contour often taken to be characteristic of conductive impairment, but there is no air-bone gap.

depend on a single test. Nevertheless, use of the ENG is essential as part of the diagnostic armamentarium for Ménière's Disease. Figure 6-4 compares a normal ENG with one obtained from a patient with confirmed Ménière's Disease.

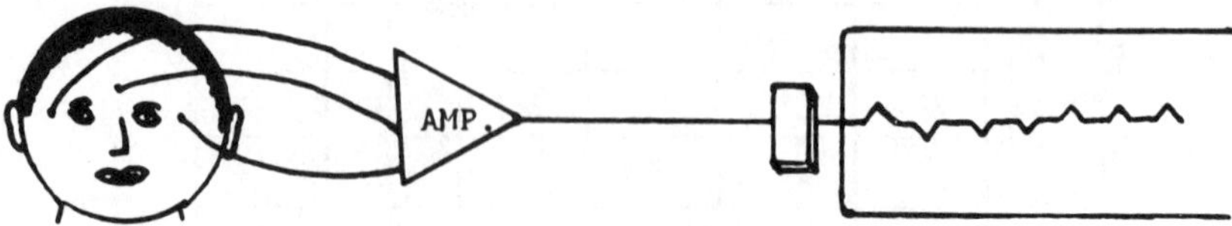

Figure 6-3. Apparatus for recording an electronystagmogram.

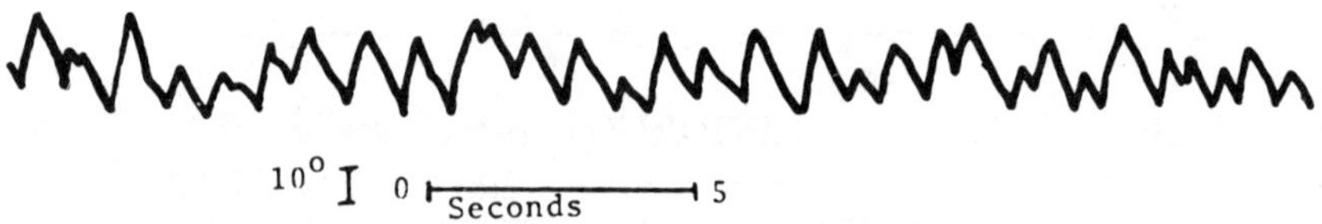

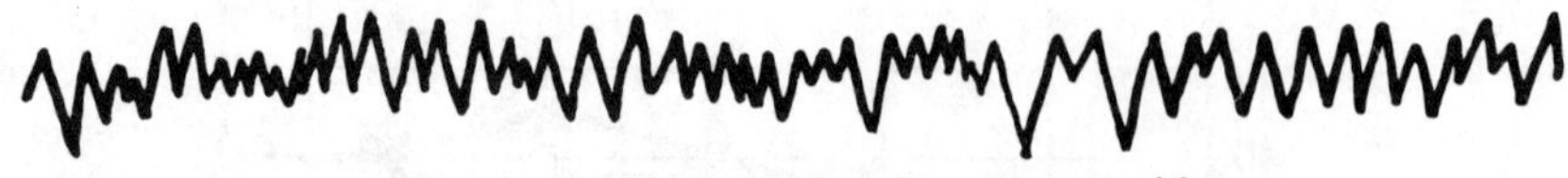

Figure 6-4. A comparison of an ENG of a normal ear (upper trace) with one displaying a vestibular lesion (lower trace). These ENGs were obtained by disturbing the vestibular system by introducing warm water into the external auditory meatus.

In all cases of adventitious hearing loss, a course of monitoring audiometry is indicated to aid in the differential diagnosis, to track any progression, and, of course, to plan rehabilitation. Unilateral hearing losses, where the other ear is normal, usually do not require intensive auditory rehabilitation, but require otological evaluation. If the better ear is not normal and/or the patient prefers, the use of a hearing aid is frequently beneficial.

Most adventitious hearing impairments, however, are not unilateral, but rather bilateral and often severe. Consequently, more than just monitoring audiometry is needed. Amplification, auditory training, speech reading, personal and family counseling are all appropriate. Special education may be required for children, as well as the services of the school audiologist and speech pathologist.

Adventitiously acquired hearing impairments may be accompanied by *tinnitus*. Sometimes this noise is loud enough to be heard by other people; then it is called objective tinnitus. All of us experience an occasional "ringing" in the ears; this is tinnitus. But many people with acquired hearing losses experience tinnitus all the time, and sometimes it is quite loud. It occurs in cases of conductive impairment as well as in sensory impairment. Tinnitus is common in presbycusis. For many patients, tinnitus is severe and handicapping; and it is usually not treatable.

In short, the entire medical, audiological, and psychoeducational armamentaria may be called upon to treat those with adventitious hearing losses. In addition, other specialists may be needed to deal with disease processes and related psychoeducational experts should be employed.

CASE STUDY 6-1:

MUMPS ENDOLABYRINTHITIS

Ms. M., age 20, stated that she has a severe hearing loss in her left ear which she acquired at age 7 following an illness which she described as swollen glands, possibly mumps. She has no family history of deafness and is in good health at the present time.

Both air and bone conduction thresholds in the right ear were within normal limits. SRT was consistent with the pure tone average: -5dB on the right and 65dB on the left. WDS was 98% at 40dB SL. Tympanometry revealed a Type A tympanogram with stapedial reflex thresholds within normal limits.

Air conduction thresholds in the left ear ranged from normal at 250Hz to profound loss at 8000Hz, with bone conduction thresholds normal at 250Hz and following the configuration of the air conduction thresholds. SRT was 65dB and WDS was 52% at 40dB SL. All testing of the left ear was done with masking noise presented to the right ear. Tympanometry revealed a Type A tympanogram; however, stapedial reflex thresholds were 35dB SL at 2000Hz, suggesting the possibility of recruitment.

It was recommended that Ms. M. return to the clinic for a follow-up evaluation in six months to be certain that her hearing is not deteriorating.

Case Study 6-1: Mumps Endolabyrinthitis

PURE TONE AUDIOGRAM

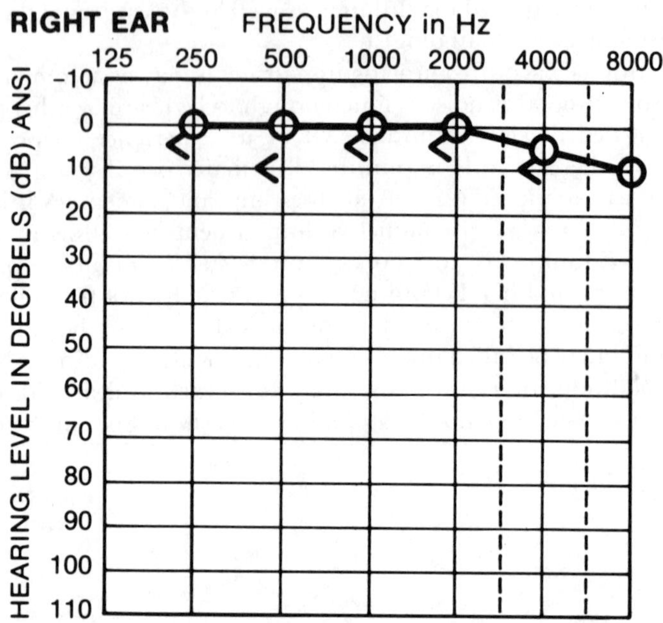

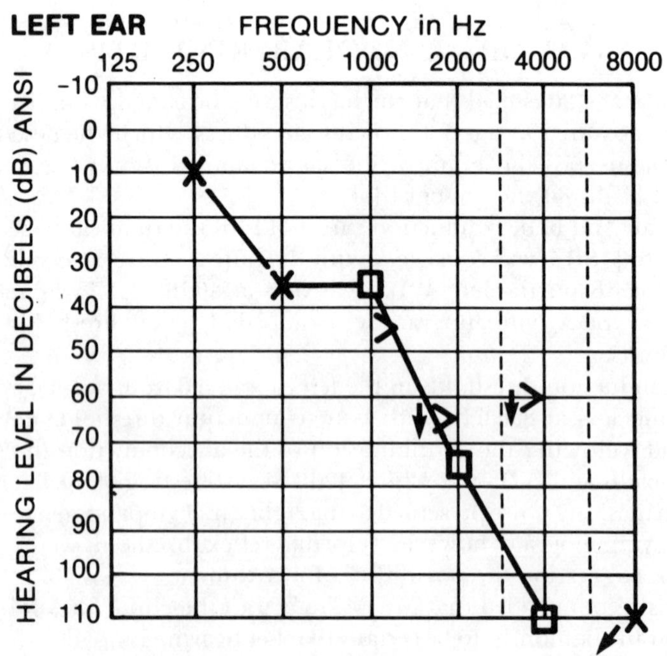

CASE STUDY 6-2: MENIERE'S DISEASE

Mr. B.D., age 35, was referred by Dr. D for a hearing evaluation. His chief complaints were tinnitus, vertigo, and hearing loss especially in the left ear. Onset of the hearing loss and tinnitus was noted in May of 1975. Vertigo appeared in October of 1978. Mr. B's mother and grandfather exhibited hearing loss with age. Previous hearing evaluations had been done but were not available.

The following tests were administered: pure tone audiometry for air and bone conduction, Speech Reception Threshold (SRT), Word Discrimination (WDS), and Tone Decay. The results of these tests showed a sloping, bilateral, moderately severe sensory-neural loss in the high frequencies. The SRT for both ears (10dB) approximated the Pure Tone Average. The WDS for the left ear was within normal limits. The score for the right ear indicates the patient may have slight difficulty in general speech discrimination ability. However, as the hearing loss is in the high frequencies, phonemes whose energy lies predominantly in the high frequencies may be more difficult to discriminate than is suggested by the WDS.

B.D. was referred back to Dr. D due to his complaint of vertigo. A hearing aid evaluation was suggested to him. It is likely that he suffers from Ménière's Disease.

CASE STUDY 6-2: MENIERE'S DISEASE

PURE TONE AUDIOGRAM

RIGHT EAR

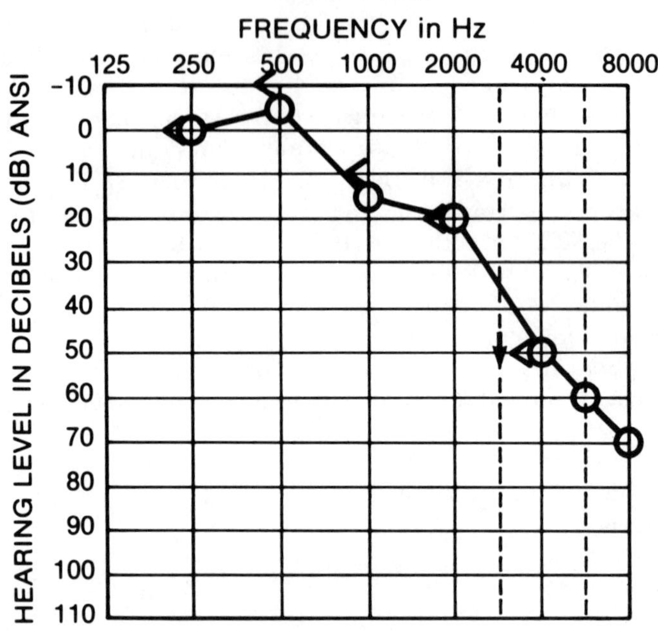

LEFT EAR

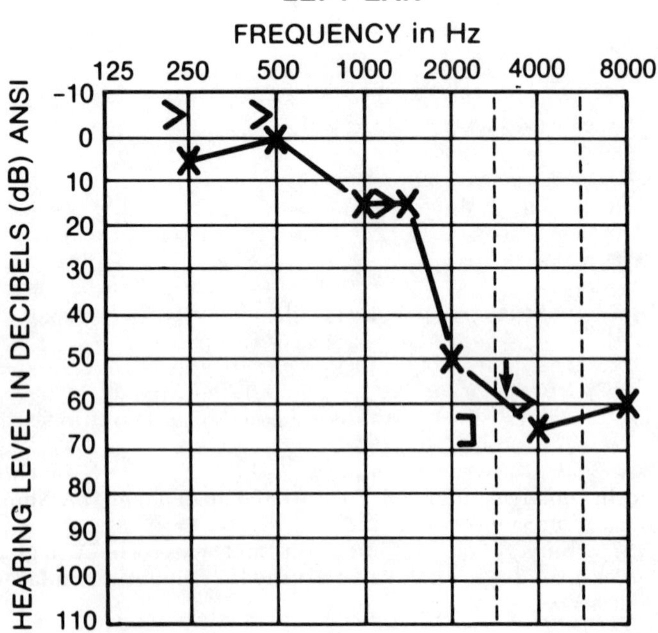

REFERENCES

Alport, A.C. 1927. Hereditary familial congenital haemorrhagic nephritis. *Br. Med. J.* 1:504-506.

Berkow, R. 1977. *The Merck manual.* 13th ed. Rahway: Dohme Research Laboratories.

Carrel, R.J. 1977. Epidemiology of hearing loss. In *Audiometry in infancy,* ed. S.E. Gerber. New York: Grune and Stratton, Inc.

Catlin, F.I. 1978. Etiology and pathology of hearing loss in children. In *Pediatric audiology,* ed. F. Martin. Englewood Cliffs: Prentice-Hall, Inc.

Cody, D.T.R. 1978. Otologic assessment and treatment. In *Audiological assessment,* 2d ed., ed. D.E. Rose. Englewood Cliffs: Prentice-Hall, Inc.

Cotton, R. 1977. Progressive hearing loss. In *Hearing loss in children,* ed. B.F. Jaffe. Baltimore: University Park Press.

Dahle, A.J., McCollister, F.P., Stagno, S., et al. 1979. Progressive hearing impairment in children with congenital cytomegalovirus infection. *J. Speech Hear. Dis.* 44:220-229.

Eichenwald, H. 1979. Rationale and efficacy of antibiotics use in ear, nose and throat practice. Presented to the Seventh Annual Meeting of the Society for Ear, Nose and Throat Advances in Children. Cincinnati.

Fraser, G.R. 1976. *The causes of profound deafness in childhood.* Baltimore: The Johns Hopkins University Press.

Gerber, S.E., Mendel, M.I., and Goller, M. 1979. Progressive hearing loss subsequent to congenital cytomegalovirus infection. *Human Communication* 4:231-234.

Glattke, T.J. 1978. Electronystagmography. In *Handbook of clinical audiology,* 2d ed., ed. J. Katz. Baltimore: Williams & Wilkins, Co.

Goodhill, V. ed. 1979. *Ear diseases, deafness and dizziness.* New York: Harper & Row, Inc.

Goodhill, V. and Harris, I. 1979. Examination of the dizzy patient. In *Ear diseases, deafness, and dizziness,* ed. V. Goodhill. New York: Harper & Row, Inc.

Goodhill, V. and Harris, I. 1979. Peripheral vertigo, labyrinthitis, and Ménière's Disease. In *Ear diseases, deafness and dizziness,* ed. V. Goodhill. New York: Harper & Row, Inc.

Goodhill, V. and Harris, I. 1979. Sudden hearing loss syndrome. In *Ear diseases, deafness and dizziness,* ed. V. Goodhill. New York: Harper & Row, Inc.

Holvey, D.N. 1972. *The Merck manual.* Rahway: Merck & Co., Inc.

House, W.F. 1975. Ménière's Disease: management and theory. In Symposium on fluctuant hearing loss, ed. J.J. Shea. *The Otolaryngologic Clinics of North America* 8:505-535.

Howie, V.M. 1977. Acute and recurrent acute otitis media. In *Hearing loss in children,* ed. B.F. Jaffe. Baltimore: University Park Press.

Konigsmark, B.W. and Gorlin, R.V. 1976. *Genetic and metabolic deafness.* Philadelphia: W.B. Saunders Co.

Lindsay, J.R. and Matz, G. 1966. The differentiation of acquired congenital from genetically determined inner ear deafness. *Ann. Otol. Rhinol. Laryngol.* 75:830-843.

McCabe, B.F. 1963. The etiology of deafness. *Volta Review* 65:471-477.

Mawson, S.R. 1967. *Diseases of the ear.* London: Edward Arnold.

Northern, J.L. 1979. Tinnitus — a continuing enigma. *Hearing Instruments* 30:11, 46.

Paparella, M.M. and Capps, M.J. 1973. Sensorineural deafness in children-nongenetic. In *Otolaryngology,* vol. 2, eds. M.M. Paparella and D.A. Shumrick. Philadelphia: W.B. Saunders Co.

Pulec, J.L. 1973. Surgery of the inner ear and retrocochlear region. In *Otolaryngology,* vol. 2, eds. M.M. Paparella and D.A. Shumrick. Philadelphia: W.B. Saunders Co.

Pulec, J.L. 1976. Ménière's Disease. In *Hearing disorders,* ed. J.L. Northern. Boston: Little, Brown and Co.

Robertson, C. 1978. Pediatric assessment of the infant at risk for deafness. In *Early diagnosis of hearing loss,* eds. S.E. Gerber and G.T. Mencher. New York: Grune & Stratton, Inc.

Rubin, W. 1968. Sudden hearing loss. *Laryngoscope* 78:829-833.

Sataloff, J. 1966. *Hearing loss.* Philadelphia: J.B. Lippincott Co.

Schuknecht, H.F. 1975. Pathophysiology of Ménière's Disease. In Symposium on fluctuant hearing loss, ed. J.J. Shea. *Otolaryngol. Clin. N. Amer.* 8:507-514.

Shulman, J.B. 1979. Traumatic diseases of the ear and temporal bone. In *Ear diseases, deafness and dizziness,* ed. V. Goodhill. New York: Harper & Row, Inc.

Shulman, J.B. 1979. Syphilis of the temporal bone. In *Ear diseases, deafness and dizziness,* ed. V. Goodhill. New York: Harper & Row, Inc.

Snow, J.B. 1973. Sudden deafness. In *Otolaryngology,* vol. 2, eds. M.M. Paparella and D.A. Shumrick. Philadelphia: W.B. Saunders Co.

Strome, M. 1977. Sudden fluctuating hearing losses. In *Hearing loss in children,* ed. B.F. Jaffe. Baltimore: University Park Press.

Vernon, M. 1969. Usher's Syndrome — deafness and progressive blindness. *J. Chron. Dis.* 22:133-151.

Visencio, L. and Gerber, S.E. 1979. Effects of hemodialysis on pure-tone thresholds and blood chemistry measures. *J. Speech Hear. Res.* 22:756-764.

CHAPTER 7

Ototoxicity

The word "ototoxicity" literally means ear poisoning. Excluded from this discussion are those ototoxic losses where the toxin itself is clearly defined as a part of a disease process (e.g., kidney disease). Discussion here is limited to those ototoxicities which are *iatrogenic;* that is, those which are medically caused. The reader should not jump to an erroneous opinion that medical practitioners cause deafness. Be assured that the medical profession knows that it should not. Unfortunately, it is the case that certain drugs are the drugs of choice when treating certain diseases—almost always in life-saving situations—and some of these drugs count deafness among their side effects. Therefore, there are instances where the aural side effects cannot be avoided; it might be a question of dead or deaf.

PATHOLOGY and ETIOLOGY

Most of the ototoxic drugs are specifically cochleotoxic, although some of them are vestibulotoxic and some are also nephrotoxic (i.e., dangerous to kidney function). The severity of these hearing impairments varies from patient to patient dependent upon the sensitivity of the individual, the size of the dosage, and/or the length of time the drug has been taken. There is strong evidence which demonstrates that the body accumulates drugs of this nature, and that it is the total accumulation effect which is the critical variable. Tinnitus is a universal precurser of ototoxic hearing loss, and is a warning sign of overaccumulation. In order to avoid overaccumulation and the associated ototoxicity, many patients are given blood tests on a regular basis to monitor the serum level of the drug. If the serum level is low enough, the drug may be reintroduced or a different drug therapy begun. But, the drug will remain in the inner ear fluids longer than in the blood, and may continue to do damage for some time. Two or more drugs sometimes may combine in the same way as additional administration of the same drug to increase the loss of hearing. Currently used ototoxic aminoglycoside antibiotics are streptomycin, kanamycin, gentamycin, neomycin, tobramycin, amikacin, and paromomycin.

In any event, the effect of ototoxic drugs on the cochlea is to destroy the hair cells directly *(Dublin, 1976).* Typically, the hair cells are destroyed beginning with the outermost row of the outer hair cells, progressing through the other two rows of outer hair cells, and finally attacking the inner hair cells. Figure 7-1 shows a cat's normal organ of Corti. Figures 7-2a and 7-2b show the organ of Corti of an animal treated with neomycin. In figure 7-2a, all sensory cells have degenerated but supporting cells are intact. Figure 7-2b, a cochlea a year-and-a-half after neomycin, shows that the organ of Corti has been completely resorbed.

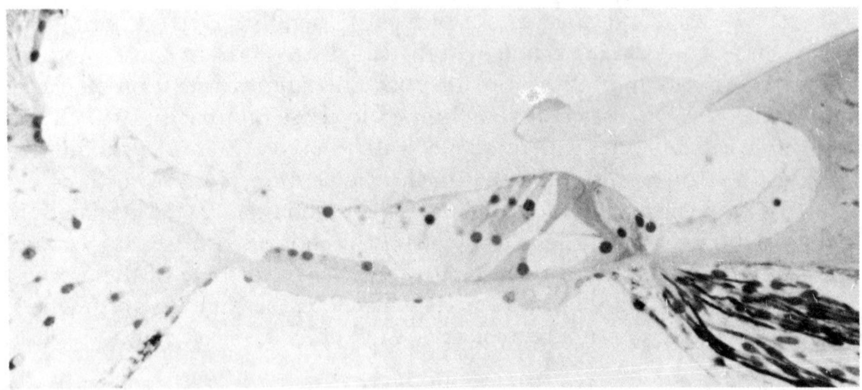

Figure 7-1. Radial section of the normal organ of Corti from the basal turn of a cat cochlea. *(Micrograph courtesy of P.A. Leake-Jones, Ph.D.)*

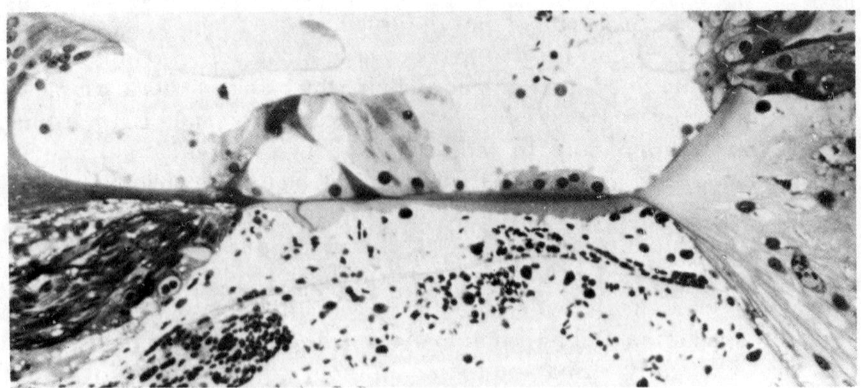

Figure 7-2a. Basal turn of cat cochlea 30 days subsequent to profound hearing loss induced by intramuscular injection of neomycin. All sensory cells have degenerated, yet supporting elements are intact. *(Micrograph courtesy of P.A. Leake-Jones, Ph.D.)*

134

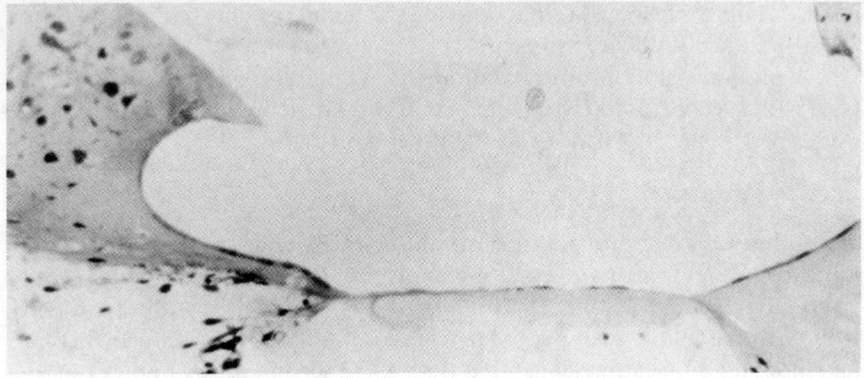

Figure 7-2b. One year and seven months following neomycin poisoning, the organ of Corti has been completely resorbed and severe loss of myelinated nerve fibers in the osseous spiral lamina is evident. *(Micrograph courtesy of P.A. Leake-Jones, Ph.D.)*

STREPTOMYCIN AND DIHYDROSTREPTOMYCIN

Probably the best known of all ototoxic drugs is streptomycin. Streptomycin has been, and still is, the usual drug of choice for the treatment of tuberculosis *(Holvey, 1972)*. Tuberculosis, still a common life-threatening disease, can occur in any part of the body except the teeth and nails. A competent program of tuberculosis therapy involves frequent monitoring audiometry to insure that the minimum amount of hearing impairment results from the use of the drug. Streptomycin, in addition to being ototoxic, is also vestibulotoxic. Consequently, the tubercular patient being treated with streptomycin may report a sensation of mild vertigo before complaining of hearing impairment. Bergstrom and Thompson (1976) observed that vestibular damage due to streptomycin is far more common than hearing loss.

Some years ago, in an effort to obviate the vestibulotoxic effect of streptomycin, a drug called dihydrostreptomycin was developed. It is just as ototoxic as streptomycin, if not more so, but does not produce vertigo. As it turns out, this is not a very good idea at all. By removing the vestibulotoxic effects, one of the early warning signs of ototoxocity was also removed. A number of people were deafened, and consequently, dihydrostreptomycin has not been utilized to any degree for many years.

Essentially all ototoxic drugs, including streptomycin, lead to tinnitus, or noise in the ear. The tubercular patient is usually warned to be especially alert to the onset of tinnitus. When tinnitus occurs, and if the patient's life is no longer at stake, the dosage is reduced or the drug is removed entirely for a period of time. In other words, the presence of tinnitus and the use of monitoring audiometry have an influence on the extent and degree to which streptomycin is used. That is the proper procedure for administration of any known ototoxic substance. Nevertheless, tuberculosis is a life-threatening disease. Tuberculosis, as well as other diseases, and patients with severe burns are still treated with streptomycin.

A program of monitoring audiometry is essential even after the drug has been withdrawn. It is likely that there will be a latent onset of hearing loss due to the persistence of the drug in the inner ear fluids.

Kanamycin and Gentamycin

Other ototoxic drugs which are in relatively wide use in pediatrics are kanamycin and gentamycin. Gentamycin is the most widely used aminoglycoside antibiotic *(Shulman, 1979)*. These drugs are frequently utilized as part of the treatment of newborn infants who are seriously ill. Once again, it should be appreciated that the pediatric community knows that the drugs are potentially ototoxic, and their use is judicious and only when necessary. It is also the case that confirmed deafness from kanamycin or gentamycin when the drug was given in very, very early life has been observed only very rarely *(Abrams, 1977)*. It may be that sensitivity to the ototoxic effects of these two drugs is something which develops later in infancy *(Hawkins, 1975)*; or it may be conjectured that the drug is not retained because of the high rate of renal clearance; or that there is a natural immunity; or methods for establishing the aural effects in newborns do not yet exist. Gentamycin is more vestibulotoxic than kanamycin *(Shulman, 1979)*. However, when used on adults, the ototoxic effects of the drugs are quite striking and, therefore, there is no point in tempting fate with babies. Kanamycin does cross the placental barrier, but affects auditory function only after development is complete *(Uziel, Romand, and Marot, 1979)*.

As a matter of fact, the ototoxicity of kanamycin is so well established and so well understood, that it is given to experimental animals as part of the ongoing investigation of the pathological effects of ototoxic drugs.

Other Aminoglycosides

Other ototoxic drugs in the aminoglycoside family include neomycin and tobramycin. There are many others, and the reader is referred to Hawkins, Johnsson, and Aran (1969) for further information. However, it should not be concluded—as some authors *(Prescod, 1978)* have done—that, because the drug has the term "-mycin" as part of its name, it is ototoxic. That is just not true; the name means that it is derived from a certain fungus. Many medications in the "-mycin" family of aminoglycosides—in fact, most of the "-mycin" drugs—have no ototoxic effect. These include terramycin and aureomycin which are drugs frequently prescribed by pediatricians, and erythromycin recommended by otolaryngologists. Furthermore, not all ototoxic drugs are members of the "-mycin" family. For example, among the most commonly used ototoxic drugs are aspirin and quinine.

Salicylates

Aspirin is a popular name for a form of salicylic acid. It appears popularly under many well-known brand names, such as Alka Seltzer,

Anacin, and Bufferin. Salicylic acid is an ototoxic drug. It is reasonable to expect that, since aspirin is so widely used, all of us should suffer some amount of ototoxic hearing loss. Clearly, that is not the case. It takes a great deal of salicylic acid for any ototoxicity to appear. The best illustration is found in a study of arthritis, a disease for which aspirin is a specific drug. Arthritics who take aspirin therapeutically consume much larger quantities of salicylic acid than those of us who take two aspirins for headaches; and, indeed, many arthritics do suffer from hearing impairment and tinnitus.

The ototoxic effects of salicylic acid appear to be temporary. If one were to stop taking the drug, the hearing loss would diminish within 72 hours *(Shulman, 1979)*. Goin (1976) reports, however, that the drug disappears rather slowly from the cochlear fluid following withdrawal.

Salicylate induced hearing loss is usually mild to moderate, peaking at approximately 40dB. There may be some decrease in speech discrimination at the peak of the toxic cycle, but this too will improve upon withdrawal.

There is no known consistent change within the hair cells or the cochlear end organ associated with salicylate toxicity. Shulman reports that it is presumed that the mechanism of the hearing disorder is related to a reversible alteration in biochemical or enzymatic function. This type of hearing loss and its results and treatment differ markedly from that associated with the aminoglycosides.

QUININE

It was thought for many years that hearing loss was a necessary result of malaria. It is the fact, though, that hearing loss resulted not from the malaria, but from the treatment of the disease with quinine and related drugs. A patient treated with quinine developed a very steep hearing loss with severe impairment limited to the high frequencies (figure 7-3). The greatest danger from the drug is not to the malaria patient, but to the pregnant patient because the drug has been known to cross the placental barrier *(Jaffe, 1977)* and to result in severe congenital deafness. Fortunately, the drug is not in common use today, as substitutes have been developed. Nevertheless, the reader should be warned that Quick (1973) reports that small doses of the drug, even in a "palatable gin and tonic" can cause tinnitus in susceptible individuals.

DIURETICS

There are other ototoxic drugs and other kinds of ototoxic drugs, but fortunately they are in rather less frequent use. An important example of one of those is ethacrynic acid, another is furosemide; they are used for pulmonary edema. These diuretics, in common with some others, do seem to have ototoxic effects.

The dispenser of any of these medications is made aware of their adverse side effects by the manufacturer. The drugs are used, most of the time, cautiously and appropriately. Nevertheless, as new drugs are developed, new problems will appear. Caution and audiometric monitoring are usually indicated.

PURE TONE AUDIOGRAM

RIGHT EAR

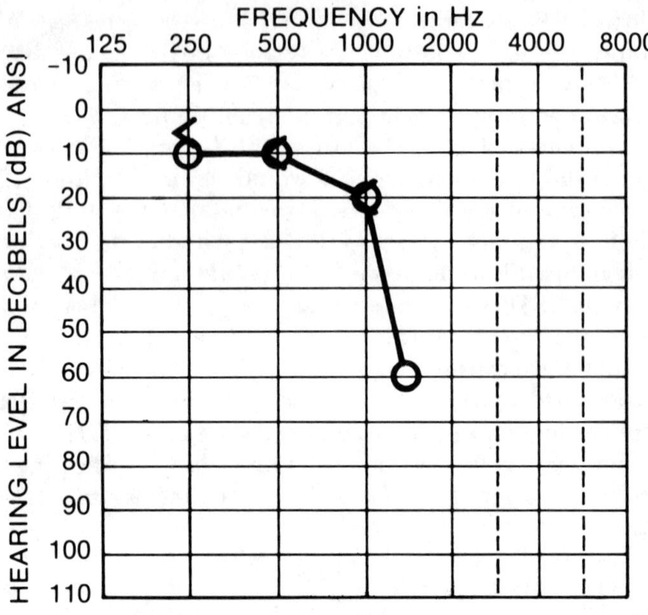

LEFT EAR

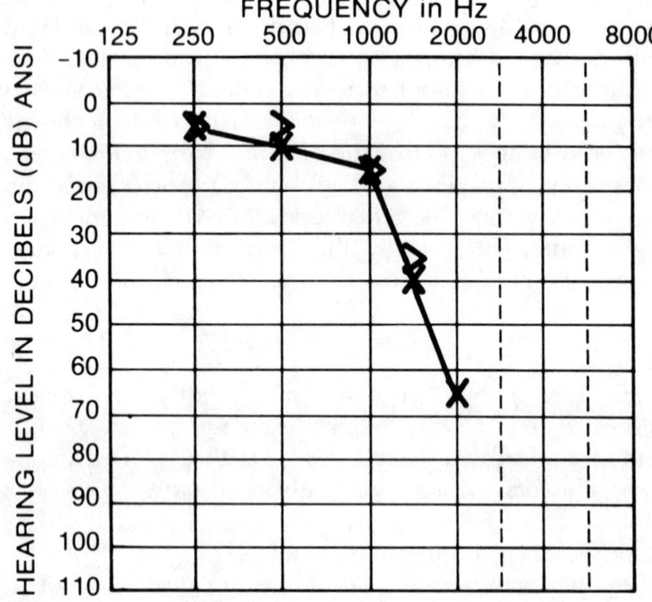

Figure 7-3. Audiograms of a patient whose malaria had been treated with quinine; there were no responses above 1500Hz in the right ear and 2000Hz in the left.

MEDICAL CONSIDERATIONS

Essentially, there is very little which the ear surgeon can do for ototoxic hearing losses. These are not correctable in the sense that hearing can be restored by some surgical procedure. On the other hand, recent innovations are arising from intense cooperation among otologists, audiologists, physiologists, and engineers. These have led to electronic devices which, some day, may be implanted within the ear to serve as substitute cochleae. At present, these cochlear implants are extremely limited in their utility, but they are useful for those persons, such as the ototoxic patient, whose hearing loss has reached the stage of total deafness. A small number of ototoxic patients have had an auditory prosthesis implanted in the cochleae. Some of them have experienced a limited degree of success. The devices, at this stage in development, seem to restore only an awareness of a few environmental sounds. The overall improvement in hearing ability is quite small, but they do seem to provide rhythm and other cues which may enhance speechreading ability, an important communication method for the hearing impaired *(Gerber, 1975)*. While individuals utilizing these devices cannot interpret specific speech sounds, they have found that the implants provide some auditory contact with the environment. Thus, while the auditory success may be considered "limited," the emotional success must be considered enormous. The development of these devices has had great psychological value for patients with severe hearing losses, notably, those who have been rendered suddenly and totally deaf by ototoxic drugs. No doubt, because that group has had prior experience with sound and is familiar with its interpretation, it will continue to be a focal point of continued research and treatment with cochlear implants. Figure 7-4 illustrates a cochlear prosthesis and how it is placed. Figure 7-5 shows the prosthesis in place with the receiver implanted into the mastoid and the electronics built into the eye-glass temple. Clearly, the implantation of such a device is an otological surgical procedure, and at present, applicable only to those who have lost their hearing because of ototoxicity.

AUDIOLOGICAL CONSIDERATIONS

In the extreme, of course, the patient rendered deaf by an ototoxic drug is about as deaf a patient as may be seen. If the individual has undergone cochleotoxicity to the extent that all of the hair cells have been destroyed, then there will be no hearing at all, at least within the limits of clinical audiometers. Insofar as the drug may have been withdrawn or refused before massive destruction of hair cells occured, the patient's audiogram will reflect it. Treatment must be based on what hearing the patient has retained, the residual hearing. Furthermore, the ototoxically impaired patient will

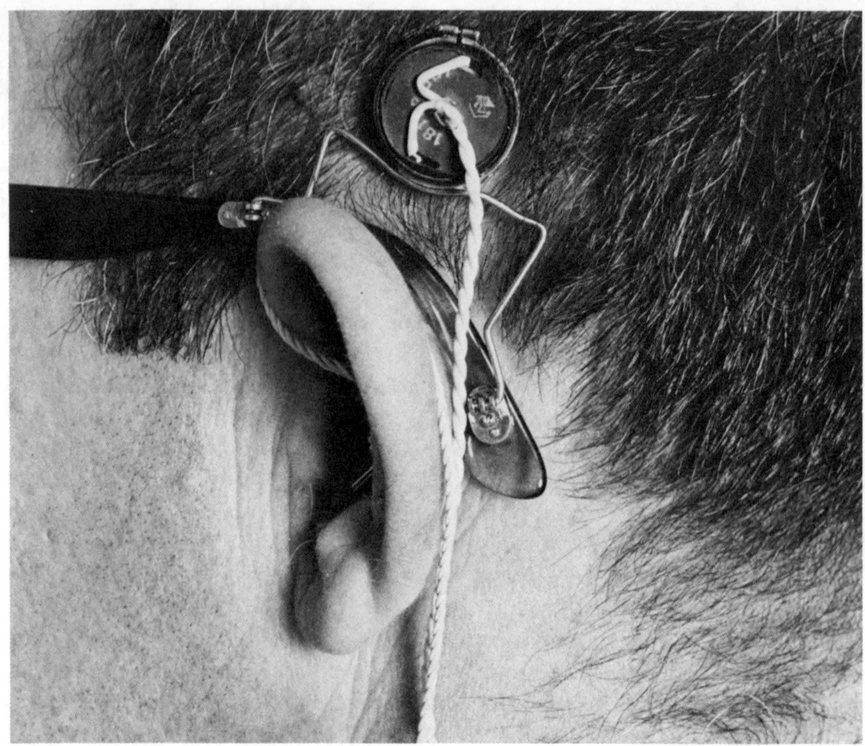

Figure 7-4a. Cochlear prosthesis in place. *(Reproduced with permission of Ear Research Institute.)*

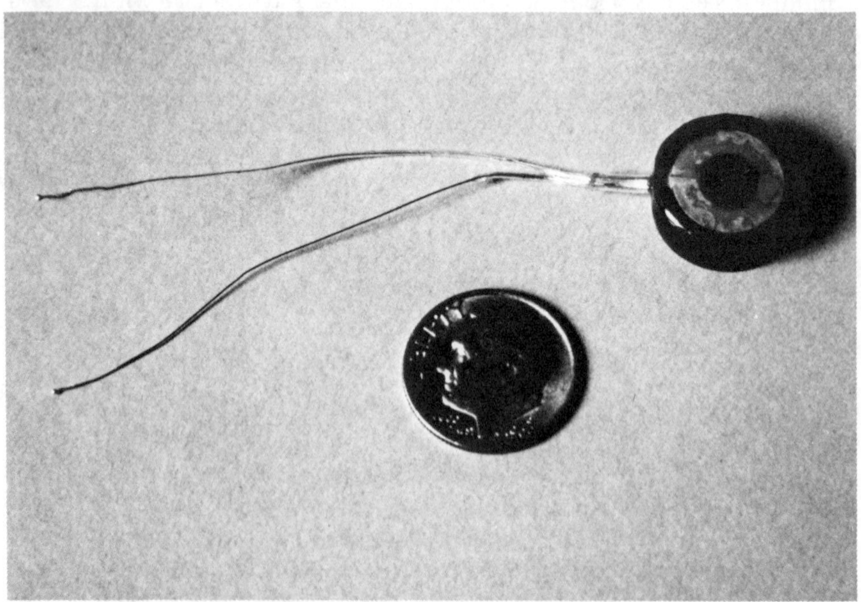

Figure 7-4b. Cochlear implant. *(Reproduced with permission of Ear Research Institute.)*

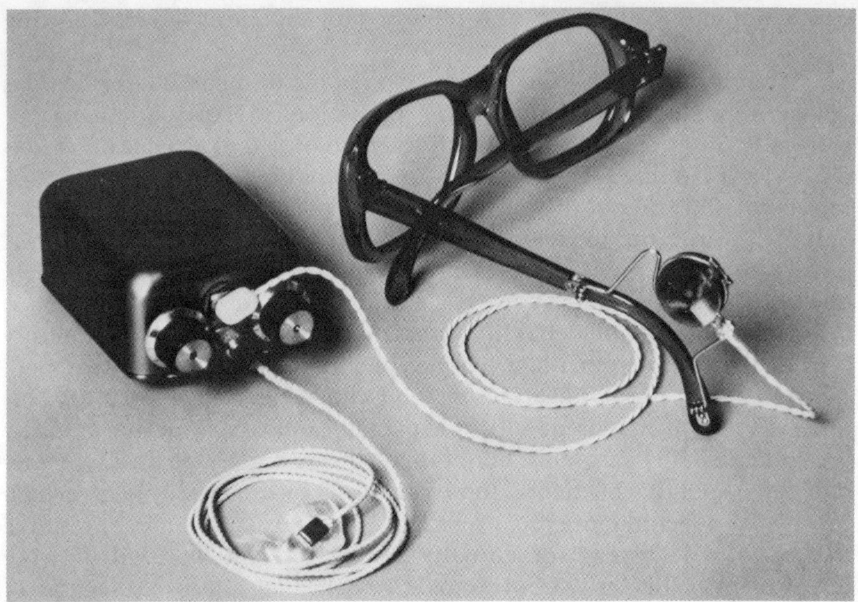

Figure 7-5. Cochlear implant system. *(Reproduced with permission of Ear Research Institute.)*

probably demonstrate tinnitus and recruitment, and those factors must also be considered.

Since the onset of hearing loss due to ototoxicity may be delayed — due both to the time over which the drug accumulates in the cochlear fluids and the relative slowness with which it disappears from the cochlear fluids — a program of monitoring audiometry is necessary. One such program monitors hearing threshold every week during administration of the drug until there is a threshold shift of 15dB at 4000Hz. Then the monitoring program is increased to twice weekly. If the threshold continues to shift, the drug is withdrawn at a shift of 25dB *(Arnst, 1980)*. Moreover, since the onset of hearing loss may be delayed, a program of monitoring audiometry should be continued after the drug has been withdrawn. A program of vestibular testing may also be employed for those drugs (e.g., streptomycin) which are largely vestibulotoxic *(Bergstrom and Thompson, 1976)*.

RECRUITMENT OF LOUDNESS

Recruitment of loudness refers to a condition of the cochlea which has the effect of making intense sounds abnormally loud to the patient who cannot hear sounds at moderate or lesser intensities. This can be an exceedingly annoying condition. The familiar story of the person who says, "Speak up, I can't hear you," and then says, "Don't shout at me!" is an excellent example of the phenomenon. The sounds of the environment tend to be either not loud enough or too loud. Recruitment is a frequent concommitant of all sensory hearing losses, but especially ototoxic hearing impairment.

What is the basis for the phenomenon of recruitment? The evidence is not entirely clear, but the following physiological explanation may be correct. In a normal ear, the sound intensity required to activate outer hair cells is less than that required to activate inner hair cells. In other words, the threshold of hearing of the inner hair cells is greater than it is for the outer hair cells. Since the tissue destruction due to ototoxicity begins with the outermost row of outer hair cells and progresses inwardly *(Dublin, 1976)*, one result is loss of outer hair cells while inner hair cells remain intact. Consequently, the patient has little or no hearing for sounds of low intensity because there are no outer hair cells to respond to them. On the other hand, the patient has normal hearing for those intensities where the inner hair cells will respond. Consequently, the patient cannot hear the low intensity (i.e., outer hair cells) sounds, but normally hears high intensity (i.e., inner hair cells) sounds. Therefore, those cochlear hearing impairments which involve the outer and inner hair cells more or less equally, such as those due to disease, will display substantially less recruitment than will hearing impairments which arise from ototoxicity and which affect specific rows of hair cells.

Another model of recruitment employs the notion of spread of excitation along the basilar membrane *(Gulick, 1971; Ward, 1973)*. This notion suggests that, when intensity is sufficient to stimulate hair cells adjacent to the damaged area, neural excitation will be initiated because healthy hair cells in the adjacent areas will fire. As signal level continues to increase, more and more of the unaffected area's sensory units will be excited as the displacement of the basilar membrane gets broader and broader. DeBoer (1967), Evans and Wilson (1977), and others lent credence to this model of recruitment when they found no evidence of lateral inhibition on the basilar membrane under various conditions.

Another model *(Davis et al., 1949)* suggests that the hair cells or ganglion cells are only relatively damaged and therefore relatively insensitive. Consequently, sufficient intensity may overcome their insensitivity and cause a sudden increase of loudness. Moreover, DeBoer and Bouwmeester (1975) found that spread of masking may extend over a wide range of frequencies in some patients with sensory hearing losses, but not in all of these patients. Hence, lack of lateral inhibition cannot account for recruitment in all patients.

It is difficult, of course, to fit a hearing aid on a patient who has recruitment. However, contrary to an unfortunately long-standing myth, it is by no means impossible to do so. The hearing aid industry is certainly aware of the phenomenon of recruitment and has provided aids with excellent compensatory response, that is, aids with peak clipping, filtering, and differential amplification for the higher and lower frequencies. Obviously, auditory training and speech reading instruction are also essential.

In summary, then, it is sometimes necessary for a physician to prescribe a life-saving drug which, among its undesirable side effects, may cause severe hearing impairment. Collectively, such drugs are called ototoxic. Hearing impairments which arise from ototoxicity are usually very severe to profound and are characterized by tinnitus and recruitment. Withdrawal of the drug may restrict the degree of the hearing loss. These losses are not otherwise subject to medical intervention except in the occasional case when there is the use of a cochlear implant. Audiological intervention is made possible by the use of special hearing aids which compress very high intensities while sufficiently amplifying lower ones. Thus, some rehabilitative relief is offered the patient. However, these types of cases require extensive counseling and support, and a great deal of patience on everybody's part during the hearing aid evaluation and adjustment period. Without that combination, success will be marginal at best.

CASE STUDY 7-1: OTOTOXICITY

Mr. W., age 53, complains that he is totally unable to hear conversational speech and that he hears only vibrations. He has no familial history of hearing impairment. His deafness dates to 1962 when he received streptomycin injections for a gunshot wound. He states he is in good health at the present time.

He has profound, bilateral, sensory-neural loss: the PTA in the right ear is 95dB and more than 100dB in the left ear. No response to any frequency was observed by bone conduction. Because of the severity of the loss, speech audiometry was impossible. Impedance audiometry showed a Type A tympanogram, normal static compliance, and absent stapedius relflex bilaterally.

Findings are consistent with profound, bilateral sensory-neural hearing loss. A hearing aid evaluation is recommended.

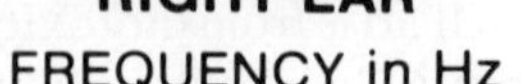

Case Study 7-1: Ototoxicity

PURE TONE AUDIOGRAM
RIGHT EAR

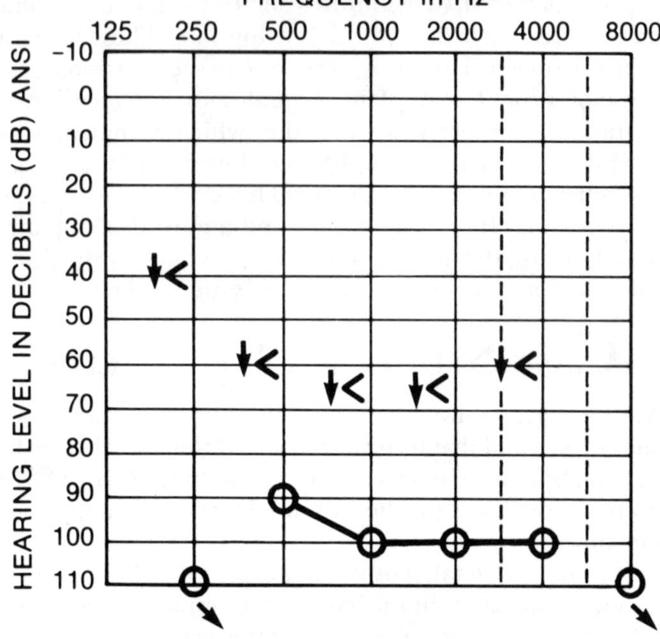

LEFT EAR

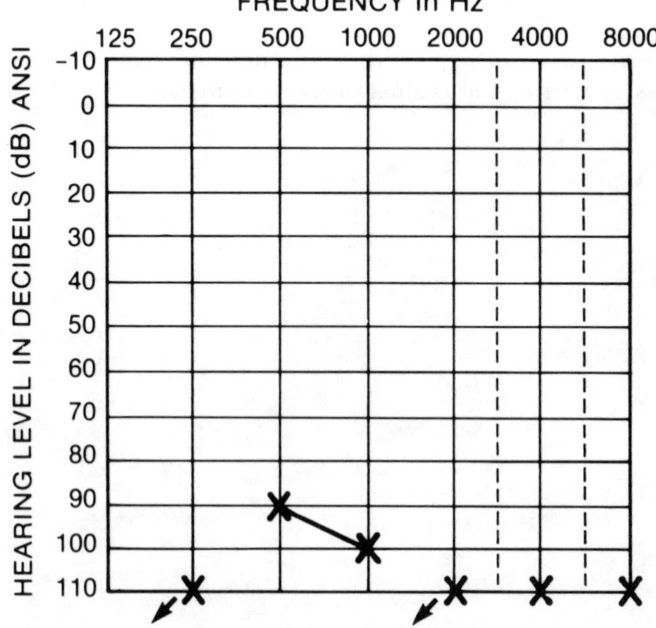

Case Study 7-2:

Cochlear Implant

L.E., age 40, contracted spinal meningitis at the age of six months; this was later cited as the cause of a profound bilateral hearing loss. Besides contracting spinal meningitis, the patient had measles at age three and rheumatic fever at age five.

Audiometric testing revealed a profound bilateral hearing loss. No responses were obtained with bone conduction tests and there was no understanding on speech discrimination testing.

The patient has not been wearing a hearing aid prior to cochlear implant surgery. An implantation of a single electrode induction coil system for his left ear was recommended.

CASE STUDY 7-2: COCHLEAR IMPLANT
PURE TONE AUDIOGRAM

RIGHT EAR

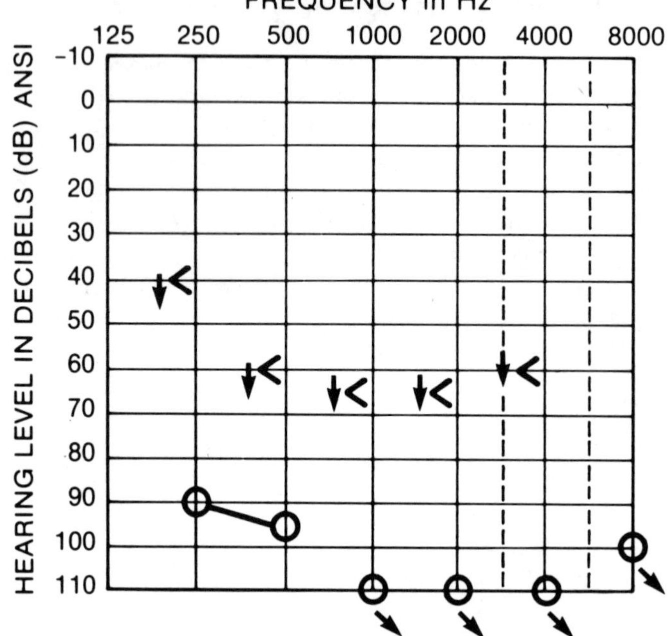

LEFT EAR

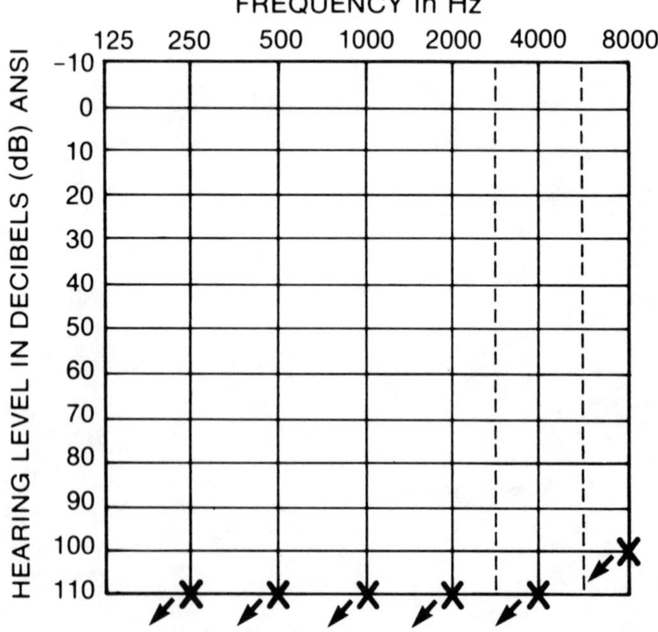

REFERENCES

Abrams, I.F. 1977. Nongenetic hearing loss. In *Hearing loss in children*, ed. B.F. Jaffe. Baltimore: University Park Press.

Arnst, D.J. 1980. Personal communication.

Bergstrom, L. and Thompson, P. 1976. Ototoxicity. In *Hearing disorders*, ed. J. Northern. Boston: Little, Brown and Co.

Davis, H., Gernardt, B.E., Riesco-MacClure, J.S. and Covell, W.P. 1949. Aural microphonics in the cochlea of the guinea pig. *J. Acoust. Soc. Amer.* 21:502-510.

DeBoer, E. 1967. Correlation studies applied to the frequency resolution of the cochlea. *J. Auditory Res.* 7:209-217.

DeBoer, E. and Bouwmeester, J. 1975. Clinical psychophysics illustrated by the problem of auditory overload. *Audiology* 14:274-299.

Dublin, W.B. 1976. *Fundamentals of sensorineural auditory pathology.* Springfield: Charles C. Thomas.

Evans, E.F. and Wilson, J.P. 1977. *Psychophysics and physiology of hearing.* London: Academic Press.

Gerber, S.E. 1975. Will cochlear implants aid childhood deafness? *Clin. Pediatr.* July, p. 623.

Goin, D.W. 1976. Otospongiosis. In *Otolaryngology: a textbook*, ed. G. English. New York: Harper & Row, Inc.

Gulick, W.L. 1971. *Hearing: physiology and psychophysics.* New York: Oxford University Press.

Hawkins, J.E. 1975. Drug ototoxicity. In *Differential diagnosis in pediatric otolaryngology*, ed. M. Strome. Boston: Little, Brown and Co.

Hawkins, J.E., Johnsson, L.G. and Aran, J.M. 1969. Comparative tests of gentamycin ototoxicity. *J. Infect. Dis.* 119:417-431.

Holvey, D.N. 1972. *The Merck manual.* Rahway: Merck & Co., Inc.

Jaffe, B.F. ed. 1977. *Hearing loss in children.* Baltimore: University Park Press.

Prescod, S.V. 1978. *Audiological handbook of hearing disorders.* New York: Van Nostrand Reinhold Co.

Quick, C.A. 1973. Chemical and drug effects on the inner ear. In *Otolaryngology*, vol. 2, eds. M.M. Paparella and D.A. Shumrick. Philadelphia: W.B. Saunders Co.

Shulman, J.B. 1979. Ototoxicity. In *Ear diseases, deafness and dizziness*, ed. V. Goodhill. New York: Harper & Row, Inc.

Uziel, A., Romand, R., and Marot, M. 1979. Electrophysiological study of the otoxicity of kanamycin during development in guinea pigs. *Hearing Research* 1:203-212.

Ward, W.D. 1973. Adaptation and fatigue. In *Modern developments in audiology*, 2d ed. ed. J. Jerger. New York: Academic Press.

CHAPTER 8

Noise Induced Hearing Loss

Noise is undoubtedly one of the world's great health problems and the single most common form of environmental pollution. Continuous or repeated exposure to high levels of noise will cause sufficient damage to the auditory system to produce a sensory hearing loss. The injury and/or hearing loss may be only temporary, lasting for just minutes or hours or even days after the exposure. It may, of course, recur chronically. That is, as exposure is repeated, the hearing loss repeats, but there is some recovery of hearing between exposures. Finally, the hearing loss may become permanent; that is, no recovery of hearing, even long after the exposure has been terminated.

Today in our industrialized western civilization no one is free from the effects of high level noise; unfortunately, noise exposure is too easily accepted as a necessary evil, a risk taken for living in a modern mechanized world. The problem is further compounded by the fact that some younger segments of our society have decided that exposure to intense noise can be enjoyable. It is a serious problem that there are those who are willing to experience more noise exposure than they should, or need to, accept. It does not matter if the hearing loss is the result of an acoustic trauma, such as that which might accompany an explosion, or if it results from an occupational exposure to intense noises over a long period of time. The eventual effect is the same: *permanent* sensory hearing loss. The amount of the loss is a function of the susceptibility of the hearer, his residual hearing, the temporal characteristics of the noise, and the duration, frequency, and/or intensity of the exposure.

Pathology and Etiology

The pathology associated with noise-induced hearing loss is quite similar, in fact essentially the same, as that which accompanies ototoxicity. The difference is that noise-induced losses tend to affect a limited region along the basilar membrane and, consequently, result in destruction of outer hair cells in restricted regions of the organ of Corti; whereas, ototoxicity tends to result in more diffuse damage and, thus, the hair cell destruction is more widespread. Except for these regional differences, the actual physical damage is quite similar; that is, loss of outer hair cells is eventually followed by loss of inner hair cells.

The area of the organ of Corti about 6 to 10 mm from the basal end, which tonotopically corresponds to 4000 to 6000Hz on the audiogram, seems to be uniquely vulnerable to the initial trauma and destruction associated with noise-induced hearing loss (NIHL). That vulnerability may be a function of excessive mechanical stress at certain frequencies during stimulation due to the response characteristics of the middle ear and the associated transmission of energy into the cochlea; or to some indigenous weakness of the structure of the organ of Corti itself *(Schuknecht, 1974)*. In any case, prolonged exposure or excessive exposure to noise is most often evidenced by a characteristic "notch" in the audiogram at 4000 and/or 6000Hz.

THE ROLE OF THE MIDDLE EAR

Unless there is a signal in excess of 160dB SPL, the middle ear will appear unaffected by the noise *(Eames et al., 1975)*. However, the middle ear does play a significant role in determining the effects of excessive noise exposure. The frequency response characteristics of the middle ear are such that low frequency tones are damped while middle to high frequency signals are transmitted to the organ of Corti with great efficiency. The end result is a human "band-pass filter" which limits the frequencies of sound which are potentially damaging to the cochlea.

For some time it was thought that the middle ear reflexes, notably the stapedius muscle reflex, provide some protection for the cochlea by stiffening the response characteristics of the conductive mechanism and, thus, preventing the transmission of sound into the cochlea. As it happens, the attenuation is primarily in the lower frequencies, at about 1000Hz and below. Further, the extent of the reflex is limited, so that its protective function is effective over only a limited range of intensities *(Dallos, 1964)*. Finally, the stapedius reflex itself is delayed in its onset by nearly 10 msec *(Salomon and Starr, 1963)*, and thus its protection is also delayed in onset.

In truth, the contribution of the middle ear structures, the pinna, the ear canal, etc., in the attenuation of excessive noise should not be taken lightly or even overlooked; but, at the same time, those structures should not be considered adequate to protect the cochlea from excessive noise or the ear from suffering a hearing loss.

DAMAGE TO THE COCHLEA

Figure 8-1 illustrates hair cell destruction in the cochlea of an experimental animal exposed to intense noise. It can be seen that there are "islands" of profound damage where the tissue is missing entirely. In noise-induced hearing loss, the site of the destruction of the hair cells is largely a function of the spectrum of the noise which produced the loss. If experimental animals are exposed to a signal which is an intense burst of a single frequency, the result will be the complete destruction of a narrow region of the organ of Corti. The region, however, will not be so narrowly restricted as to be limited exclusively to that place along the basilar membrane which corresponds directly with the stimulating frequency. Rather, the damaged region will be somewhat broader than that, and will extend more toward the basal end (high frequencies) than toward the apical end (low frequencies) of the cochlea. This is because the spread of energy along the basilar membrane distributes frequency information from high to low. Since, in the presence of intense noise, the basilar membrane is displaced continuously from the base to its maximum point, it is only natural that hearing loss should occur at some frequencies close to, and higher than, the stimulating frequency.

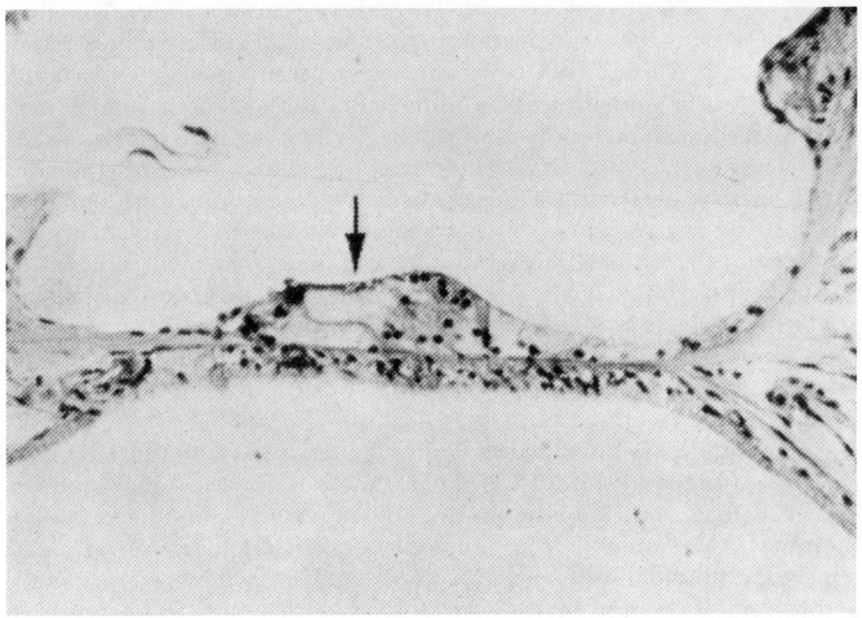

Figure 8-1. Noise induced hearing loss in the cochlear region corresponding to 4000 to 8000Hz. *(Courtesy of Harold F. Schuknecht, M.D., Massachusetts Eye and Ear Infirmary.)*

Acoustic trauma, which may be caused by an explosion, a blast, gunfire, etc., will result in pathology nearly identical to that seen in an occupationally based hearing loss. The major difference is that in the one case the hearing loss is obtained cumulatively at work, while in the other it is sudden in onset, directly the result of trauma to the auditory mechanism. What is more important is that occupational hearing loss has the same effect histopathologically as trauma. Repeated exposure to noise in either industry or the environment results in permanent loss of hair cell tissue. The hair cells are themselves tissues of the central nervous system, and since central nervous system tissue does not have the property of regeneration, as do most of the other tissues of the body, such a loss is irreversible. For an excellent description of the progression of the degeneration within the organ of Corti as a result of noise trauma, the reader is referred to Bohne (1976), Spoendlin (1976), and Durrant (1978).

We did a series of interviews with workers who had been employed in a lumber yard for as long as 15 years and who exhibited a lack of knowledge about industrial hearing loss. Analysis of the answers to our questions suggested that an unsophisticated interviewer questioning a worker who has been exposed to occupational noise for a considerable period of time may be led to a false impression about the effects of noise. That is, when queried about the effects of noise exposure, the response "it doesn't bother me anymore" was most often heard. There are two curious things about that response. First is the fact that it is not true, and second is that the workers believe that it *is* true. They believe it is true because they have incurred sufficient hearing impairment over time so that the noise of the lumber yard does not seem very loud to them. However, loudness is not the relevant issue. The relevant problem is the effect of excessive sound pressure reaching the basilar membrane, irrespective of the listener's perception of the loudness. The hearing impairment is caused by sound pressure indirectly "beating" on the hair cells through the excessive force of the movement of endolymph and perilymph in the cochlea. If some of the hair cells are destroyed, then the apparent loudness is diminished. The sound pressure, however, has not been diminished; unfortunately its effect continues. Due to the loss of loudness, however, the worker is not fully aware of the effect the noise is having on his remaining hearing.

Exposure to occupational noise usually tends to result, initially, in a *temporary* threshold shift (TTS). That is, after a work day, the employee knows there is a hearing loss; however, the hearing is better the following morning. A common fallacy among workers is that recovery from a temporary threshold shift is always complete and total. It is true that there is a considerable amount of auditory fatigue which results in a temporary hearing loss for which the worker often does, initially, completely recover. Eventually, however, the price is paid and permanent hearing loss occurs. It is as though someone borrowed a dollar overnight and repaid only 99¢ the next day. The loss of 1¢ would cause very little suffering. However, if the procedure continued . . . imagine the end of the 100th day. The analogy holds for occupational hearing loss. That is, the amount of hearing loss which occurs from day to day may be negligible, but it does accumulate every day, and eventually there is a *permanent* threshold shift (PTS).

Most workers exposed to excessive noise will suffer a TTS, but some will have greater permanent threshold shifts than others. While there is some direct correlation between the amount of temporary threshold shift and the amount of permanent threshold shift *(Jerger and Carhart, 1956),* there is no clear evidence or rationale to explain why some people are more susceptible than others to a permanent noise-induced hearing loss. There seems to be no effective means of predicting who the most susceptible persons might be so that they can be offered extra protection from occupational noise *(Burns, 1969; Kryter, 1970)*.

MEDICAL CONSIDERATIONS

There is no specific medical treatment for noise-induced hearing loss *per se*. Nevertheless, the disorder is a prime illustration of how the medical community, in this case usually through otology, can play a significant role in the prevention (rather than the treatment) of a physical disability. For example, the Research Center of the Subcommittee on Noise in Industry* surveyed large companies and published noise data about them *(Glorig, Ward, and Nixon, 1961)*. A direct result of that work was a series of published guidelines for industry and government which have formed the basis for some of our current anti-noise regulations. These may be seen in figure 8-2, and are discussed in detail later in this chapter.

Another major contribution by the medical profession is a set of criteria which have been developed by the American Academy of Otolaryngology and the American Council of Otolaryngology (1979). In an effort to place industrial hearing screening programs in a proper sequence of events which includes prevention, monitoring, and treatment, a series of guidelines is offered to industrial hearing screening technicians so that they will know when to refer employees with apparent industrially caused hearing losses to specialists. According to the new guidelines, workers whose audiograms show a change of more than 15dB at 500, 1000, or 2000Hz, more than 20dB at 3000Hz, and more than 30dB at 4000 or 6000Hz, should be referred to an ear specialist for investigation of a probable hearing problem. When comparing previous or baseline audiograms, the elapsed time between testing should be no more than two years.

Other criteria which would indicate the need for referral to a specialist include: average hearing level greater than 30dB at 500, 1000, 2000, and 3000Hz; a single frequency loss greater than 55dB at 3000Hz, or greater than 30dB at 500, 1000, or 2000Hz; a difference in average hearing level between the better and poorer ear of more than 15dB at 500, 1000, and 2000Hz, or more than 30dB at 3000, 4000, and 6000Hz; and unusual hearing loss curves or inconsistent responses.

All testing should be performed by a properly trained and certified industrial hearing screening technician utilizing equipment which meets ANSI Standard S3.6-1969. Further, all testing should be done in a proper environment and, if a problem is confirmed, the worker should be referred to

---

*The members of this subcommittee of the Committee on the Conservation of Hearing of the American Academy of Ophthalmology and Otolaryngology were otologists, psychologists, audiologists, and statisticians. The Director of the Research Center was an otologist.

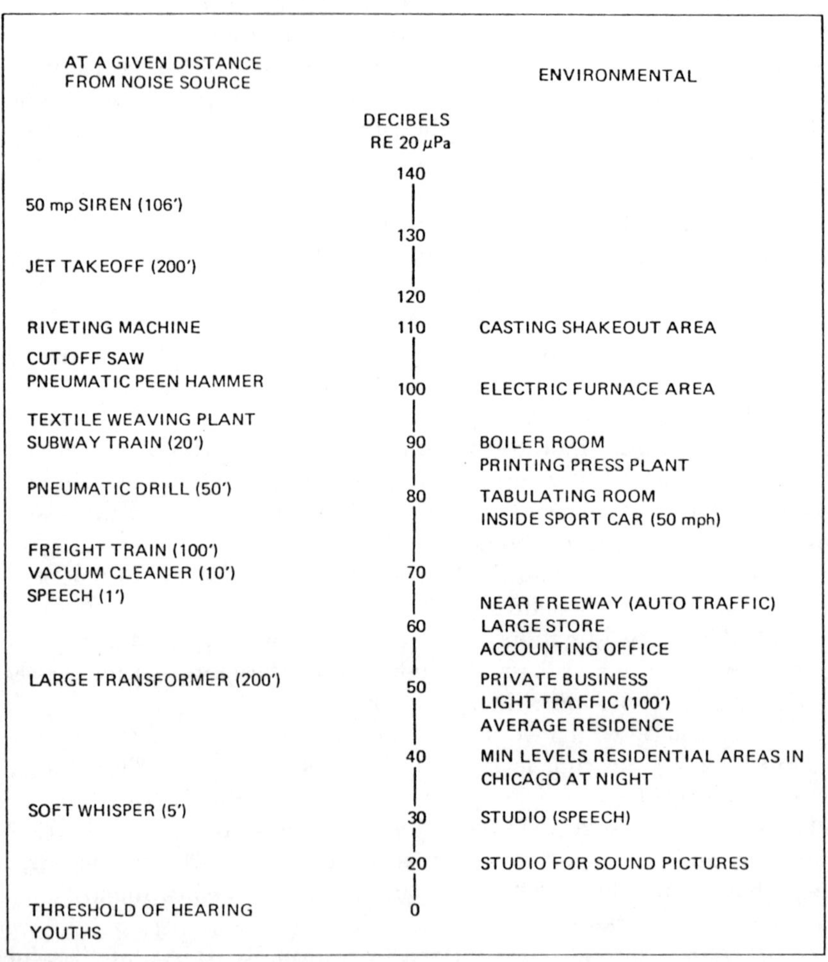

Figure 8-2. A-weighted sound levels from familiar sources. *(Reprinted with permission of Peterson and Gross, 1972.)*

an otolaryngologist for evaluation.

In addition to the items on the ACO guidelines, audiometric screening technicians will also refer directly to an otologist if any of the following symptoms are present, regardless of the employee's status on the hearing screening test:

1. Active drainage from the ear within the previous 90 days,
2. Sudden or rapidly progressive hearing loss,
3. Acute or chronic dizziness, or tinnitus,
4. Unilateral hearing loss of sudden or recent onset,
5. Significant air-bone gap,
6. Visible evidence of cerumen accumulation or a foreign body in the ear canal.

There is one final comment regarding medical care for the patient with a noise-induced hearing loss which must be considered. Many of these patients may demonstrate tinnitus, recruitment, and even vertigo. Medical treatment for those symptoms will usually provide relief for the patient, even if only until he/she mistakenly reenters the noisy work environment. The physician's counsel and advice is also certainly critical, especially where job change or reorientation becomes a forced choice for the worker. It is important that the audiologist not underestimate the role of the medical profession in dealing with the patient with a noise-induced hearing loss.

AUDIOLOGICAL CONSIDERATIONS

Hearing loss resulting from exposure to noise is not really a new problem. Pliny the Elder, who lived from about the year 23 to about 79, described a village near one of the cataracts of the Nile in which artisans (probably coppersmiths) became deafened as they plied their trade. No doubt gunpowder, modern warfare, the Industrial Revolution, and the machine age have thrust the problem into modern society's attention. Audiology as a profession can trace its origins to the effects of noise and its interference with communication. Thus, it is not surprising that it is the audiologist who plays the major role in the diagnosis of the problem, its prevention, and its treatment.

AUDIOLOGICAL DIAGNOSIS

Industrial noises tend to contain little low frequency energy relative to the amount of middle and high frequency energy. Consequently, when noise-induced hearing loss does occur, in the main it is restricted to the high frequencies, typically one-half to one octave above the frequency of the exposure noise. The handicapping effects of noise-induced hearing loss vary with the level and/or duration of exposure, susceptibility of the individual, and the previous amount of permanent hearing loss. Some individuals exposed to large doses of noise suffer little trauma at all. If a worker is susceptible to the effects of noise and then is removed from further noise exposure, there is usually no additional hearing impairment. Those who have been exposed to high levels of industrial noise for many years, and some of those who have been exposed to extreme noise for shorter periods, may have hearing losses sufficiently severe to significantly interfere with their ability to communicate. Specifically, the critical factor is the audiometric contour. That is, interference with communication depends upon the frequency regions in which the hearing impairment is significant. Experience has shown, in fact, that industrial hearing losses tend to occur most significantly around 4000Hz or at least in the octave between 3000 and 6000Hz. Also, since industrial noises do not usually occur at very high frequencies, and since the amount of displacement of the basilar membrane at its base is not particularly great, the typical audiometric contour of a noise-induced hearing loss will show more severe impairment at around 4000Hz than at either 2000Hz or 8000Hz (figure 8-3). One thing which audiometrically distinguishes noise-induced hearing loss from other sensory losses is the characteristic notch in the air conduction audiogram at 4000Hz*. This notch might be quite narrow and deep, or it may be broad, depending upon the spectrum of the noise producing the loss and the amount of time the ear has been exposed to that noise. Further, noise-induced hearing impairments occur in the company of other things — such as diseases or age — which also affect our hearing. Audiometrically, then, an audiogram such as the one shown in figure 8-3 may have quite a marked dip, even as great as 40dB or 50dB, in the affected frequency range, and some other low or high frequency components related to the other pathology.

As one might expect, the severe and restricted threshold shift seen in noise-induced hearing loss can have quite a marked effect on speech discrimination, even in ears where the speech reception threshold is nearly normal. This is because there is normal or nearly normal hearing for most frequencies, and the ability to receive speech is only mildly affected compared to the impairment of the ability to understand speech. Most of the information of speech is carried by consonants, and they are characterized by high frequency information *(Gerber, 1974)*. The information pertinent to sorting one phoneme from another may be lost in the presence of a noise-induced hearing loss. Thus, employees who work in noisy situations do, in fact, have more difficulty communicating than even they appreciate. Not only because of the noise, however, but also because of an ever increasing reduction in their own auditory acuity.

The site of lesion for a noise-induced hearing loss is the cochlea. Therefore, results of special audiometric tests will often indicate recruitment and, as already indicated, reduced speech discrimination. By contrast, results of tests of the central auditory system are usually normal as are tests of cortical function. The audiometric configuration, the case history, and the difficulty in communication usually make an audiological diagnosis of noise-induced hearing loss relatively straight forward.

Rehabilitation involves making maximum use of residual hearing (auditory training) and the use of clues in the environment to assist with

---

*Remember: Carhart's Notch, indicative of otosclerosis, appears at 2000Hz and only in the bone conduction audiogram.

PURE TONE AUDIOGRAM

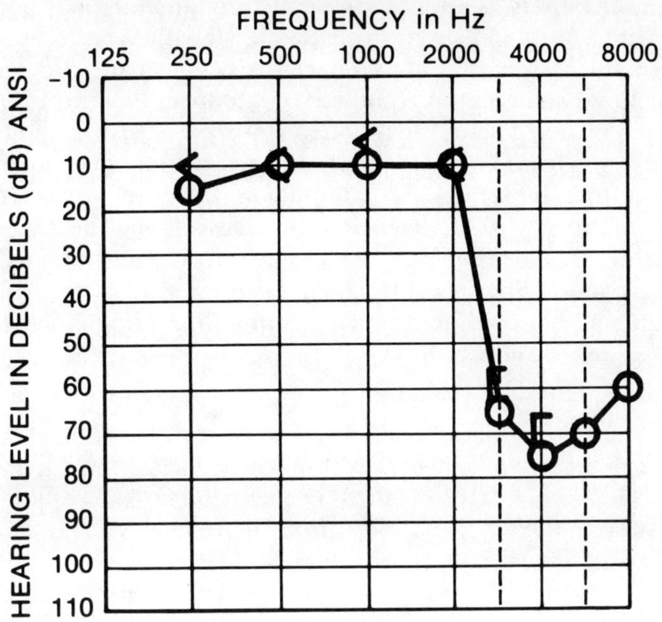

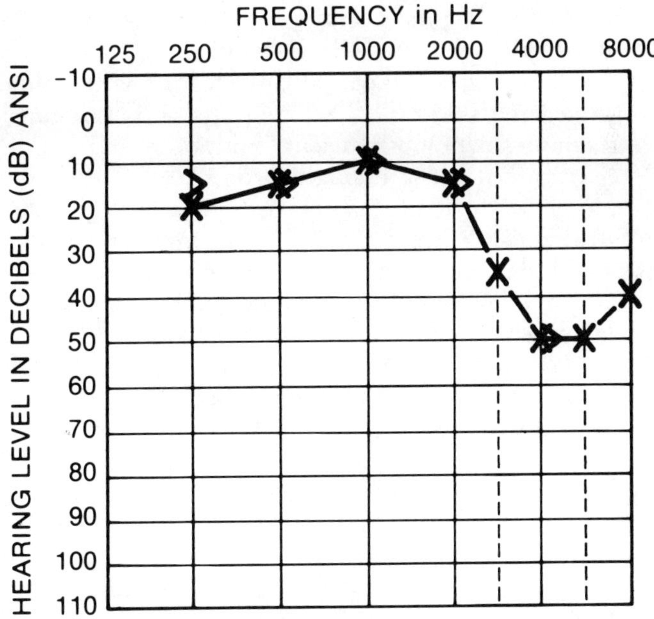

Figure 8-3. Audiogram displaying a noise-induced hearing loss.

understanding speech. Speech reading training is usually very helpful as well.

If the hearing loss is severe enough to merit use of a hearing aid, the same considerations as apply to the patient with ototoxicity apply to the patient with a noise-induced hearing loss. That is, the hearing aid should be chosen on the basis of response characteristics which are frequency shaped for the contour of the loss and compressed so as to prevent excessive loudness at high intensities. These patients often require extensive counseling in the proper use of a hearing aid and a significant amount of encouragement as they adjust to it. Incidental background noise often seems to accentuate the patient's tinnitus, while, if the patient has relatively good hearing in the low frequencies, the hearing aid itself may cause some discomfort. The audiologist must be particularly sensitive to the patient's work environment and social and personal needs during counseling. The challenge is one of the biggest for the clinician.

PREVENTION

REGULATIONS. Noise-induced hearing losses can and *must* be prevented. In the United States three federally funded agencies, the Environmental Protection Agency (EPA), the Occupational Safety and Health Administration (OSHA), and the military, have imposed regulations upon the makers of industrial, occupational, and/or community noise. In the years just prior to the introduction of the regulations, the number of people reporting industry related hearing losses was increasing rapidly, as was the severity of the losses being reported. The Federal agencies have the authority, usually employed with insufficient frequency or force, to prevent employers from subjecting their employees to too much noise. To be sure, OSHA has fined and even closed the plants of individual manufacturers.

The military has expressed particular concern over this situation, but has demonstrated the sincerity of its concerns with varying degrees of success. For example, in the most extensive study of its kind ever undertaken, Gerber (1965) examined 82,000 audiograms on 59,000 different military and civilian employees of the United States Air Force and found that it was not possible to distinguish between those who claimed to wear ear protection and those who did not. Certainly, one might conclude from the investigation that, even though the Air Force exposes more people to more noise than anyone else and is very much aware of government regulations, it does not thoroughly enforce its own regulations about the use of ear protection. Such a conclusion is sad indeed, especially because occupational noise control is easy to affect and it is inexcusable to fail to employ it.

Table 8-1 displays the OSHA standards for hazardous noise exposure, the damage risk criteria. It is interesting and unfortunate to note that they permit rather extreme levels of noise exposure. Regulations allow for a trade-off between sound intensity and the duration of a continuous exposure. That is, they permit exposure to high intensity noises only for brief periods of time, as opposed to a longer exposure to lower intensity sounds. The more intense the noise, the briefer the exposure must be.

158

Duration per day, hours	Sound level dBA slow response
8	90
6	92
4	95
3	97
2	100
1½	102
1	105
½	110
¼ or less	115

Table 8-1. Permissible noise exposures.

NOISE CONTROL. Perhaps the most important role the audiologist plays in noise-induced hearing loss is in prevention. In fact, the role is so great and so critical that an entire branch of the field called Industrial Audiology has developed. The audiologist's effort is directed toward what is called an Industrial Hearing Conservation Program. The program has five basic components:

1. Noise measurement and identification of those work areas where the sound level is in excess of regulations and hazardous to hearing.
2. Development of a reliable system for monitoring employee exposure to noise in terms of both time and the intensity of the signals.
3. Determination of the hearing of employees before they begin employment or baseline audiograms for those employees already working.
4. Engineering programs to eliminate noise in excessive noise areas.
5. Provide ear protection for employees and train them in its use.

1. Noise measurement and identification of high risk work areas. The ear is one of the best measuring devices for detecting excessive noise. Unfortunately, one must endanger the ear if it is to be used as a measuring system. Furthermore, "excessive noise" is really a subjective term. What may be an important sound to one man may be unpleasant and excessive to the next; symphonies and tractors both make beautiful music to some listeners and a racket to others. Finally, the frequency components of the signal, which affect the pleasantness or unpleasantness of the signal, are not as important as the intensity characteristics. Intensity can be objectively measured on a device called a sound level meter. Containing a microphone to detect sound and to convert it into an electrical signal, an amplifier to boost the electrical energy to the point where it can drive a meter, and a meter to reflect signal intensity, the sound level meter can provide a precise measure of the pressure of the signal. Most sound level meters have built in weighting networks, labeled A, B, and C (figure 8-4), which are utilized to change the responsivity of the meter to low frequency noise and thus, to view the noise in a manner similar to the human ear. Furthermore, intensity

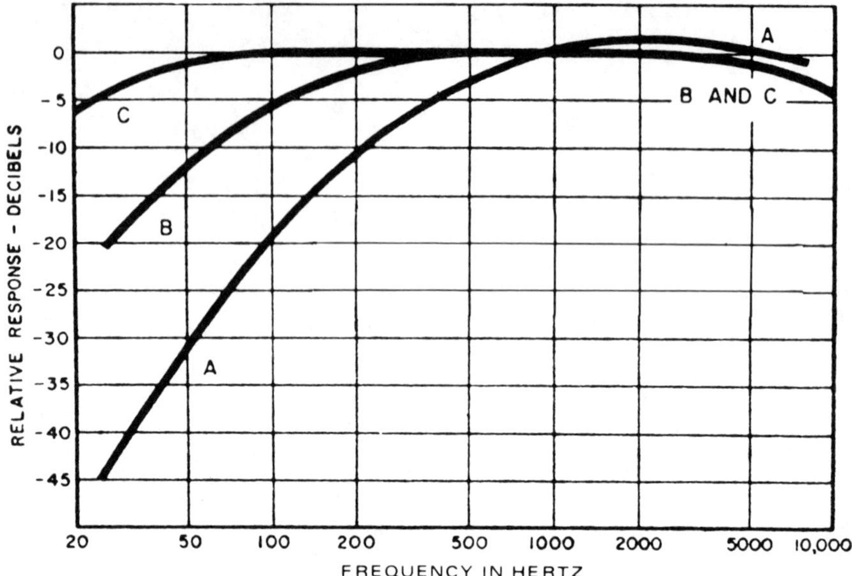

Figure 8-4. The A, B, and C weighting characteristics for sound level meters.

measures in specific frequency bands may also be examined if an octave band filter is attached to the meter. Suffice it to say, with a good sound level meter and a number of appropriate attachments, noise levels can be measured and high risk work areas can be easily identified. Industrial audiologists, engineers, architects, acousticians, health and safety officers, and many others can perform these measures accurately and rapidly.

2. Monitoring employees' exposure to noise. Once high risk areas have been identified, a noise control program would determine the schedule of each employee within the area and set up procedures to ensure that time and intensity exposures were reduced to non-hazardous levels and/or that protection was provided. There are a number of commercial devices available to assist in the monitoring program (e.g., Dosimeter). Enforcement procedures must be an integral part of the program.

3. Pre-employment audiograms. All new employees should be screened before starting work and monitored regularly thereafter. Employees who have been with a company for a number of years will also require audiometric tests. However, the program should be structured in such a way as to allow for testing only after a rest from noise exposure. This often means testing before work begins in the morning. Records need to be kept on all employees. When hearing changes from one examination to the next, the employee needs to be seen for in-depth audiological and otological evaluation.

4. Engineering programs to eliminate noise. In a hypothetical program of noise control, the highest priority is to stop making the noise, or to abate it at

160

its source. While this is obvious, it is not always possible, particularly in most industrial situations. If it is necessary to accept a certain amount of noise as a risk normally attendant upon the benefits of an industrial society, the problem is then to protect the workers in the environment.

If the noise cannot be eliminated, the second level priority would be to make less noise. This is not as improbable a solution as it may seem at first glance. For example, some manufacturing processes can be done electrically rather than pneumatically. Lower speed machines can be utilized. The result is a concommittant reduction in the noise which is generated.

The third priority in a noise control program would be to separate workers from the noise either by putting the noise source in some kind of a box or by having the workers perform the job remotely. Manufacturing equipment which is noise producing can be enclosed in containers made of absorbing material. They can be installed in such a way as to permit the worker to operate the machine while outside the enclosure. In addition to, or instead of, covering the noise, it may be possible for the worker to be located away from the source of the noise. This is routinely done in other hazardous occupations; for example, workers who handle nuclear material are completely removed from exposure.

5. Ear protection for employees. The least desirable alternative in a program designed to prevent noise induced hearing loss is personal ear protection; that is, to require the worker to protect himself with ear muffs or ear plugs. Those devices are effective, but less so than making less noise in the first place. Certain kinds of occupations, of course, do demand that form of protection. For example, ground crews at airports are pretty well limited to the use of ear muffs to attenuate aircraft noise as the mobility of both the workers and the noise source dictates that a portable, lightweight method is required. In most industrial settings, however, one of the other alternatives of noise control is usually a better choice. That is true because many workers resist wearing ear plugs, claiming that it is uncomfortable or not "manly" or that it is important that they be able to communicate with their fellow workers. There is the fear that the wearing of ear plugs will prevent workers from hearing their comrades. That fear is falsely based. The wearing of sun glasses offers a good explanatory analogy. It is well known and accepted that it is easier to see objects in bright light while wearing sun glasses because the glasses filter out certain light rays which interfere with vision. The same is true for the ability to communicate in noise. That is, certain sounds are filtered out by the wearing of ear plugs and it is actually easier to communicate in the presence of most noise. It is ironic that most industrial workers, if asked to stare at the sun for some period of time, would insist, and justifiably so, that they could not for fear of hurting their eyes. However, the effect on vision is completely analogous to the effect on audition incurred by having the ears continually exposed to high level noise. Noise-induced hearing loss is cumulative and irreparable and, more importantly, in most cases it is unnecessary. The audiologist's responsibility in public education, particularly with workers in noisy industries, is self-evident. One area of education is to teach that noise exposure does not produce immunity to additional noise-induced hearing loss.

COMMUNITY NOISE.Community noise is also a major problem, be it at home or out on the street. For example, one aspect of noise that some people consider acceptable is in the use of certain kitchen appliances. The electric can opener, mixer, garbage disposal, dishwasher, and/or blender, often do a much better job of making noise than of doing their assigned tasks. The Environmental Protection Agency, for some time, has been looking into home appliances as a source of noise and, therefore, as a potential source of noise-induced hearing impairment. There is now an EPA regulation on that subject which provides manufacturers with specific controls. However, that does little for what happens in the home.

Surveys of general community noise levels reveal some interesting data. Apparently, listeners are bothered more by barking dogs than by motorcycles. Noisy vehicles, among them motorcycles, defy the basic laws of physics: specifically, the law of the conservation of energy. In the case of motor vehicles, fuel is being converted into motive force. A certain amount of noise is required to do this. Any noise beyond that certain amount is gasoline converted into noise and not into speed. This is obviously wasteful energy, not to mention wasteful of one's patience and temper. Quiet motorcycles go as fast as noisy ones.

Sometimes, however, economics really overrides common sense. Farmers purchase tractors by the number of horsepower. That is, the higher the horsepower, the higher the price tag. Mufflers which reduce noise levels also reduce effective horsepower. Many farmers, therefore, will purchase a smaller tractor than required and remove the muffler, thus beefing up the power of the unit and defeating noise control regulations. There are other similar behavior patterns in other industries.

Some municipal agencies, such as the City of Boulder, Colorado, and Santa Clara County in California, have imposed community noise regulations. The states of California and Connecticut have highway safety noise regulations. However, the few scattered reports are not encouraging, suggesting that the regulations are not well enforced. Law enforcement agencies claim that they have neither the time nor the personnel to pursue violators of noise ordinances, which are generally considered nuisance ordinances and not health ordinances. The police maintain that there is simply not enough public outcry to merit the financial and time commitment necessary for the enforcement of these regulations.

There are many, many considerations when discussing community noise controls, all of which are relevant to the daily living and good health of our citizens. Noise pervades our homes as well as our jobs, and often pervades our enjoyment of nature. It is still possible, at least in most parts of the world, to escape from air and water pollution but, even with camping in the mountains, noise cannot be avoided. Overflying commercial aircraft, chain saws, and off-the-road vehicles (notably snowmobiles) destroy quiet and hair cells. Even in those times and places when we think we can escape environmental pollution, it follows us everywhere. Virtually all of us are affected by excessive noise, and many of us are being impaired unnecessarily. That is unfortunate and unnecessary as prevention of noise-induced hearing loss is possible. The relevant technology exists.

CASE STUDY 8-1: NOISE EXPOSURE

S.M., age 47, was sent for an evaluation of his hearing status upon referral from Workmen's Compensation. According to the referral, there is a history of progressive sensory-neural hearing loss considered to be due to noise exposure. There is a long history of work-related noise exposure. Mr. M. also reported that he had been exposed to gunfire over the years, mostly associated with hunting on weekends.

The results of pure tone air conduction and bone conduction testing revealed essentially normal hearing sensitivity for the frequency range 250 to 1000Hz, above which there was a significant high frequency drop down to a maximum of 65dB at 4000Hz in the right ear, and 75dB at 4000Hz in the left ear. The high frequency drop in the left ear was more significant above 1000 Hz.

Speech reception thresholds were found to be approximately 10dB in each ear. Formal speech discrimination testing at 40dB SL revealed a score of 84% for the right ear, and only 52% for the left ear.

Electroacoustic impedance measurements for middle ear function showed essentially normal middle ear function bilaterally. Acoustic reflexes were elicited at levels consistent with pure tone findings. With stimulation of the left ear, probe right, there were no reflex responses at 2000 and 4000 Hz, again in agreement with pure tone findings.

Mr. M.'s bilateral sensory-neural hearing loss is typical of noise-induced hearing loss. However, considering his previous exposure to gunfire, it is felt that attributing the hearing loss solely to work-related noise exposure is somewhat questionable. It should be pointed out that the hearing loss is more significant in the left ear. Mr. M. is right handed, which makes the left ear more vulnerable to acoustic trauma caused by gunfire. Unfortunately, it is impossible to isolate the two proposed etiologies.

Case Study 8-1: Noise Exposure

PURE TONE AUDIOGRAM

RIGHT EAR

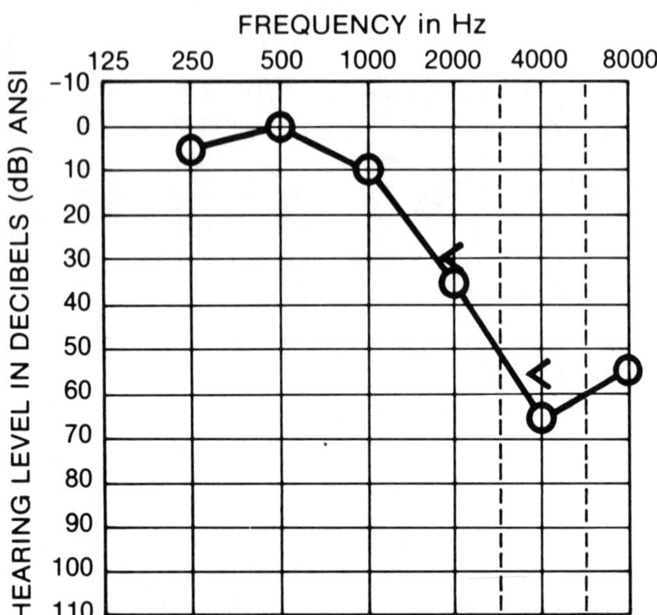

LEFT EAR

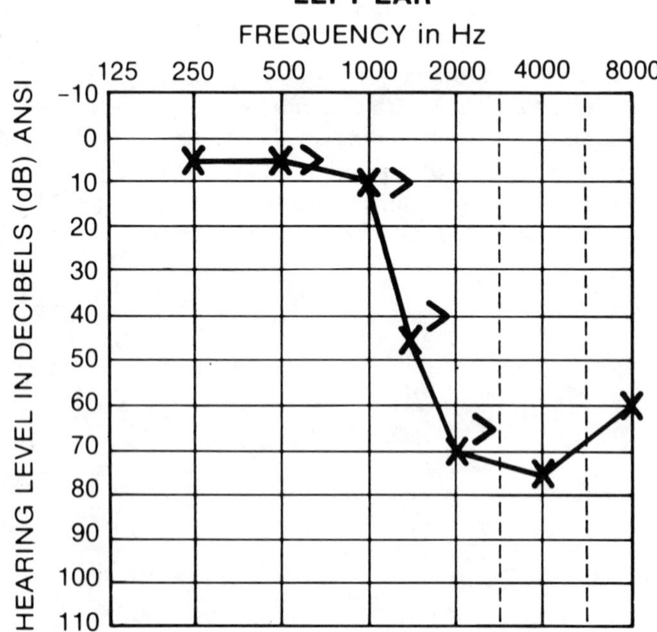

CASE STUDY 8-2:
NOISE INDUCED HEARING LOSS

Upon referral from Workmen's Compensation, Mr. H., age 58, was seen for a complete evaluation of his hearing status. He has worked for his present employer for approximately 20 years. Nine of those years he worked in the log room, which he reports had very high noise level. For the past 11 years, he has worked there as a tinsmith and wears ear protectors intermittently.

Pure tone air conduction and bone conduction testing revealed normal hearing bilaterally for the low frequencies, sloping to a moderate high frequency, sensory-neural loss in the left ear.

Speech discrimination testing at 40dB SL indicated that his ability to discriminate selected one syllable words was 88% bilaterally.

Electroacoustic impedance measurements of middle ear function revealed normal middle ear function, bilaterally.

References

AA00 Committee on Conservation of Hearing 1959. Guide for the evaluation of hearing impairment. *Trans. Am. Acad. Ophthalmol. Otolaryngol.* 63:236-238.

ANSI S3.6 1969, American National Standard Specifications for Audiometers.

Bohne, B.A. 1976. Mechanisms of noise damage in the inner ear. In *Effects of noise on hearing*, eds. D. Henderson, R.P. Hamernik, D.S. Dosanjh, and J. Mills. New York: Raven Press.

Burns, W. 1969. *Noise and man*. Philadelphia: J.B. Lippincott.

Dallos, P. 1964. Dynamics of the acoustic reflex: phenomenological aspects. *J. Acoust. Soc. Amer.* 36:2175-2183.

Durrant, J.D. 1978. Anatomical and physiologic correlates of the effects of noise on hearing. In *Noise and audiology*, ed. D. Lipscomb. Baltimore: University Park Press.

Eames, B.L., Hamernik, R., Henderson, D. and Feldman, A. 1975. The role of the middle ear in acoustic trauma from impulses. *Laryngoscope* 85:1582-1592.

Gerber, S.E. ed. 1974. *Introductory hearing science*. Philadelphia: W.B. Saunders Co.

Gerber, S.E. 1965. *Evaluation of air force hearing data*. Fullerton: Hughes Aircraft Co., Ground Systems Group.

Glorig, A., Ward, W.D. and Nixon, J. 1961. Damage risk criteria and noise induced hearing loss. *Arch. Otol.* 74:413-23.

Jerger, J.F., Carhart, R. 1956. Temporary threshold shift as an index of noise susceptibility. *J. Acoust. Soc. Amer.* 28:611-613.

Kryter, K.D. 1970. *The effects of noise on man*. New York: Academic Press.

Salomon, G. and Starr, A. 1963. Electromyography of middle ear muscles in man during motor activities. *Acta. Neurol. Scand.* 39:161.

Schuknecht, H.F. 1974. *Pathology of the ear*. Cambridge: Harvard University Press.

Spoendlin, H. 1976. Anatomical changes following various noise exposures. In *Effects of noise on hearing*, eds. D. Henderson, R. Hamernik, D.S. Dosanjh, and J. Mills. New York: Raven Press.

CHAPTER 9

Presbycusis

Presbycusis, a reduction of auditory sensitivity with age, is the only hearing disorder which occurs more often than those associated with noise exposure. The term "presby-" means elder. The word *presbycusis* literally means the acuity of the old. The longer we live, the more subject we are to it. Presbycusis is a normal concomitant of aging and, although it affects all of us, it will affect some of us at a younger age than others.

It is difficult to separate the effects of presbycusis from the effects of the noise of the society in which we live. In an attempt to do so, Rosen et al. (1962) studied a rather noiseless society, the Mabaans of the Sudan. It was the specific purpose of the investigation to determine the relative contribution of age to hearing loss in a society where noise would have been practically a non-contributory factor. Of course, many things affect the Mabaans which do not affect western society, and many things other than noise affect our civilization which do not affect them. Nevertheless, on the basis of audiometric test results, the study indicated that the Mabaans hear better than North Americans at any given age. An 80-year-old Mabaan hears much better than an 80-year-old New Yorker, but not as well as a 20-year-old Mabaan, suggesting that there is a loss of hearing with age. But, those of us who live in a so-called civilized society suffer hearing impairment along with the benefits of our civilization, and not surprisingly, not all of what we have called presbycusis is due to age alone. Whether or not our society hastens the onset of presbycusis or increases its effects through environmental noise, or whether the two have a cumulative result has not been determined. Conjecture suggests that either or both may be true, but only continued research will truly tell.

PATHOLOGY and ETIOLOGY

The histopathology of presbycusis is one of tissue change as well as tissue loss. Noise-induced and drug-induced hearing impairments involve destruction of hair cell and nerve cell tissue. In some cases of ototoxicity the tissue has disappeared entirely. Not so with presbycusis. Apparently, as a function of aging, there is a reduction of cell production and an accumulation of other materials such as cholesterol and lipids *(Naunton, 1973)*.

Schuknecht (1964) studied the histology of presbycusis and described four different types: 1) *sensory,* characterized by atrophy of the organ of Corti at its basal end; 2) *neural,* characterized by a reduction of the number of neurons in the auditory pathway; 3) *metabolic,* typified by atrophy of the stria vascularis which, of course, affects the contents of the cochlear duct; and 4) *mechanical,* identified by a calcification and stiffening of the basilar membrane and a consequent alteration of cochlear mechanics. The audiometric effects of the four types of changes are essentially the same — hearing loss in the higher frequencies. There may be slightly different audiogram contours associated with each type which may or may not affect rehabilitative efforts.

The specific etiology of presbycusis is unclear. The problem is further compounded in that there are several factors contributing to its progress and effects. If any specific element is causative, *per se,* the evidence has yet to be presented. Normal life involves a continuous process of cell death and replacement by new cells. This process slows down with time, eventually stopping and culminating in death. Aging of all tissue is characterized by the gradually increasing loss of cellular production. Surely, the origin of presbycusis must be found in such a normal process.

There is probably also a genetic component to presbycusis. When sensory hearing impairment occurs in a person in middle age in the absence of any evident cause, the paradoxical term "early presbycusis" is often invoked. Usually, this "early" presbycusis has occurred elsewhere in the family as well. Thus, it seems evident that some individuals seem to be more susceptible to the hearing loss which accompanies aging than others.

No doubt other factors play a major role in presbycusis. There are metabolic effects due to the individual's lifetime diet, environment, and habits. Further, arteriosclerosis due to dietary habits is a frequent adjunct of aging in western society. The consequent interference with blood supply throughout the body, particularly to the auditory nervous system, may play a significant role in presbycusis.

Rosen and his associates demonstrated that people who live in relatively quiet environments seem to display less presbycusis than the rest of us. Although Rosen did not explain why one aged Mabaan may hear better than another (a genetic factor?), he certainly did implicate noise as a contributing factor in our society.

168

MEDICAL CONSIDERATIONS

There is nothing which can be done medically or surgically to treat presbycusis *(Goodhill, 1979)*. It is the physician's role, of course, to assure that the presbycusic patient does not acquire ear disease which could result in additional handicap. What is perhaps more important for the physician is to properly counsel the patient concerning the disorder, contributing factors (e.g., noise exposure, poor diet, etc.), and what can be done about it. The patient must be taught that some presbycusis derives from the ailments which affect all of us as we get older, and therefore such things as the routine monitoring and regulation of blood pressure may help to alleviate it. The patient must be taught to avoid excessive noise exposure so as to preserve residual hearing. The patient should be made aware of the fact that, although there is no medical or surgical treatment for the problem, a competent audiologist can alleviate the communicative symptoms. It is important for the physician to know, and convey to the patient, that the elderly can benefit from hearing aids only with proper fitting and only if the aid is part of a total auditory rehabilitation program.

The elderly are also handicapped by visual impairments, primarily those which are called by a name similar to the auditory problem, presbyopia. As an individual ages, he doesn't hear as well as he did, he doesn't see as well as he did, he doesn't walk as well as he did, and many other of his bodily functions don't do as well as they did. The older the individual, the more handicapping the presbycusis and the visual deficits. Whatever else may be happening with the patient, it is also well known that decrease in these two critical sensory modes contributes markedly to aging. The physician must not only counsel his patient, he must provide ongoing ophthalmological and otological care (e.g., removal of cerumen) to ensure that the patient does not suffer from additional handicap. In short, the principal role of the physician becomes that of an educator, a counselor, and a provider of resource services and health care. Admittedly, some people are more adversely affected by aging and its handicaps than others. The physician's role is to treat those who need medical treatment and to guide the others to proper rehabilitative services. The elderly are not exempt from ear disease. Goodhill (1979) has cautioned that many disorders and diseases which produce hearing losses can be mistaken for presbycusis. Suggesting the term *pseudopresbycusis* as a useful concept for differential diagnosis of those diseases of the ear which cause hearing losses, particularly in the sixth, seventh, eighth, and ninth decades of life, he recommends careful consideration of genetic diseases, otomastoiditis, otosclerosis, ossicular fixations, temporal bone dystrophies, tumors, direct trauma, barotrauma, acoustic trauma, ototoxic drugs, syphilis, labyrinthine membrane ruptures, viremias, vascular lesions, and other causes before a specific diagnosis of presbycusis is applied. He added,

> Because of the potential multiple causality inherent in hearing losses, it is important to avoid a simplistic stance in considering

diagnostic and management aspects of hearing losses in older people. The label 'presbycusis' is tenable only when no other specific cause for older adult hearing loss . . . can be found. . .

AUDIOLOGICAL CONSIDERATIONS

Presbycusis differs from other hearing disorders in that its pathology is far more widespread. First of all, presbycusis has to be bilateral: after all, one ear is the same age as the other. The hearing loss may be truly sensory-neural because the auditory nerve in a given ear is the same age as the cochlea of that ear, but it may be sensory and not neural because the organ of Corti may be affected first.

Recruitment is usually less than in noise-induced or drug-induced losses. This is true, again, because the inner hair cells are the same age as the outer hair cells in the same ear, and change and/or destruction is equal for both sets of cells. Hearing impairments which accompany aging tend to develop from the high frequencies to the lower ones. Consequently, presbycusis is characterized by a high frequency hearing loss, and not by a low frequency loss. It is also characterized by a slowly progressive nature in which the high frequencies are more and more affected with time, and the lower frequencies become involved more gradually. Von Békésy (1956) calculated that auditory sensitivity is reduced 80Hz from the higher end of the frequency spectrum every six months of life. Audiometric tests at very high frequencies are not usually done; but, if they were done on children, the results would undoubtedly confirm von Békésy's notion.

Since presbycusis seems to first affect the high frequencies and then progress to the low frequencies, the description of a specific pure tone audiogram is difficult, as the different stages of the process will reflect differences in hearing. It has been reported *(Corso, 1963)* that there is an apparent increase in the rate of presbycusis around age 43 in American males and about age 48 in American women. That increased process of degeneration seems to slow down in the decade of the fifties. Figure 9-1 summarizes audiograms we expect in our society as a function of age for each decade of life. Clearly, the median audiograms of our society are affected by noise, diet, and life style, but they also reflect the changes which occur within the auditory system which are purely a function of age.

The audiogram accompanying presbycusis may be quite similar to one which accompanies noise-induced hearing loss, with the notable exception that, instead of a notch indicating a frequency-specific hearing loss, sensitivity continues to decrease as frequencies increase (figure 9-2). Since, however, most of us are subject to both age and noise, it is not always easy to make a distinction between the types of hearing losses. In fact, the distinction between presbycusis and noise-induced hearing losses sometimes can be made only on the basis of family and occupational history.

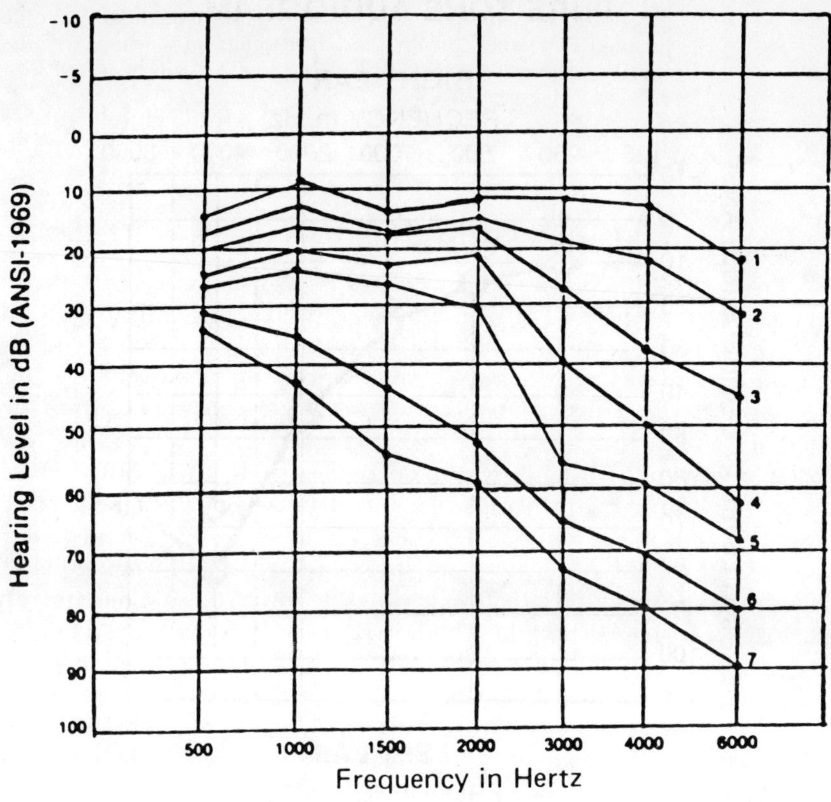

Figure 9-1. Median hearing levels per decade from age 10 (curve 1) through age 79 years (curve 7). *(These data are adapted from those reported by Glorig et al., 1957.)*

PURE TONE AUDIOGRAM

RIGHT EAR

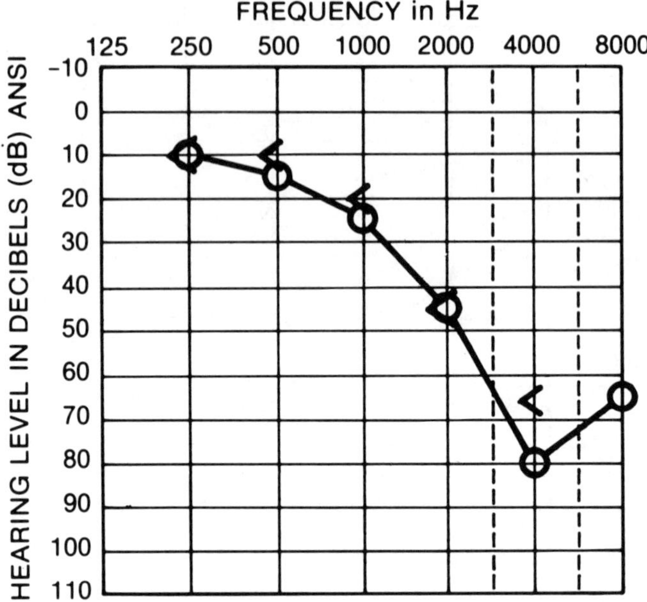

LEFT EAR

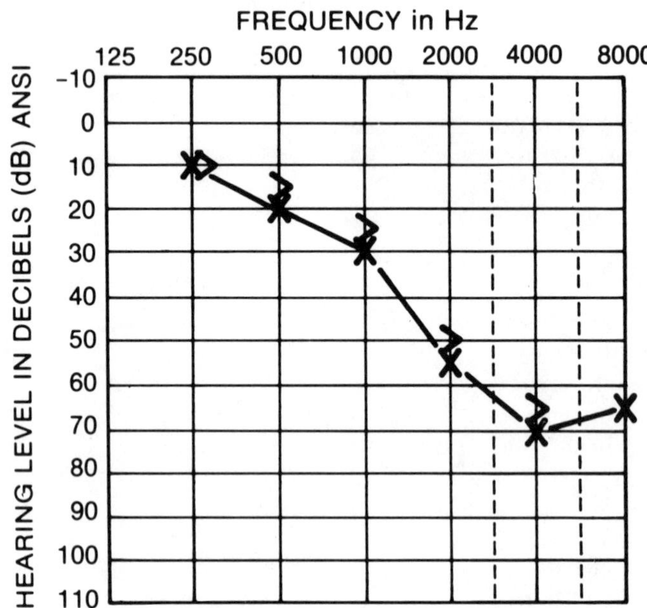

Figure 9-2. Audiogram of a gentleman in his eighties displaying clear evidence of presbycusis.

In the absence of a history of occupational noise exposure, the typical presbycusic audiogram will show an increased hearing loss, continuous with frequency, up to an extreme of 15dB per octave at advanced age.

Speech discrimination is generally worse than would be expected from the pure tone audiogram (figure 9-3). In some cases it is so markedly reduced as to be a significant problem for the patient. This phenomenon has been called *phonemic regression*. The reduction of speech discrimination seems to bear no relationship to mental capabilities, appears more frequently in persons over 50 years of age, and is limited to a yet undefined sub-group of persons suffering from presbycusis.

Site of lesion audiometric testing yields inconsistent results from patient to patient. Recruitment may occur, but it is rare in pure presbycusis and is usually less severe than in drug or noise-induced hearing losses. Tinnitus may occur with presbycusis, even though the origin of the disorder is not irritative.

Tests of higher auditory function will usually yield poorer results for the presbycusic than for the younger individual with the same audiogram. That result, coupled with the unusual speech discrimination problems seen with this pathology, suggest that the disorder involves higher auditory centers. It is difficult to determine how much of presbycusis is of cochlear origin — whether due to noise or age — and how much is the result of pathology in higher auditory centers.

The principal audiological considerations for presbycusis are rehabilitative. Old people can and do benefit from rehabilitative audiology. It is a fallacy, often perpetrated, that the aged can receive only limited benefit from amplification. Indeed, they can benefit dramatically from amplification, given that it is appropriate and correctly fitted, and that they are properly educated in the use of the hearing aid. It must be understood that a hearing aid is exactly what it says it is, an *aid*. Just as they should find vision improved with properly fitted lenses, they should find their hearing improved with properly fitted hearing aids and education. Unlike eye glasses, however, the hearing aid does not suddenly restore hearing to its former or normal function. Its purpose is to maximize use of residual hearing. Those suffering from presbycusis will rarely find hearing aids, alone, to be totally satisfying. But, that must not prevent a patient from using an amplification device.

Group rehabilitation sessions for the aged are very, very useful, and are usually seen by that clientele as a highly valuable experience. In addition to auditory training and speechreading sessions, as well as information regarding successful hearing aid usage, the sessions usually focus on daily living and communication. The social and counseling aspects of rehabilitation groups cannot be overstressed. It is important for the hearing-impaired aged person to encounter other hearing-impaired people and to communicate with them. It is inexcusable for there to be any failure to provide treatment for the aged that denies that inter-communication. The aged person should not be required or allowed to assign himself the

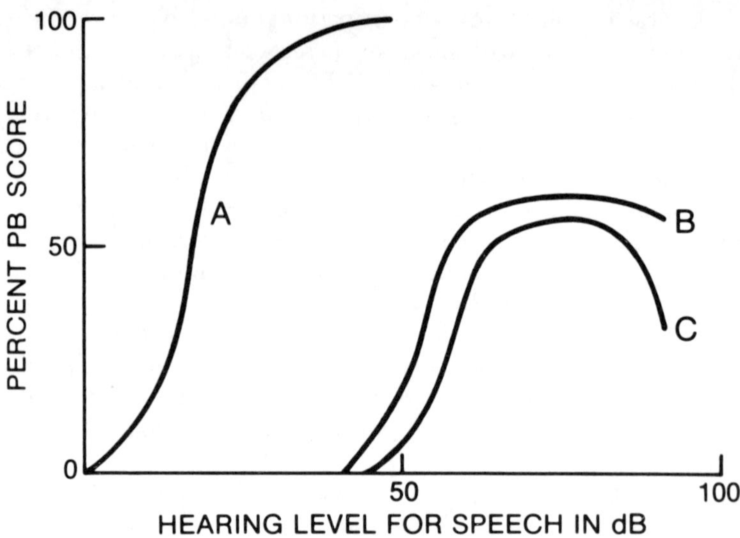

Figure 9-3. Curves showing how PB Max is displayed in a normal ear (A) and with a roll-over effect in sensory-neural impaired ears (B and C).

remainder of his life, alone, without communication with his peers. At a time when people are living longer lives, and those lives are productive much longer, the audiologist has an obligation to insure adequate auditory rehabilitative services for the presbycusic patient.

Presbycusis is the most common form of hearing loss. The longer we live, and the more of us who live longer, the more presbycusic patients there will be. It is encumbant upon each individual to do all the acoustical and environmental things possible to minimize presbycusis. It is especially important that each of us be acutely aware of the fact that the presbycusic patient can be helped. It is also important that the elderly person be made to understand that the hearing problem can be alleviated by amplification and education and rehabilitation.

CASE STUDY 9-1: PRESBYCUSIS

Mrs. B, age 57, was referred to the clinic by her daughter. Mrs. B reports that it is becoming difficult to hear conversations or to hear the telephone ringing. Both her father and brother acquired a hearing loss late in life and presently wear hearing aids.

Standard pure tone air and bone conduction tests were administered. Results reveal a sensory-neural loss in the high frequencies for both ears. The SRT and speech discrimination test results confirm the pure tone air and bone tests of her loss in the high frequencies which causes her inability to hear consonants. Also, an unaided discrimination test revealed difficulty understanding low conversation levels.

It was suggested to Mrs. B that she be evaluated for a hearing aid.

174

CASE STUDY 9-1: PRESBYCUSIS

PURE TONE AUDIOGRAM

RIGHT EAR

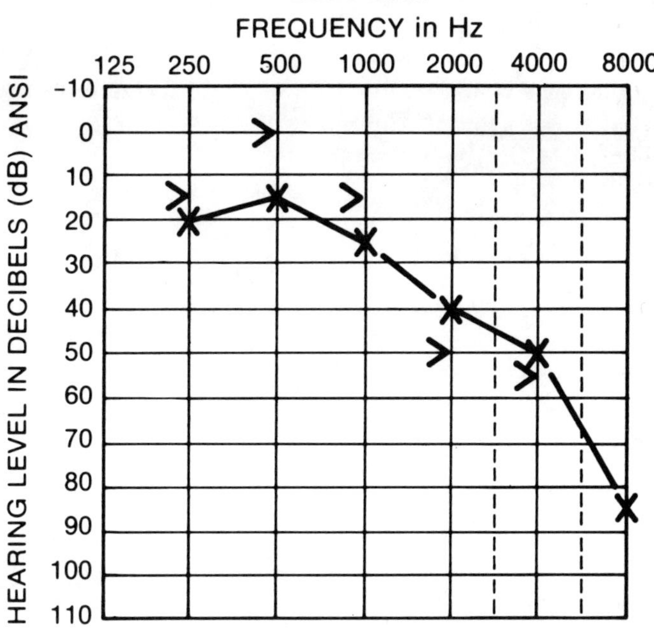

CASE STUDY 9-2: EARLY PRESBYCUSIS

Mrs. K, age 38, felt that she had trouble hearing normal conversation. She noted this problem especially when talking to members of her family. She reported a history of hearing problems among female members of her family.

Pure tone thresholds were normal for air and bone conduction except for slightly depressed air conduction thresholds of 25dB at 2000Hz and 30dB for 4000Hz. SRT and pure tone averages were in agreement. Word discrimination was excellent. SISI tests were negative and tone decay was absent except for mild tone decay for the left ear at 4000Hz. Impedance results revealed a normal tympanogram in the right ear, and an "A deep" tympanogram in the left ear. Stapedial reflexes were within normal limits.

It was recommended that Mrs. K see an otologist due to the abnormal tympanogram in the left ear. It was also suggested that she be seen annually for audiologic evaluation due to the presence of hearing difficulties in her family history, slightly depressed threshold in her left ear, and her present problem hearing her family. She may be showing early signs of presbycusis.

Case Study 9-2: Early Presbycusis

PURE TONE AUDIOGRAM

RIGHT EAR

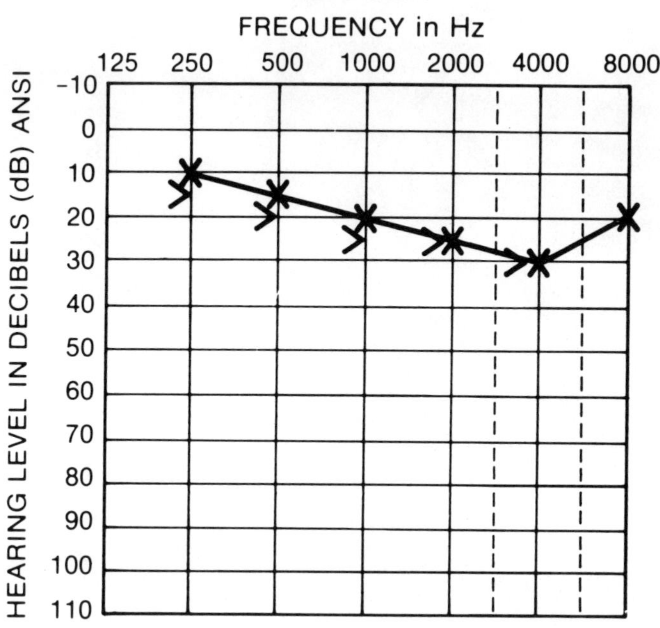

LEFT EAR

REFERENCES

Corso, J.F. 1963. Age and sex differences in pure-tone thresholds. *Arch. Otolaryngol.* 77:398-399.

Glorig, A., Wheeler, D., Quiggle, R., et al. 1957. 1954 Wisconsin State Fair hearing survey. *Am. Acad. Ophthalmol. Otolaryngol. Monograph.*

Goodhill, V. ed. 1979. *Ear diseases, deafness and dizziness.* New York: Harper & Row, Inc.

Hull, R.H. 1978. Assisting the elderly client. In *Handbook of Clinical Audiology,* ed., J. Katz. Baltimore: Williams & Wilkins Co.

Jerger, J. 1973. Audiological findings in aging. *Adv. Otorhinolaryngol.* 20:115-124.

Naunton, R.F. 1973. Presbycusis. In *Otolaryngology,* vol. 2, eds. M.M. Paparella and D.A. Shumrick. Philadelphia: W.B. Saunders Co.

Rosen, S., Bergman, M., Plester, D., et al. 1962. Presbycusis study of a relatively noise free population in the Sudan. *Ann. Otol. Rhinol. Laryngol.* 71:727-743.

Schuknecht, H. 1964. Further observations on the pathology of presbycusis. *Arch. Otolaryngol.* 80:369-382.

Von Békésy, G. 1956. Current status of theories of hearing. *Science* 123:779-783 (539-547).

PART 3

Neural

Hearing

Impairment

When discussing neural hearing impairment, the topic shifts to less clearly defined disorders, and thus to hearing problems which are not so easily diagnosed and/or treated. For the purpose of this text, neural hearing impairments are defined as those which have the site of pathology central to the cochlea. Included in that definition are those disorders historically called retrocochlear lesions, as well as those which have been called central lesions. A useful distinction is the one, drawn by Davis and Silverman (1978), which employs the following terms: 1) *anacusis*, deafness; 2) *hypoacusis*, loss of sensitivity; and 3) *dysacusis*, referring to all those auditory impairments which "are not simple losses of sensitivity of hearing." This section is concerned primarily with dysacusis. However, as Davis and Silverman stressed, a loss of sensitivity certainly can accompany dysacusis. Consequently, some of the things discussed in this section will be characterized by both dysacusis and hypoacusis and the differential diagnosis may be one of relative degree.

The causes of dysacusis may appear anywhere in the auditory nervous system; that is, the central nervous system itself, the brainstem, along the auditory nerve, or in the sensory end organ. More importantly, unlike hypoacusis, dysacusis cannot be relieved by the use of a hearing aid. In fact, as in the case with central lesions, there may not even appear to be a hearing loss present. The problem is not one of receiving the signals, rather, it is one of processing them.

REFERENCES

Davis, H. and Silverman, S.R. (1978), *Hearing and Deafness* 4th ed., New York: Holt Rinehart, and Winston.

CHAPTER 10

Disorders of the Auditory Nerve and Brainstem

Disorders of the auditory nervous system, other than those which are due to congenital dysplasia or malformation (e.g., a Michel Anomaly), are of three kinds: 1) tissue degeneration, 2) invasion by tumor, and 3) lues. Presbycusis is the primary disorder in which there is tissue change and marked degeneration within the cochlea and the auditory nerve, as well as the brain itself. As indicated, those changes are a part of the normal aging process. The reader is referred to chapter 9 for a discussion of that disorder, and to chapter 6 for a discussion of lues. The other significant disorder of the auditory nerve is called the acoustic tumor. Tumors bearing that descriptive title may appear anywhere along the VIIIth cranial nerve or within the brainstem.

PATHOLOGY and ETIOLOGY

Tumors which arise in the acoustic branch of the auditory nerve (figure 10-1) are almost always benign and are rarely seen before the third decade of life *(Weaver and Northern, 1976)*. The affix "-oma" refers to tumor; so, neuroma means a tumor of a nerve. Thus, when the tumor invades the region of the auditory nerve, it is usually called an auditory neuroma or neurinoma. To be even more narrowly accurate, if a tumor arises on the acoustic branch of that nerve, it is called an acoustic neuroma. Similarly, if it arises on the vestibular branch, it is more properly called a vestibular neuroma. Further, when the tumor actually arises from the Schwann cells of the myelinized nerve sheath, to be completely accurate, it should properly be called a schwannoma or a neurilemoma. Nevertheless, the most frequent term in the audiology literature is an "VIIIth Nerve Tumor," called so because of its involvement with that cranial nerve.

The etiology of acoustic nerve or brainstem tumors has been extremely

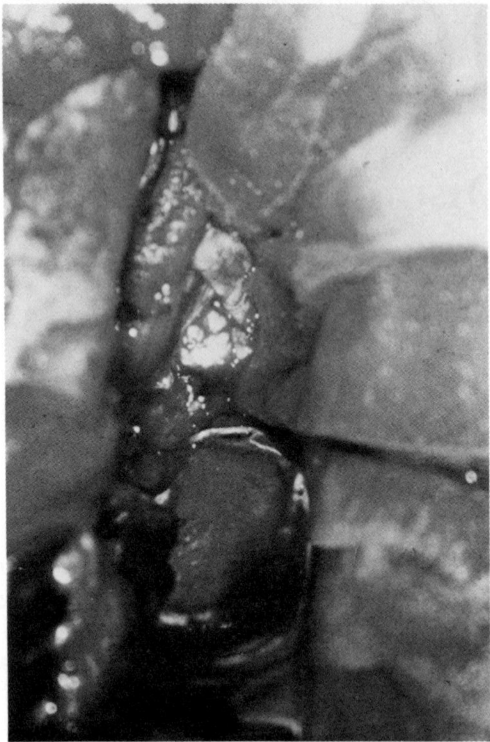

Figure 10-1. Acoustic nerve tumor in situ.

difficult to determine. In the main, they are neoplastic growths which are considered to be idiopathic; that is, the actual cause is unknown. Von Recklinghausen's Disease, characterized by multiple brain tumors, is known to run in families and often to have similar effects and symptoms to VIIIth nerve tumors. In fact, the two conditions are often confused. Further research is needed to determine if the origin of tumors of the VIIIth nerve is also familial.

Because VIIIth nerve tumors characteristically originate within the internal auditory meatus, one of the more reliable diagnostic signs of the presence of such a lesion is a radiologically apparent enlargement of that space. This is because, as the tumor grows, it may erode and expand the bony internal meatus. Sometimes, however, these tumors appear sufficiently medial to the internal auditory meatus so that an expansion does not occur, or at least does not occur to such an extent that it is apparent in an x-ray. In any event, since acoustic neuromas are benign, the problem is not that they invade and destroy the surrounding tissue, but rather that they displace it. A large tumor may lead to compression of the brainstem with the attendant risk of cardiac and respiratory complications.

A tumor of the VIIIth cranial nerve may invade or involve other nearby cranial nerves as well, particularly the VIIth or facial nerve. The Vth cranial nerve, the Trigeminal, may also be involved. The effect of invasion of the Vth and VIIth cranial nerves is a loss of sensation to the face and the eye, and, potentially, a loss of the motor functions of the muscles of the face. In fact, a frequent presenting complaint of VIIIth nerve tumor patients is that of a sense of numbness of the face. Hence, even though it is the auditory nerve which is involved, the chief complaint is often not an inability to hear.

Because the VIIth (facial) nerve courses along the internal auditory meatus, another common post-surgical problem occurs when that nerve is involved during surgery (figure 10-2). It is sometimes compressed by the expanding tumor — particularly those of the cerebello-pontine angle. As a result, during the surgery the nerve may be damaged or even sacrificed, and, thus, the patient may be left with some visible sign of the experience. Results are much better now than when MacKenzie (1965) reported that fewer than half of the 130 patients who had undergone surgery to remove VIIIth nerve tumors in his center were able to return to the way they had lived pre-operatively. Presumably, this was due more to damage to the facial nerve than to profound hearing impairment in one ear.

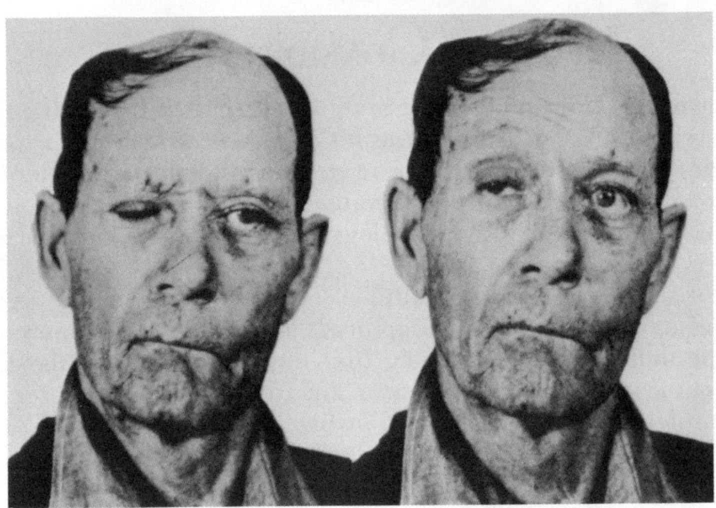

Figure 10-2. Hemifacial paralysis due to involvement of the seventh cranial (facial) nerve. (*Reproduced with permission of Year Book Medical Publishers, Inc.*)

Occasionally, tumors which are difficult to diagnose appear in the brainstem at levels superior to the VIIIth cranial nerve. Unfortunately, because of the current state of the art a patient with this type of lesion may occasionally go to his death with the tumor undiagnosed. As with the VIIIth nerve patients, the form of the disorder is that of a neuroma or neurilemoma.

The tumor may be situated at the level of the cochlear nucleus or anywhere above, with one of the most common sites being the inferior colliculus. As with most VIIIth nerve lesions, the etiology of the brainstem neuroma is unknown and, thus, it is usually called idiopathic.

Obviously, in spite of the fact that most of these tumors are benign in structure, there is always the danger that a large enough lesion may eventually lead to death. Or, if the tumor is recognized and surgical intervention is attempted, there is always the possibility of a post-surgical handicapping effect. Naturally, the larger the tumor, the greater the risk of a post-surgical deficit.

A tumor of the brainstem at a region higher than the level of the auditory nerve will usually result in handicapping effects not appreciably different from those of VIIIth nerve lesions. If the tumor has grown to an extensive size there may be hearing loss, facial nerve involvement, and respiratory or cardiac difficulty. Occasionally, during the course of the operation, the surgeon finds it necessary to destroy the cochlea as he removes the tumor. Obviously, such an action results in a total loss of hearing in the ear involved (figure 10-3). In some cases where the cochlea is preserved, there may be difficulty processing speech in the absence of any clear signs of hearing loss.

Medical Considerations

There are no ear problems, *per se*, which are specific to VIIIth nerve disorders. When the patient presents his complaint to a physician, because of dizziness or tinnitus, he may be referred to an otologist, a neurologist, and/or a neurosurgeon for further evaluation. Several otologists now limit their surgical practices to "neurotology," that is, surgery for these neural disorders of hearing.

The surgery to remove VIIIth nerve tumors is truly *neuro*surgery. A prerequisite to the actual procedure itself is the gathering of information from the audiologist about hearing, from the radiologist about the size and shape of the internal auditory meatus, and from the neurologist regarding the neurological signs suggestive of involvement of other cranial nerves or areas of the brain. All of the material is combined to provide information regarding location and estimated size of lesion. Once aware of the location, and having decided to operate, the surgeon must apply his skill. The actual surgical procedure itself is fairly straightforward. A piece of bone is removed from the skull, a section of the cerebellum is pushed aside so that the tumor may be visualized and cut away from its attachments to the auditory nerve. Sometimes this may be achieved only by severing the nerve and removing it. If the tumor is small (i.e., less than 3 cm. in diameter), it may be removed through the ear, rather than by drilling a hole in the skull. In such a case, though, part of the inner ear must be removed in order to gain access to the internal auditory meatus. That is the typical case in which the hearing must be sacrificed *(Pulec, 1973)*.

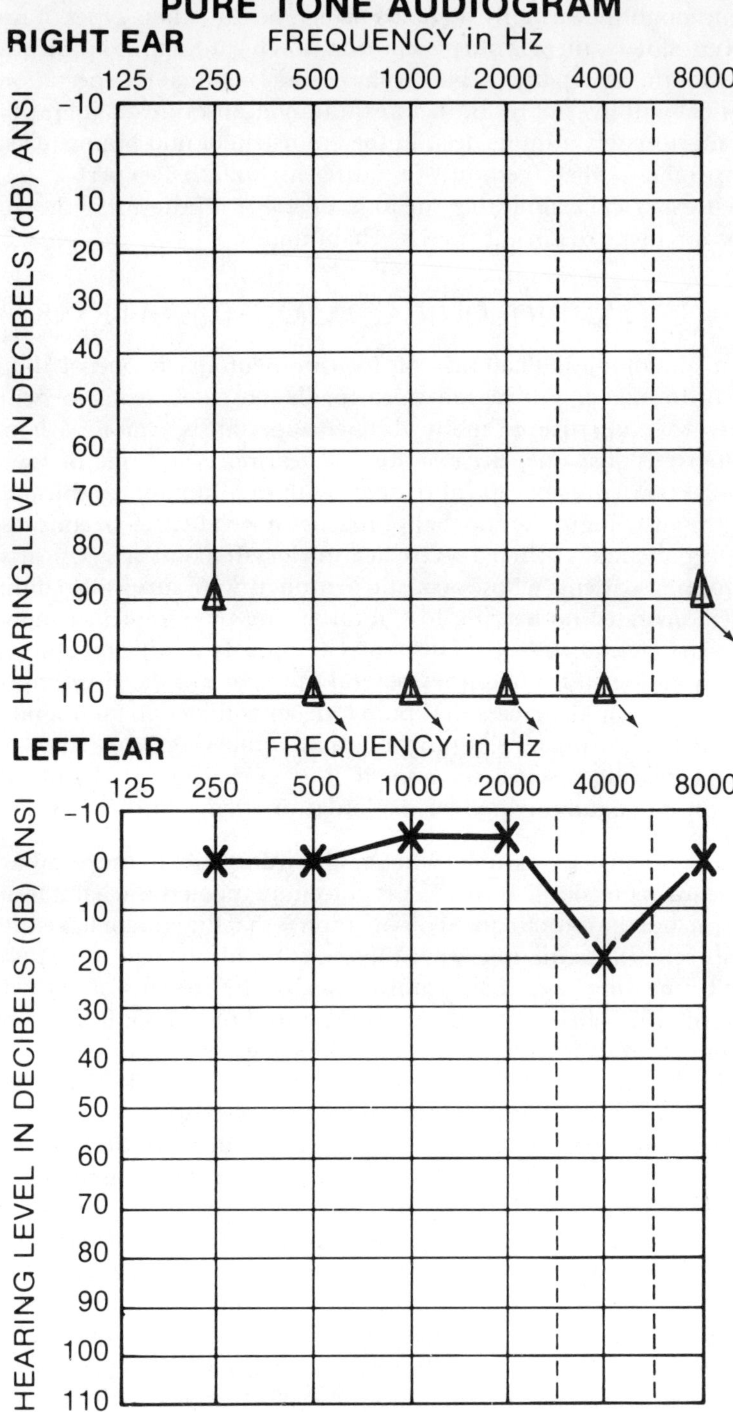

Figure 10-3. Dead right ear.

It is true that tumors occasionally stop growing as mysteriously as they start, although they usually do not. Further, because these types of tumors grow very slowly, there is often some question regarding the application of surgery for the aged patient. There may be some reasonable expectation that the patient will live out his life before the tumor causes any major problems.

Unfortunately, tumors deep in the brainstem or mid-brain are usually not operable. They certainly require all of the expertise of the oto/neurosurgical team if they are to be operable. The result of the surgery may be a patient requiring speech rehabilitation.

Audiological Considerations

An audiological diagnosis of acoustic neuroma is one of the most difficult to make. Furthermore, early diagnosis of acoustic neuroma requires the expertise of many different specialists, among whom the audiologist is just one. Because loss of hearing is not one of the most common complaints of typical patients with small tumors of the auditory nerve, the audiologist may not be approached for evaluation or consultation until the patient has suffered severe hearing loss. In point of fact, nearly half of a group of patients whose acoustic neuromas were surgically confirmed had demonstrated no hearing loss at all during pure tone air conduction audiometry *(Johnson, 1968)*. This is an enormously significant observation for the audiologist. It underlines, several times, one of the most important concepts to learn: the fact is that pure tone air conduction audiograms are not sufficient hearing tests. A pure tone audiogram is only one small part of the total hearing assessment; and, if it is normal in a patient who is complaining of auditory and/or vestibular problems, further tests must be done.

The patient often exhibits what has been described by the peculiar term "phonemic regression." It is difficult to accurately describe what is meant by that term, but the most frequent observation is that the patient has extremely poor speech discrimination, especially inexplicable in view of the results of the other hearing tests. For example, one of the patients of Weaver and Northern (1976) had a speech reception threshold of 35dB but a speech discrimination score of only 34%. Phonemic regression does occur in other pathologies, notably presbycusis (chapter 9), lues (chapter 7), and cerebral arteriosclerosis; so the investigator needs to be careful.

There are audiometric signs suggestive of neuroma, but they are easily confused with signs of Ménière's Disease, which were discussed earlier (chapter 6). These include vertigo, tinnitus, and hearing loss. Recruitment is less likely to occur with VIIIth nerve pathology than in patients with Ménière's Disease, but tinnitus is common even in the absence of hearing impairment. Among the five VIIIth nerve patients who were described by Weaver and Northern (1976), one presented with a complaint of tinnitus, and two others did not complain of hearing loss at all.

In a typical case, the audiologist should expect to find a patient complaining of a progressive hearing loss of gradual onset, perhaps extended over as long as one or two decades. The hearing impairment will usually be unilateral and further characterized by marked difficulty understanding speech in the involved ear. The patient may report tinnitus, numbness of the face, and sometimes a sense of fullness in the ear. The audiological considerations include performing all possible tests to eliminate from the differential diagnosis those things which may be confused with acoustic neuroma, such as brain disease, Ménière's Disease, cerebral arteriosclerosis, etc.

Recently, there have been studies of the electrical activity of the auditory brainstem as a potentially diagnostic discriminant of VIIIth nerve tumors. The use of the auditory brainstem response (ABR) in diagnosis has been described at length by Davis (1976) and Mendel (1977). Notable differences between the two ears may appear in the auditory brainstem response due to the presence of a tumor in one ear. In general, these take the form of relative latency shifts which are different between the two ears (figure 10-4). Thomsen, Terkildsen, and Osterhammel (1978) claimed that the "main indicator of retrocochlear versus cochlear disease" is this latency difference. Most of the research in this area is in a very early stage, and surgical confirmation of its accuracy is awaited.

Frequently, the operated patient is left with a "dead" ear, and thus audiological consultations must also be rehabilitative in nature. If the cochlea is destroyed as a necessary concommitant of the surgery, and there is no hearing at all on that side, the patient may find the unilateral loss significant. In the case report appended to this chapter, the patient is a police officer for whom the ability to localize sound was critical, certainly far more important than it is for most of us. The patient's auditory rehabilitation program consisted of two hours per week for over one year, during which time he relearned localization.

If the patient has no obvious loss of auditory sensitivity, what are some of the more subtle audiological considerations? A report by Bocca and Calearo (1963) revealed that patients with tumors of the brainstem suffer a disability of binaural fusion. To be sure, one does not appear at the otologist's office complaining of a difficulty with binaural fusion. How, then, is such a phenomenon discovered, and what does it mean to have a deficit in that function?

Binaural fusion is the normal process within the auditory nervous system which makes it possible for us to function in a reverberant world. Our ears are bombarded by multiple reflections of sound in any live acoustic space. A signal, speech or otherwise, generated in or into that space reflects off walls, floors, ceilings, furniture, other people, etc. The result is that, at any given moment, the acoustic waveform at one ear differs from the acoustic waveform at the other ear. Yet, we as individuals are never conscious of that difference. That is because of our skills at binaural fusion. The auditory nervous system, due in part to its bilateral representation, renders a single percept from the two acoustic events. If pathology exists, a test for binaural fusion may reveal it. The test is quite simple (see chapter 11).

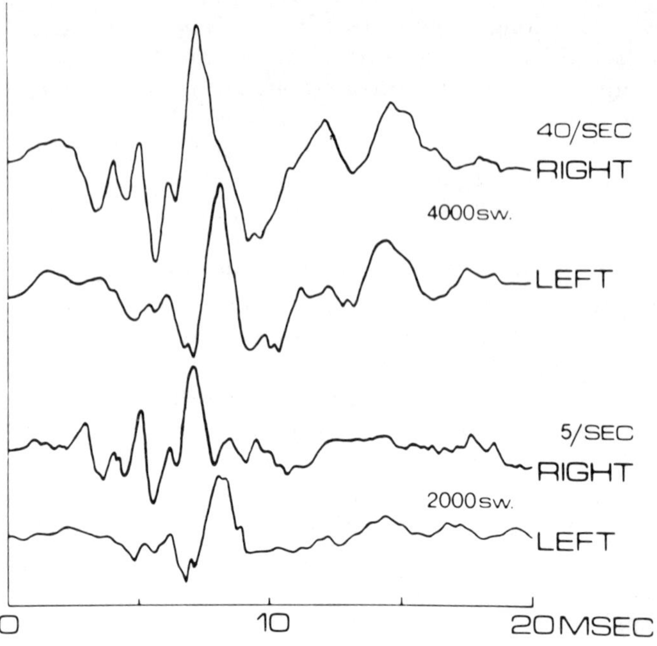

Figure 10-4. Electric response audiograms displaying the phenomenon of IT-5; that is, the two ears show different latencies of the fifth peak. This is clear at two click repetition rates. *(From J. Thomsen, K. Terkildsen, and P. Osterhammel, Auditory brainstem responses in patients with acoustic neuromas. Scandinavian Audiology 1, 7:179-183, 1978. Reproduced with permission of J. Thomsen.)*

If a recording of speech were played to a normal listener through earphones in such a way that all the information below a certain frequency was presented to one ear while all the information above that frequency was presented to the other ear, only one signal would be perceived. That is, the two entirely different signals would be heard as one and render 100% discrimination for speech processed in that way. One would not notice that one ear had differed from the other. Not so with the patient who has a lesion to the upper brainstem. If that patient were to listen to either one, but not both of the signals, the result would be a speech discrimination score consistent with the information received in only one ear. When the patient is required to respond to both ears with the signal filtered as described above, his speech discrimination score drops markedly. Probably due to the failure of binaural fusion, the two signals interfere with one another rather than add to each other.

The patient rarely complains of hearing problems, or for that matter, of vestibular problems. As a result, unless referred for specific advanced audiological tests with a referral indicating the suspected diagnosis, most audiological centers will not routinely administer binaural fusion procedures. As a result, a mid-brain or upper brainstem tumor may go undetected until it is too late. All suspect patients should receive a screening for binaural fusion at every audiological visit. The great extent and vast detail required of audiology in these kinds of cases have been discussed elsewhere (e.g., Katz, 1978).

In summary, then, it is appropriate to quote Davis (1978):

> We must expect that the effects of brainstem lesions will not be clearly predictable and will often be quite bizarre. This very feature may distinguish lesions of such a small, compact, complicated piece of nervous tissue in which so many neuro-physiological functions are carried out.

CASE STUDY 10-1:

ACOUSTIC NEUROMA

Mr. W., age 39, complained of having a hearing loss and tinnitus in his right ear for the past twenty years; however, in the last two or three years, hearing in his right ear worsened.

In the right ear, masked bone conduction thresholds were beyond the limits of the audiometer. When white noise masking was introduced contralaterally, SRT could not be obtained due to poor speech discrimination. Unmasked speech discrimination at 10dB SL was fair (70%); discrimination scores at 20, 30, 40, and 50dB SL were good. However, at 40dB SL with effective contralateral masking, the score was 28%. At 10dB SL with 0dB S/N the score was 20%; and at 10dB SL with -10dB S/N, the score was 12%. Threshold tone decay testing with masking showed 35dB of decay at 2000Hz and 30dB of decay at 4000Hz.

In the left ear, audiometric testing revealed hearing of pure tones to be within normal limits. SRT was consistent with pure tone audiogram. Speech discrimination was good.

Mr. W. was referred to his physician for further evaluation. Studies by Dr. P determined that Mr. W did indeed have an acoustic neuroma. It was surgically removed, but it was necessary to destroy the cochlea. Mr. W made a remarkable recovery from the surgery, had virtually no dizziness afterward, and was fitted with a CROS hearing aid. Auditory training was very effective, and Mr. W's localization ability approximates normal. He has returned to a successful career as a police officer.

CASE STUDY 10-1: ACOUSTIC NEUROMA

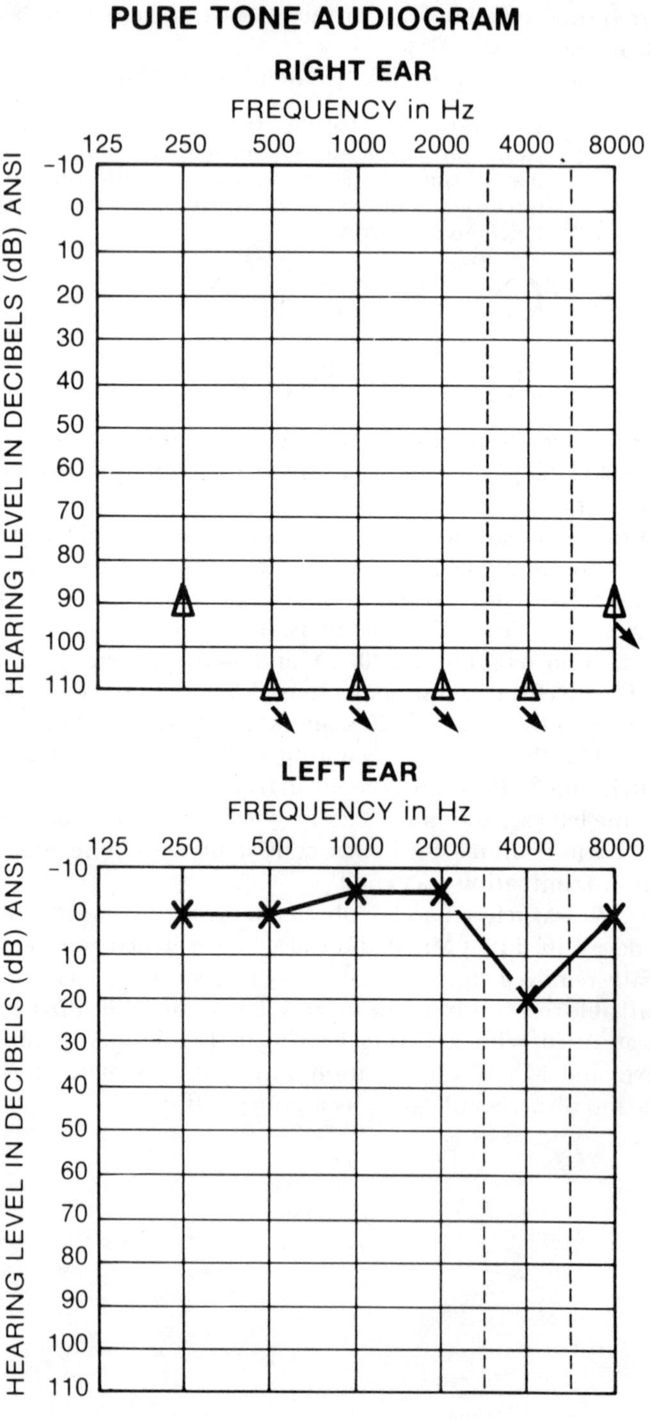

PURE TONE AUDIOGRAM

RIGHT EAR

LEFT EAR

REFERENCES

Bocca, E. and Calearo, C. 1963. Central hearing processes. In Modern developments in audiology, ed. J. Jerger. New York: Academic Press.

Davis, H. 1976. Principles of electric response audiometry. *Ann. Otol. Rhinol. Laryngol.* Suppl. 28, 85: No. 3, part 3.

Davis, H. 1978. Audiometry: other auditory tests. In *Hearing and deafness.* 4th ed., eds. H. Davis and S.R. Silverman. New York: Holt, Rinehart and Winston.

Johnson, E.W. 1968. Confirmed retrocochlear lesions. *Arch. Otolaryngol.* 88:598-603.

Katz, J. ed. 1978. *Handbook of clinical audiology.* 2d. ed. Baltimore: Williams & Wilkins.

MacKenzie, I. 1965. Consequences of removing an acoustic neuroma by conventional surgical means. *Proc. R. Soc. Med.* 58:1071.

Mendel, M.I. 1977. Electroencephalic tests of hearing. In *Audiometry in infancy,* ed. S.E. Gerber. New York: Grune & Stratton, Inc.

Pulec, J.L. 1973. Surgery of the inner ear and retrocochlear region. In *Otolaryngology,* vol. 2, eds. M.M. Paparella and D.A. Shumrick. Philadelphia: W.B. Saunders Co.

Thomsen, J., Terkildsen, K., and Osterhammel, P. 1978. Auditory brain stem responses in patients with acoustic neuromas. *Scand. Audiol.* 7:179-183.

Weaver, M. and Northern, J.L. 1976. The acoustic nerve tumor. In *Hearing disorders,* ed. J.L. Northern. Boston: Little, Brown and Co.

CHAPTER 11

Auditory Processing Disorders

Historically, several more or less equally confusing terms have been employed to label those kinds of situations in which the patient seems to sense the signal adequately, but is unable to process it. Davis (1978) likes the broad term "central dysacusis," while others have employed central deafness, auditory agnosia, word deafness, receptive aphasia, and autism, to name just a few. The fact is that these may or may not be terms which describe the same behavior.

In general, experimentally induced lesions at certain locations within the brain result in specific peculiarities in behavior *(Penfield and Roberts, 1959)*. It is also generally true that, the more narrowly restricted the lesion, the more narrowly restricted the aberrant behavior. However, clinical lesions can rarely be so specifically and clearly defined as to give these statements diagnostic meaning. It is necessary to consider the pathology and etiology in each case to be able to discriminate among the several possible behavioral sequelae. It is a clinical irony that in practice it may not be important to be so discriminating. The effects or symptoms of many central pathologies are overtly similar, as are the treatments regardless of the site or etiology of the disorder. Sometimes, only the fine nuances of a test for central auditory pathology can tell them apart.

Assessment of the patient with a central auditory deficit is not an easy task. The patient will usually pass all of the conventional audiometric tests, and it is often only the astute clinician who pursues the problem further. The case history is the key, not the audiogram. The young patient in educational difficulty, the hyperactive child, the adult with a headache, the dizzy patient, and sometimes as little as a statement such as "I keep forgetting what I am told," should be enough to trigger an investigation.

PATHOLOGY and ETIOLOGY

In general, auditory processing disorders arise from cerebral lesions with the site of the pathology often being the temporal lobe. Sometimes these disorders are due to improper connections between the auditory area of the temporal lobe and some other sensory, motor, or integrating area of the brain. Auditory processing disorders may also arise from a pathology in those structures which connect the two hemispheres of the brain. Figure 11-1 is a simplified drawing illustrating the location of the principal areas of the auditory nervous system. There are connections between the two hemispheres which indicate the flow of acoustic information from one side to the other. There will be differences in behavior as a function of which of these areas is damaged and to what degree, and at what age or stage in development the lesion occurred.

Two generalizations which can be made about the effects of pathology upon the central auditory system are: 1) lesions occurring after language development will usually result in specific and identifiable language deficits; while 2) lesions occurring prior to the onset of language development will result in more subtle and generalized deficits which are not so easily identified. Deficits will also be a function of the severity of any lesion, regardless of the age of onset.

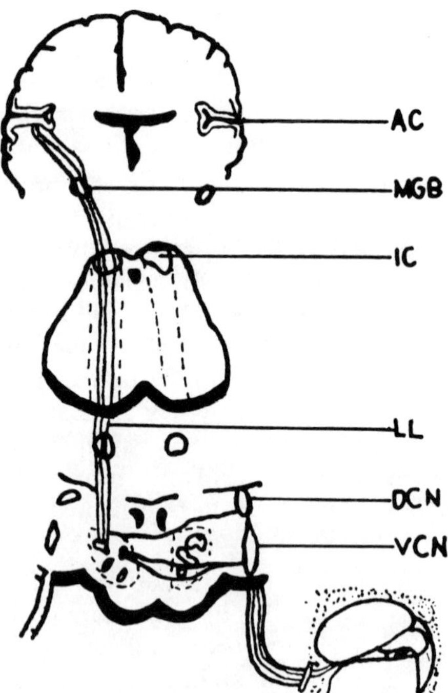

Figure 11-1. The ascending auditory pathways: VCN, ventral cochlear nucleus; DCN, dorsal cochlear nucleus; LL, lateral lemniscus; IC, inferior colliculus; MGB, medial geniculate body; AC, auditory cortex.

For purposes of discussion here, the various disorders are considered in terms of their pre- and post-linguistic onset. In effect, the difference is a congenital versus an acquired pathology. Hopefully, that artificial and arbitrary division will facilitate the students' understanding of a very complex subject, and not result in any misconceptions regarding central auditory pathologies.

Pre-Lingual Disorders

Congenital malformations and/or disorders of the central auditory system may be so subtle that they go unnoticed for a lifetime, or they may be so dramatic as to cause severe retardation, seizures, and/or what appears to be a total agnosia (cortical deafness). Aside from the intellectual and scientific knowledge gained from associating a site of lesion with a specific pathological behavior, if one could be found, information concerning the locus of a congenital central disorder is of minimal clinical treatment value.

Chief among the prenatal and natal factors associated with central deficits have been toxoplasmosis, hyperbilirubinemia, trauma at birth, a prolapsed cord and/or the umbilicus tightly wrapped around the throat causing a severe or prolonged oxygen deprivation (asphyxia). Asphyxia seems to have the greatest potential to produce damage to the brain, including the auditory nervous system. In fact, Robertson (1978) singled out oxygen deprivation as a major cause of hearing impairment and motor disability in the newborn. Deprivation of oxygen associated with environmental toxins may also have widespread neurological sequelae. It should also be noted that asphyxia is one of the high risk items from the register for early detection of congenital sensory and neural hearing losses.

Almost all of the things which cause congenital deafness are likely to produce processing difficulties, even in the absence of an actual hearing loss *(Gerber, 1977)*. For example, Tooley (1973) has indicated that infants with hemolytic disease and respiratory distress in the early neonatal period often have somewhat lowered I.Q.s when measured at age three years and mild to moderate language disturbances when examined at age seven years. Leopold (1979) found that neonatal asphyxia had occurred frequently in the histories of children with language delay.

Mencher et al. (1978) reported that a significant number of children on the high risk register for hearing loss, who had failed the high risk screening but who had normal hearing, demonstrated physical and mental anomalies, as well as decreased performance in the school environment. Some people who have difficulty reading or spelling have an inability to make the connection between auditory input and verbal output. Certainly, that type of processing disorder, while not a hearing loss in the customary sense of the word, is an auditory system processing deficit. The audiologist must be aware of the relationship between hearing and auditory processing and, of course, the possibility that some learning disorders are really disorders of auditory processing.

For auditory stimuli to be meaningful, there must be an intact auditory perceptual system which transmits, processes, stores, and retrieves information provided by the peripheral hearing mechanism. It is the perceptual system which permits focusing on specific stimuli while blocking out irrelevant auditory information. It is the perceptual system which enables identification of a voice or which permits recognition of "sit" as one of the "it" words that rhymes with "hit."

Auditory perceptual disturbances involve the entire communication cycle, interfering with the complex interdependence of auditory sensitivity, auditory perception, language, and speech. The acoustic world is not perceived normally by children with deficits in these areas. The end result is that the delicately balanced relationships between cognition and language and between language and subsequent academic behavior are disturbed.

The general term auditory perception, utilized for lack of a better one, encompasses a number of sub-areas: auditory discrimination, auditory association, auditory closure, auditory memory, auditory localization, and auditory figure-ground perception *(Mencher and Stick, 1976)*. Disruption of any one or more of these perceptual skills may result in a moderate to severe learning disability. For purposes of discussion here, the sub-areas are reviewed independently; however, they are interdependent and deficits rarely appear in one sub-area alone.

AUDITORY DISCRIMINATION. Auditory discrimination is the ability to recognize acoustic similarities and differences. Phoneme combinations are meaningless or confusing to the child with an auditory discrimination deficit. A disorder may be manifested by the inability to differentiate contrasting vowels and consonants (e.g., set from sit, peg from keg, and pick from pit). This disorder must not be confused with the reduction of speech discrimination ability which results from cochlear pathology involving the destruction of the hair cells of the organ of Corti (see chapter 9). It should be noted that this problem is quite similar, if not identical, to that seen as phonemic regression in the presbycusic patient. Abnormal auditory discrimination due to central deficit is the consequence of a distortion of speech sounds at the cortical level which creates internal chaos, so that the child is unable to learn the correct association of visual and auditory symbols, and, as a result, has difficulty learning to read aloud.

AUDITORY ASSOCIATION. Auditory association is the ability to relate meaning to particular environmental sounds and/or spoken words. A child with this problem may recognize the sound of a bird (auditory discrimination and auditory sensitivity) and be able to differentiate between a bird whistle and a human whistle; however, he is unable to recognize the significance of either signal. Similarly, he may be able to hear speech, but be unable to relate a combination of specific sounds to an appropriate referent. Abstraction ability is hampered, and thoughts are visually concrete. The ultimate result is a reduction in the ability to manipulate symbolic ideas. When an auditory stimulus cannot be linked to previous experience, the individual frequently responds in an inappropriate manner, or fails to respond at all.

196

AUDITORY CLOSURE. The ability to complete the missing part of a verbally presented message is called auditory closure. For example, ". . . uper . . . arket" may be difficult for a child with a closure problem to recognize aurally as "supermarket." Good auditory closure is necessary for the development of the phonetic skills required in sound blending, and is thus closely tied to the child's ability to read, spell, speak, and write. Further, such a child may not be able to fill in a word missing in a sentence (e.g., Answer the . . . when someone knocks on it). Auditory closure enables correct analysis of the signal and filling in when a portion of the message is not heard or perceived. Without closure skills, the sequencing of events becomes extremely difficult and auditory imagery either will be distorted or will be impossible to achieve. Relationships between concepts often become irrational or non-existent. The patient's speech may become dysfluent and hesitant, and it becomes difficult to use oral language as a medium for thought.

AUDITORY MEMORY. The ability to recall a sequence of information presented acoustically is called auditory memory. Short term memory is concerned with retention over a period of seconds, or, at the very most, a few minutes; while long term memory refers to storage of auditory information over an extended period of time. The capacity for storage is usually quite variable, dependent upon the uniqueness of the material, the frequency of exposure, and the individual's interest and skill. Typically, deficits are manifested by an inability to recall previous events and to associate them with current experiences. There may also be a parallel deficit in auditory sequencing. That is, the person may be unable to correctly order events. The result of these multiple problems will be a variety of order errors in sound blending (e.g., *fist* becomes *fits*) and a marked number of letter reversals when writing.

AUDITORY LOCALIZATION. Spatial orientation, or auditory localization, refers to the ability to locate the source of a sound in the environment. Skill in that area is expected as early as three or four months of age. Even children as young as one day will shift their eyes in the direction of a sound *(Brazleton, 1969)*. Most children with auditory perceptual localization difficulty remain undetected because their audiograms and general auditory behavior are normal. Only in specific situations, often involving physical safety where the direction of a danger is critical, does the handicap become evident. Rapid changes in the direction of a sound generate anxiety, creating chaos in the learning situation.

AUDITORY FIGURE-GROUND PERCEPTION. The ability to isolate relevant sounds from background noises and to separate them meaningfully requires figure-ground perception. The cocktail party effect *(Cherry, 1966)*, the ability to tune into a conversation when there may be another, perhaps closer and louder competing conversation nearby, illustrates this skill. Because they are unable to satisfactorily screen out irrelevant stimuli, those with inadequate auditory figure-ground balance often appear distractable.

They react to both important and unimportant auditory stimuli. Such children are often deemed to be hyperactive and poorly disciplined, and are often classed as having behavior problems.

SUMMARY. The child who has even a little trouble with comprehension, attention, distractability, perception, or language needs help. It is inadequate to examine only for a peripheral auditory disorder. The possibility of a deficit in central auditory processing must also be considered. A treatment regime in which other avenues of input are employed and special teaching devices and methods are utilized is necessary in order to compensate for the impaired auditory channel. Such a child must be, and can be, allowed to develop to her or his fullest potential.

POST-LINGUAL DISORDERS

The etiologies which produce acquired central auditory pathology are as diverse as the processing disorders themselves. These may range from tumors to debilitating disease processes to head trauma, either intrinsic (e.g., cerebrovascular accidents or strokes) or extrinsic (e.g., a blow to the head). The problem is even further compounded in that the results of cortical lesions will vary depending upon their location and severity. That is, lesions in the temporal lobe will have more serious effects on audition than lesions of the occipital or parietal lobes. Further, lesions of the left cerebral hemisphere will have more serious effects on audition than lesions of the right hemisphere; and, of course, a lesion affecting both hemispheres is far more serious than a unilateral problem.

NEOPLASMS. The most dramatic and feared lesion of the central system is a tumor. Neoplasms, both malignant and benign, which appear anywhere within the cranial space are popularly called "brain tumors." Fortunately, those neoplasms that are self contained, or that are restricted to the meninges (therefore, meningioma) or covering of the brain and spinal cord, frequently can be removed with limited residual effect.

A meningioma located on the temporal lobe may cause seizures and/or auditory hallucinations. In addition, it is extremely likely, if the tumor is on the left side, that there will be an interference with speech and language production or reception. One patient reported hearing a Beethoven symphony during a seizure, while another recalled radio broadcasts first heard as a child 30 years earlier. Just what mechanism triggers this auditory memory is not known. Surgical intervention — which involves opening the skull and literally peeling the tumor off the surface of the brain — will usually relieve the symptoms.

Tumors within the structure of the brain tissue itself may result in behavior similar to that seen with meningioma; however, the prognosis is usually guarded. Named after their cellular structure, these lesions are often called by such names as glioma, astrocytoma, blastoma, etc. Generalizations are very difficult where brain tumors are concerned, but, if the patient survives, invasion of cortical tissue by disease will usually result in some permanent deficit.

DISEASES. Chief among the diseases causing auditory deficits are meningitis, encephalitis, lues (syphilis), and many kidney disorders. Those have been considered earlier (chapter 6), and need not be reviewed here. Suffice it to say, these disease processes can result in deafness in the usual sense, and an auditory perceptual deficit as discussed here, or in some combination of the two.

Multiple sclerosis (chapter 6) is an excellent example of the type of disorder likely to be seen when a disease process invades the central auditory pathways. In general, this disease is characterized by plaques or islands of demyelination throughout the central nervous system. Lesions are most frequently found on the optic nerve, in the brainstem, the cerebellum, and/or the pyramidal motor system. Early signs of the disease may include transient weakness, minor gait disturbances, vertigo, and/or visual involvement (diplopia and blurring). If the temporal lobe and/or other auditory areas become involved, the patient may demonstrate an apathy and lack of judgment not previously seen, seizures, and alterations in speech. There may be scanning speech, dysarthria, and a very slow speaking rate. These may be accompanied by word finding difficulties; sometimes the pattern resembles stuttering. Speech discrimination and perception become markedly reduced when there is a great deal of background noise present; that is a typical sign of central auditory pathology. It often requires very sophisticated audiometric procedures to pinpoint such a disorder, a discussion for later in this chapter.

HEAD TRAUMA. Any serious head trauma, whether intrinsic or extrinsic, can result in an auditory processing disorder. Intrinsic trauma is more common and is frequently accompanied by aphasia, loosely defined as an inability to employ language in the normal manner. If the language system is seen as a flow of processed information from interacting auditory, sensorimotor, and visual systems, and an associated feedback mechanism for each of these channels, it is easy to conceptualize aphasia as an inability to utilize one or more of the information systems in conjunction with the others *(Schuell, 1965)*. The more specific and singular the damage to a particular sensory system, the more clearly defined is the linguistic disorder; and the more restricted are abstractions, generalizations, and discriminations.

The same is true with varying degrees if the lesion is unilateral or bilateral. Of course, if the lesion is unilateral, the nature of the handicap depends on which hemisphere of the brain is involved. For most people (whether right-handed or left-handed), language function predominates in the left cerebral hemisphere *(Wada and Rasmussen, 1960)*. Consequently, the processing of speech is more severely impaired by left-side lesions than by right-side lesions. Damage to the left hemisphere leads to those disorders which are classically and traditionally described as aphasia, that is, the loss or diminution of the ability to process and/or produce meaningful spoken language.

It is not clear what happens to auditory processing in the case of lesions to the right cerebral hemisphere. It is thought that damage to the right side of the brain will lead to auditory processing difficulties for acoustic events which are not related to speech. Currently, research is being directed toward that question *(Duane, 1977)*.

A more generalized disorder related to aphasia is auditory agnosia. The patient with auditory agnosia is unable to discriminate acoustic events from one another, whether or not they include speech. That is, the ear can hear the sounds, but the brain cannot decode them. In the extreme, a pure auditory agnosia would involve a total word deafness in which the ear receives and transmits a signal, but the brain cannot relate it to auditory memory, to previous linguistic experience, or to clues from other sensory modes. Inability to monitor one's own verbal output through one's own auditory channel, an extremely critical factor in verbal interaction, is destroyed; and, consequently, so is aural/oral communication.

IATROGENESIS. Some trauma to the brain may be *iatrogenic,* that is, doctor-caused. These lesions usually result from brain surgery performed to alleviate other problems and/or symptoms. For example, removal of a cyst or tumor which has grown within the head may necessitate the loss of or damage to cortical tissue and/or may result in the development of scar tissue. An excellent example for study was a child who developed a large cyst (the size of a man's fist) on the left parietal lobe. In order to remove the cyst, and in subsequent operations to remove scar tissue, most of the parietal lobe and much of the left temporal lobe were removed. In fact, eventually the entire left hemisphere was removed. The child's language function was disturbed in a very peculiar way. After recovering from the surgery and returning to school, he greeted all of the teaching and the rehabilitative staff by title. He went from room to room in his wheelchair identifying each person by occupation; for example, "You are physical therapy." He was right, too. However, he knew no one's name after the surgery, even though he had known them all quite well before the operations. This interesting case serves to illustrate two points: 1) that the child's anomaly and peculiar verbal behavior are not as important as the concepts that this language disturbance was iatrogenic, and that the surgery was a life-saving procedure; and 2) it suggests that a significant proportion of the children discussed earlier in this chapter, who were described as "learning disabled" or as suffering from an "auditory processing disorder," have language difficulty similar to that child. The etiology and age of onset may be different, but the overt problems are quite similar. This further illustrates that the decision to separate central auditory processing disorders into categories based on age of onset (e.g., pre-lingual vs. post-lingual), type of trauma (e.g., intrinsic vs. extrinsic), or location of lesion (e.g., temporal lobe vs. parietal lobe) is purely an arbitrary one. Be advised: it is the patient's behavior which is most important therapeutically and not the diagnostic label.

MEDICAL CONSIDERATIONS

In dealing with auditory processing disorders, it is important to recognize that the discussion is not concerned specifically with ear disease, the principal domain of the otologist. However, that does not mean that the otologist should not be involved or attend to central problems. Psychiatrists, pediatricians, and neurologists have dealt with these problems for a long time.

Since the otologist is the medical specialist most concerned with hearing, he is frequently the first to have contact with a patient who has a central processing disorder. These central disorders, exclusive of those related to disease and surgical intervention, are a new area for most medical practitioners but one which is worthy of attention and demanding more and more of it. At present, medical treatment is primarily drug oriented to control seizures, motor disorders, and aberrant behavior. Since this topic is somewhat apart from auditory dysfunction, we do not consider it further; the reader is referred to other texts such as Bartram (1975).

AUDIOLOGICAL CONSIDERATIONS

It is the educational, speech-language, and audiological centers which carry the primary clinical burden for the majority of these patients. The primary care provider sends the patient to the people who specialize in the patient's particular problem, but speech and hearing centers still need to know and do more.

Hearing testing is appropriate and important but may not be fruitful. Patients in this group may not suffer from impairment of auditory sensitivity. It is only on special tests designed to probe auditory perceptual skills under varying conditions that patients with central deficits will display their special disabilities. Most procedures for differential diagnosis of these types of disorders involve analysis of a patient's ability to process verbal signals which have been distorted by filtering, speeding them up, slowing them down, competing with them, alternating them between the ears, or delaying the normal feedback channel to the ears. The patient with a central auditory lesion will have difficulty processing any one or all of these combinations, depending on the type, extent, and location of the lesion. Most of the common procedures have been described in detail in other sources *(Katz, 1968, 1977; Keith, 1977)*, and the interested reader is urged to begin exploration there.

Tests for central auditory pathology may be grouped into four main categories each aimed at detecting lesions in a fairly limited area of the brain. The first category involves techniques of binaural fusion, a procedure Matzker (1959) related to lesions in the brainstem. In a typical test sequence, the patient will be asked to integrate high frequency information presented to one ear with low frequency information presented to the other ear. That is, some high frequency components of a spondee will be received in one ear, while some low frequency components of the same word will be presented simultaneously to the other ear (figure 11-2). Neither portion of the word carries enough information to make the word meaningful to a normal listener, but normals can easily understand the word when both halves are presented. Patients with brainstem lesions cannot do so easily *(Ivey, 1969)*.

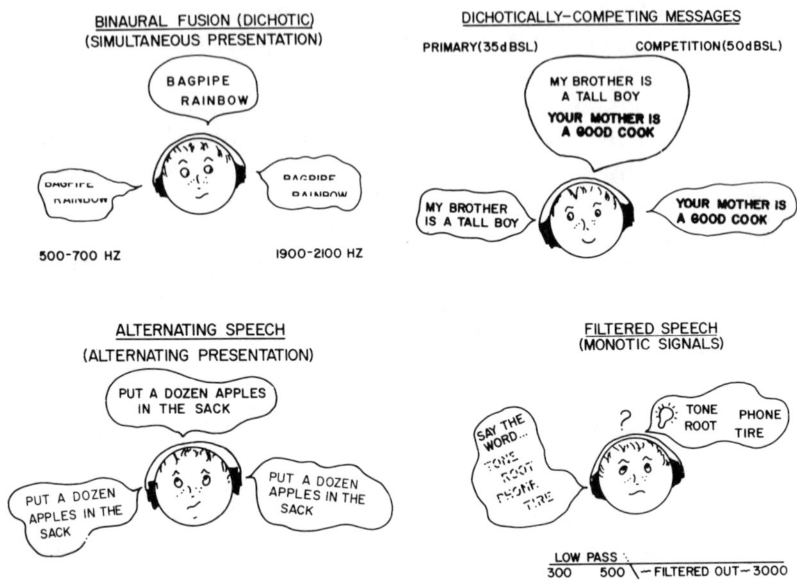

Figure 11-2. Tests for assessing central auditory behavior. *(Reproduced with permission of Grune & Stratton, Inc.)*

The second category of tests involves techniques of alternation. A sentence is presented to the patient via earphones, with the signal alternating between the ears every 300 milliseconds (figure 11-2). Patients with diffuse central pathology, as may be seen in children with auditory perceptual disorders or those with brainstem lesions, do not perform well on this type of task. That is, they cannot interpret a signal presented to the two ears into a single message *(Willeford, 1977)*.

The third category of tests involves techniques of filtering (figure 11-2). In one such test, the patient is presented with a sequence of words in only one ear. The filter attenuates frequencies above 500 Hz at a rate of 18 dB per octave. Patients unable to identify and repeat words presented in this fashion may have lesions in the temporal lobe. Willeford (1977) has developed age norms up to nine years for this task.

The tests reviewed here are presented only as samples. The important concept is not the tests *per se*, but rather how similar the tests are to the disorders considered under both the headings pre-lingual and post-lingual disorders. For example, the section on post-lingually acquired disorders contains a discussion of a problem called auditory figure-ground perception. One of the test procedures, dichotically competing messages (figure 11-2), is clearly going to be useful in identifying the child with a figure-ground deficit. In this type of test, competing messages are presented one to each ear at different sensation levels. The patient is asked to repeat both messages, a task which requires separate interpretation of the competing signals. That procedure is put to excellent application when utilized to evaluate an adult patient suspected of having a temporal lobe tumor. As indicated earlier, neither the age of onset of the disorder nor the medical terminology is as important as the behavior of the patient.

An additional example is the Staggered Spondaic Word (SSW) test first described by Katz in 1968. Basically, it is a competing message test: a spondee is presented to each ear at 50dB sensation level and the patient is required to repeat both of them. A great deal has been written about the interpretation of SSW test data. We are not going to summarize all that information here, but observe that Katz (1977) "found peculiar response bias pattern in our patients to have diagnostic significance . . ." These patterns seem to reflect surprisingly specific sites of brain lesions. The SSW is now "an effective, standardized, and versatile test of central auditory function" *(Katz, 1977)*. It is sufficiently complex in its interpretation, however, so that one requires special training to employ it.

What about treatment and management? For the young child, the burden of responsibility has fallen to the educational audiologists, psychologists, teachers of the hearing-impaired, teachers of the learning disabled, speech pathologists, pediatric neurologists, and militant parents who have grown tired of having their children shuffled back and forth among the specialists. With the exceptions of a few centers, treatment and management are limited. Educational approaches include use of alternate sensory modes (visual versus auditory), drug therapy, reduction of motor activities during communication, limited expectations and educational goals (sometimes in spite of above average intelligence), repetition of messages via recorded programs, and other similar methods. In fact, Rapin and Ruben (1979) have proposed that children with "auditory verbal agnosia" be educated as though deaf, that is by total communication. Some of these children are already in classrooms for the hearing-impaired. Some are given amplification via auditory trainers in the classroom, and some even get hearing aids. Unfortunately, that sometimes occurs because the child's lack of auditory response is mistaken for a peripheral hearing loss.

The adult fares no better. If the problem is medically based, and it usually is, treatment is usually surgical. The resulting deficit frequently goes untreated unless it is displayed as something as dramatic as aphasia or agnosia. Treatment by a speech-language pathologist will then usually follow. If the problem is subtle, treatment is typically non-existent.

Summary

This chapter has only touched on the question of auditory processing disabilities. This is a new area for the audiologist, but one which is worthy of our attention and is demanding more and more of it. At present, it is the educational audiologist who carries the primary responsibility for treatment of these types of cases. While that is a good step, it is also unfortunate as it suggests that these patients are being missed in the standard audiological facility. That is particularly true where adults are concerned. It is important that audiologists and otologists become increasingly involved with the diagnosis and treatment of auditory processing disorders, and that audiology centers have available a complete procedure for diagnosing these disabilities in both children and adults. Equally important, there should be programs for their treatment and management. As continued research develops new procedures for diagnosis and treatment, more and more of the audiologist's time will be spent in dealing with these types of patients.

CASE STUDY 11-1:

CHILD WITH CENTRAL

AUDITORY PROCESSING DISORDER

K's speech clinician referred him to the clinic for a hearing evaluation. He has articulation and language problems. He has no history of ear infection or injury. He has never been hospitalized or had any of the childhood illnesses. His family has no history of hearing problems.

Pure tone air conduction thresholds were obtained at 500, 1000, 2000, and 4000 Hz. The results in both the left and the right ears show normal hearing. The speech reception thresholds obtained were 0dB in the left ear and 10dB in the right ear. The speech discrimination test was done in the sound field first with no noise, then with masking noise coming out of one speaker (behind K). He did just as well repeating the words in noise as he did in silence. He was not distracted by the background noise.

The sound recognition subtest of the G-F-W Sound-Symbol Tests was administered. K was to point to the picture of the stated word. The word was pronounced with each phoneme stated separately. He did not correctly respond to any of the 6 words presented. The Auditory Sequential Memory Test and the Auditory Memory Span Test were given. For the former, numbers were presented (first 2 numbers and then 3 numbers). K was to repeat them in correct order. He could repeat them correctly only when there were 2 numbers. The Auditory Memory Span Test presents words rather than stated numbers and the response does not have to be in correct order. Out of 3 pairs and 3 sets of 3 words presented, K got only the first pair correct. The results on these tests show that K is performing below the level of threshold of adequacy.

K's hearing is within normal range. His auditory processing is delayed and he needs remediation in this area.

REFERENCES

Bartram, J.B. 1975. Cerebral dysfunction (learning disorders). In *Nelson's textbook of pediatrics*, eds. V.C. Vaughan, R.J. McKay, and W.E. Nelson. Philadelphia: W.B. Saunders Co.

Brazelton, T.B. 1969. *Infants and mothers: differences in development.* New York: Delacorte.

Cherry, E.C. 1966. *On human communication.* Cambridge: The M.I.T. Press.

Davis, H. 1978. Audiometry: other auditory tests. In *Hearing and deafness.* 4th ed., eds. H. Davis and S.H. Silverman. New York: Holt, Rinehart and Winston.

Duane, D.D. 1977. A neurologic perspective of central auditory dysfunction. In *Central auditory dysfunction.* ed. R.W. Keith. New York: Grune & Stratton, Inc.

Gerber, S.E. 1977. Prevention of handicap by early detection. Keynote address presented at Interprofessional Forum on Learning. University of Santa Clara.

Ivey, R.G. 1969. *Tests of CNS auditory function.* Unpublished Master's Thesis, Colorado State University, Fort Collins.

Katz, J. 1977. The staggered spondaic word test. In *Central auditory dysfunction.* ed. R. Keith. New York: Grune & Stratton, Inc.

Keith, R.W., ed. 1977. *Central auditory dysfunction.* New York: Grune & Stratton, Inc.

Leopold, R.E. 1979. *A retrospective study of the relationship between perinatal anoxia anoxia and communicative disorders.* Unpublished Masters Thesis, University of California, Santa Barbara.

Matzker, J. 1959. Two new methods for the assessment of central auditory functions in cases of brain disease. *Ann. Otol. Rhinol. Laryngol.* 68:1185-1197.

Mencher, G.T., Baldursson, M.S., Tell, L., and Levi, C. 1978. Mass behavioral screening and follow-up. Presented to the meeting of the National Research Council-National Academy of Sciences, Assembly of Behavioral and Social Sciences Meeting of the Committee on Hearing, Bioacoustics and Biomechanics. Omaha.

Mencher, G.T. and Stick, S.L. 1976. On beyond the cochlea: auditory perceptual disorders. In *Early Identification of Hearing Loss*, ed., G.T. Mencher. Basel: S. Karger.

Penfield, W. and Roberts, L. 1959. *Speech and Brain Mechanisms.* Princeton: Princeton University Press.

Rapin, I. and Ruben, R. 1979. Clinical appraisal of auditory function. Paper presented to the symposium on Developmental Disabilities in the Preschool Child. Chicago.

Robertson, C. 1978. Pediatric assessment of the infant at risk for deafness. In *Early diagnosis of hearing loss.* eds. S.E. Gerber and G.T. Mencher. New York: Grune & Stratton, Inc.

Schuell, H. 1965. *Differential diagnosis of aphasia with the Minnesota test.* Minneapolis: University of Minnesota Press.

Tooley, W. 1973. *Hyperbilirubinemia and respiratory distress syndrome.* 65th Ross Conference. Columbus: Ross Laboratories.

Wada, J. and Rasmussen, T. 1960. Intracarotid injection of sodium amytal for the lateralization of cerebral speech dominance. Experimental and clinical observations. *J. Neurosurg.* 17:266-282.

Willeford, J. 1977. Assessing central auditory behavior in children: a test battery approach. In *Central Auditory Dysfunction*, ed., R. Keith. New York: Grune & Stratton, Inc.

4

Assessment

of the

Handicap

After all is said and done, what really matters is the extent of the handicap. The audiogram, the X-ray picture, the otoscopic examination, and the special tests for central disorders, etc. measure hearing and auditory function, but they really do not assess the handicap. It is known, for example, that a patient with a sensory-neural hearing loss of 50dB can sometimes have more difficulty in his daily living than another patient with a hearing loss of 75dB. It is also known, as was illustrated by the case of the child who had had a hemispherectomy (chapter 11), that some massive insults may result in less handicap than smaller lesions. While it is true that the diagnostic strategy of audiology is directed toward identifying the anatomical site of an impairment of hearing — whether in the middle ear, inner ear, auditory nerve, or the central nervous system — it must always be understood that audiology is not only a diagnostic profession. It is a (re)habilitative profession. While planning for (re)habilitation is based on assessment, it must be directed toward alleviation of a handicap, and not limited to an assessment or alleviation of a hearing loss.

CHAPTER 12

Handicapping Effects

of a

Hearing Loss

The essential distinction between "deaf" and "hearing-impaired" is the ability to learn and to effectively use residual hearing in a particular environment, regardless of the configuration of the audiogram. If, with special help, a child with a loss of hearing can learn in a normal school environment, that child is "hearing-impaired" and not "deaf," irrespective of the amount of hearing loss. If, on the other hand, the use of amplification and special teachers is not sufficient to produce a normally functioning human being, then the child is "deaf," even if the audiogram says otherwise. The important distinctions between deaf and hearing-impaired should be based only on the ability to acquire language — language, not speech.

It is the working professionals (audiologist, otologist, teacher of the deaf, etc.), who want and need the structure of such terms as mild, moderate, severe, and profound when describing a hearing loss. There seems to be a constant need to assign numbers to these words, something which is not an easy task. Numbers seem to mean very little, however, in terms of the actual handicap. For example, what does it mean to say that a hearing impairment of less than 25dB is or is not significant? Many people *(e.g., Northern and Downs, 1978)* are concerned about the ability of some children to learn when suffering from a continuing "mild" hearing loss due to recurrent otitis media. In virtually every area studied, children with recurrent or chronic otitis media have had poorer achievements than their well-matched controls.

For adults, the issue is similar. Think of elderly patients who withdraw from society and are thereby profoundly handicapped by a hearing loss which, in reality, may not be very severe by numerical standards. Imagine a 60-year-old woman with a high frequency hearing loss due to vascular disease and aging. She may comment on how noisy things have become, particularly in the supermarket. She may stop going to new movies because she has heard the records or seen the plays from which older movies were made, but when newer ones come along she no longer knows the material and is no longer entertained by the films. Playing cards, going to church, and visiting friends have become chores. In short, this imaginary, but all too real, woman has become "deaf" and a dropout from society. On the other hand, if that same woman is fortunate and is properly treated medically and audiologically, she will have a good understanding of the nature of her disorder and the rehabilitation program designed to overcome it. If she is properly counselled and guided, and applies her own native intelligence and abilities, she may retain her articulatory skills, make maximum use of amplification, and become a good speech reader. Given those conditions, this "deaf" patient may find that her handicap is really not so severe.

There are, of course, medical-legal problems associated with acquired hearing loss, particularly where compensation is involved. Some hearing losses may be the result of the use of ototoxic drugs, while others are occupationally caused, and others are due to accident or injury. How much is that worth? Do the numbers actually tell the story? Do they tell of the wages lost? The social deficits? The family trauma? The assessment of a handicap, then, simply does not rest on auditory tests alone, nor does it rest on medical-legal standards. Obviously, however, some quantifiable scale is necessary so that compensation can be made to those who have lost their hearing occupationally or accidentally, or so that professionals can agree as to what they mean when they say a patient has a hearing loss.

Percentage of Hearing Loss

A number of years ago there was an effort to generate standards for calculating a percentage of hearing loss (figure 12-1), so that the courts could render proper and adequate financial compensation to those suffering losses through noise and trauma (AA00, 1959). Unfortunately, the notion of "percentage of hearing loss" makes little sense. Suppose, for example, it is said that someone has a 50% hearing loss. What does that mean? Does it mean that he hears half of each word? Does it mean that he hears alternate syllables? It means none of these, and, more importantly, no one is quite sure what it does mean. It had been hoped, therefore, that the per cent concept would disappear. It didn't. In fact, just recently the American Academy of Otolaryngology joined with the American Council of Otolaryngology to develop a new mathematical formula (1979). There are three steps in the calculation:

1. The average of the hearing threshold levels at 500, 1000, 2000, and 3000 Hz should be calculated for each ear.
2. The percentage of impairment for each ear should be calculated by multiplying by 1.5% the amount by which the average hearing threshold level exceeds a low fence of 25dB. The impairment should be calculated up to 100%, reached at a high fence of 92dB.

3. The impairment then should be calculated by multiplying the percentage of the better ear by 5, adding this figure to the percentage from the poorer ear, and dividing the total by 6

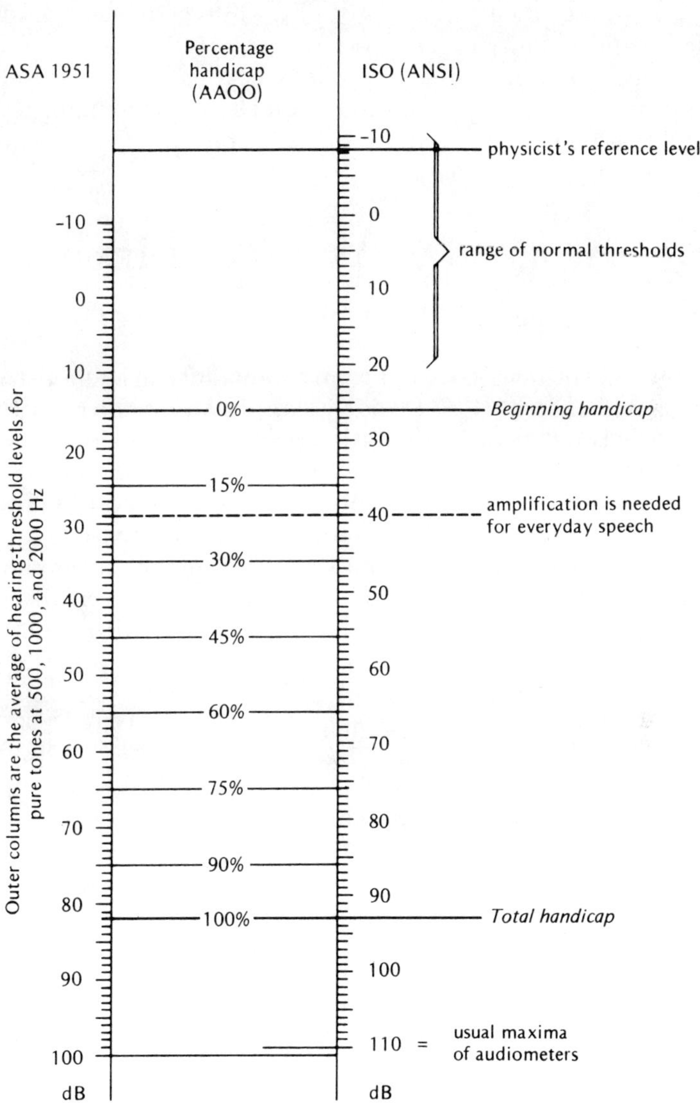

Figure 12-1. The center column shows the percentage handicap as defined by the AA00 in 1959. The other two columns are the old and new audiometric references. *(Reproduced with permission of Holt, Rinehart, & Winston.)*

The difference between this formula and the earlier procedure is the inclusion of 3000Hz in the calculation*. Definitions of impairment, handicap, and disability are also provided. Permanent impairment is defined as a change for the worse in either structure or function which is outside the range of normal. The loss should not be evaluated until maximum rehabilitation has been achieved and there is no progression of the impairment. Permanent handicap is defined as an impairment that affects a person's efficiency in daily life, while permanent disability is specified as the inability to remain employed at full wages.

Any decision concerning a worker's hearing disability and/or his entitlement to worker's compensation should be based on complete medical evaluation, using national uniform standards for assessment, regardless of how the disability was acquired.

SCALES FOR ASSESSING HEARING LOSS

In 1948, in an attempt to more formally quantify an auditory handicap as compared to a hearing loss, Davis developed a Social Adequacy Index for hearing. Based on the assumption that a given patient will hear the words of every day speech correctly and then, through a simple formula averaging that assumption over all possible speech events, Davis concluded that the threshold of social adequacy should be 55dB (ANSI), given that discrimination is perfect (100%) and the speech reception threshold is at 10dB or better. That decibel level seems quite high, and actually suggests that any individual, much less one who is hearing-impaired, is not socially adequate in normal quiet conversation. Since that is not true, the Davis scale does not seem to really define a hearing handicap very well.

A number of other scales and indexes have evolved since 1948 *(Noble and Atherley, 1970; Ewertsen and Birk-Nielsen, 1973; Ward, 1976; Newby, 1979)*. Most attempt to assess performance in typical listening situations. However, most are really limited indicators in that they do not explore all aspects of the patient's performance. Recently a procedure somewhat different from all the others was developed by Giolas, Owens, Lamb, and Schubert (1979). Called the Hearing Performance Inventory (appendix A), it attempts to assess the difficulty a patient experiences in all aspects of everyday listening. The inventory utilizes a self-report response style in which the hearing-impaired person is asked to judge how often he experiences difficulty in specific situations. The patient marks a scoring sheet with "Practically Always, Frequently, About Half The Time, Occasionally, or Almost Never."

The 158 items include questions in six categories of auditory performance: Understanding Speech, Intensity, Response to Auditory

---

*Copies of the new formula may be obtained by writing to the American Academy of Otolaryngology, 15 Second Street S.W., Rochester, MN 55901.

Failure, Social, Personal, and Occupational. The "Understanding Speech" questions are designed to assess a variety of areas representative of everyday conversation; speech discrimination and understanding are stressed both with and without visual clues. The "Intensity" questions, on the other hand, aim at determining the degree of the hearing loss. Respondents judge whether they are aware of specific auditory stimuli in specific situations (e.g., how often are they aware of a doorbell). "Response to Auditory Failure" queries particular behavior in designated listening situations (e.g., asking for repetition or adjusting a hearing aid); while at the same time the "Social" cluster of questions stresses social interaction outside of occupational settings. The "Personal" questions deal with how a patient may feel about his hearing impairment and its influence on self-esteem and social interaction. Finally, the "Occupational" section explores listening skills at work.

The items are presented in random order, and the respondent is merely checking off replies to a series of questions, without regard for categorization. Nevertheless, when the results are scored, an overall profile of the patient's difficulty is obtained.

While the format and procedures outlined by Giolas et al. (1979) have been presented here in some detail, and the Hearing Performance Inventory appears to be an excellent tool for assessing some hearing handicaps, the reader should recognize that it is not a panacea. It has some fundamental weaknesses. For example, some patients may not have language sophisticated enough to fill out the questionnaire. Furthermore, the questions are structured in such a way as to make the information obtained from a profoundly impaired patient of minimal value. In other words, this inventory appears to be superb where it can be utilized, but limited in use to only the mildly or moderately hearing-impaired. Furthermore, as Giolas et al. indicate, the methodology is fraught with pitfalls:

> Such a self-report approach was selected because we are convinced that rehabilitative programs must take into account areas of difficulty as perceived by the hearing-impaired even though the accuracy of their judgments regarding the effect of their hearing impairment on their everyday life can be questioned. In the absence of validity criteria we are merely using the judgments as a starting point for rehabilitation, mindful of the findings of Silverman et al. (1948). These investigators were forced to conclude that responses from hearing-impaired respondents reflected too heavily the person's attitude toward the difficulty rather than the actual magnitude of the communication problem. These two aspects must be measured separately so that one knows which rehabilitative measures are needed. The question of which aspect we are measuring is one facet of the validity of these items. Thus, as refinement of the inventory proceeds, we are eager to correlate the responses with other criteria including the clinician's own observations of the hearing-impaired person's behavior, and observations of a critical informant such as a spouse or close friend.

Clearly the lesson to be learned from this brief discussion of scales and inventories is that no single quantifiable assessment method exists which truly reflects the degree of handicap caused by any particular hearing loss. Perhaps what is needed is a multi-dimensional approach to each individual which considers every relevant aspect of the problem. That is an impossible task.

The Department of Social Services of the Province of Nova Scotia called together a group of professionals to deal with exactly this problem. The group represented audiology, speech-language pathology, psychology, social work, community resources, medicine and others. Its charge was to develop procedures for evaluating the disability of each patient applying for pension or financial support because of a hearing loss, regardless of the etiology of the disorder, the degree of the hearing loss, or the extent of the handicap. The model which was developed is still in its formative stages, but it certainly appears to have promise. It is predicated on the philosophy that the definition of degree of hearing loss is not translatable into any meaningful term which reflects the degree of handicap or disability. Further still, it recognizes that the definition of disability shifts constantly; subject to the progression of the hearing loss, the advancements of modern science, and the social, financial, and psychological milieu of the hearing-impaired individual. Edwards (1979) placed the issue in a proper prospective when she summarized the deliberations of her group as they developed their assessment program and tried to provide a universal definition of deafness:

> By deafness we knew we were discussing an *effect* of disease, injury or genetic failure. But did we mean almost any degree of hearing impairment or an "exact measure" such as "82dB or more across the speech frequencies"? And were we talking of disability, a concept for a data base, as a one dimensional definition of a permanent condition? If so, how would we measure this? For example: Was the measure a metric one (for financial calculations?), or was it for a policy definition (who is eligible for services or a pension?), or for some other purpose, (such as statistical research concerning epidemiology)? Would one definition serve all those purposes?
>
> The pure tone average, which we all agreed was necessary, was at least measurable, and had an administrative advantage, as did the definition: "Does not understand speech through the ear." However, we had to think in terms of "handicap" - which has a *social* value, and which would shift in degree from one situation to another, and which did not necessarily show a correlation between the end organ measurement and the self evaluation of the individual. Moreover, deafness does not occur in isolation. It coexists with a wide constellation of other factors: psychological, physical (especially vision and balance), financial background, and so on. Thus, from the beginning we had found that we could not confuse the measurement of the disability with the assessment of the handicap and that each would, of necessity, be incomplete.
>
> Much time and effort was spent on this basic dilemma — which is also probably the reason deafness appears to be among the least understood and least assisted of the handicaps. Other handicaps have traditional methods of measurement and obvious limitations of function which allow the professional to be both efficient and sympathetic. Not so with hearing loss.

The method of evaluating hearing-impaired persons which was developed in Nova Scotia, through the guidance of Dr. Joyce Edwards of the School of Human Communication Disorders at Dalhousie University, involves a team approach during which each of the specialty areas evaluates the patient individually. These should include a psychologist's statement about intellectual and personality function; a speech-language pathologist's consideration of linguistic skills; an audiologist's report on sensory, neural, and central auditory skills; a social worker's evaluation of social, economic, and interpersonal skills; a physician's report of physical health; a vocational counsellor's assessment of job-oriented skills and limitations; and a report by the patient about his own strengths, weaknesses, and needs. Each of the reports is considered by itself, each is weighted in terms of all of the others, and then they are all taken together and the patient is considered as a whole at a team staffing. For example, a patient who is profoundly deaf may receive a low score from the audiologist, but that may be counterbalanced by the speech-language pathologist if the patient has good speech and language because the loss was of late onset. By the same token, a patient with a moderate hearing loss from birth who has not developed adequate oral language or vocational skills will not score any better because the audiologist reports that hearing is only moderately impaired. One of the keys to the success of this model is a document called the "Aural Rehabilitation Questionnaire." It is offered here (appendix B) only as a sample document so that the reader may understand some of the parameters involved in patient assessment and classification.

CONCLUSION

It is a well established fact that persons whose hearing impairment is acquired after the age of six years have higher median incomes throughout their lives than those who were born congenitally deaf (figure 12-2). This has been stressed repeatedly by Downs (1976; 1978) who estimates that hearing handicaps cost society 1.75 million U.S. dollars per year for education, rehabilitation, and the result of lost labor. In contrast, the economic gain which may be incurred by early, thorough, correct diagnosis and rehabilitation, runs into billions of dollars. The cost of detecting a single case of congenital deafness is substantially less than the cost of failing to detect it. Derbyshire (1970) calculated that, if an audiologist was hired to work in a newborn nursery, and that audiologist was to discover only one deaf infant per year, the difference between the cost of the salary and the money saved by early identification would ensure that society would benefit financially. The cost of later habilitation greatly exceeds the cost of early habilitation. The difference may be measured in hard dollars and cents as a marked increase in the amount of taxes paid by the working and productive hard-of-hearing person in a lifetime as a constructive member of society.

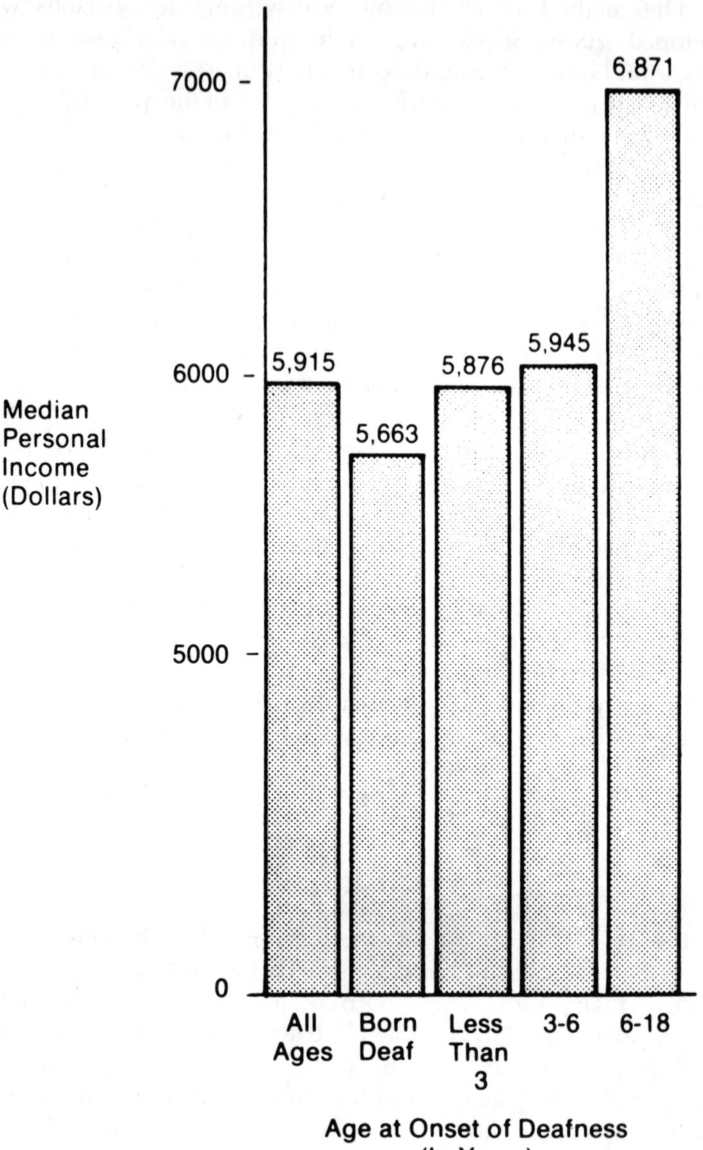

Figure 12-2. Median personal incomes in 1971 of employed deaf persons in the United States by age at onset of deafness. *(From Schein and Delk, The Deaf Population of the United States. Silver Springs: National Association of the Deaf, 1974. Reproduced with permission.)*

All of us are handicapped by our own failure to vigourously search out, diagnose, and rehabilitate the hearing-impaired. As new diagnostic, therapeutic, and rehabilitative techniques develop, it is important that they be explored and implemented whenever and wherever possible. Hopefully, those methods will soon be forthcoming. In the meantime, we offer the simple mnemonic of table 12-1 for consideration.

Table 12-1. Some A B C D E's of the Deaf

S -	Skull Fracture	Primary
O -	Ototoxic Drugs	Causes of
M -	Meningitis	Acquired Loss
E -	Encephalitis	
A -	Affected Family	Primary
B -	Bad Breath (asphyxia)	Causes of
C -	Congenital Rubella	Congenital
D -	Defect of Ear, Nose & Throat	Loss
E -	Elevated Bilirubin Level	
S -	Small at Birth ($<$ 1500 grams)	

OF THE

D -	Detection & Medical Care	Primary
E -	Education	Causes of
A -	Auditory (Re)Habilitation	Success in
F -	Family Guidance	Management

CASE STUDY 12-1:

MODERATELY IMPAIRED WOMAN

J.D., a 38-year-old woman, has had a hearing loss since very early childhood, perhaps even since birth, although there are no data to support that conclusion. She has had some difficulty developing speech, although her language is excellent. She has attended regular schools, but she has had to wear a hearing aid for many years. There is no family history of hearing loss, and no known etiology for the present problem.

In spite of the fact that she has had a hearing loss since early childhood, J.D. had not been severely handicapped by it. Recently, however, she suffered with a case of mumps, which has caused her further problems.

J.D. first came to our clinic in July, 1975. At that time her audiogram indicated a moderate to severe hearing loss on the left side, and a severe loss on the right (the result of the mumps). Speech discrimination score on the left was 72%. Discrimination was so poor on the right that a score could not be obtained. Speech Reception Threshold for the left was 55dB. No valid result was obtained for the right. Threshold of discomfort on the left side is 105dB. Impedance results suggested normal middle ear function, but the presence of stapedius muscle reflexes at slightly elevated levels suggest recruitment is present in both ears.

Initial hearing aid evaluation suggested that a **BICROS** hearing aid might be useful. However, J.D. was unable to obtain a satisfactory fitting and elected to switch to a monaural aid on the left side. The patient has a 35dB SRT while wearing her hearing aid. Speech discrimination is unaffected by the aid, remaining at 72%. The patient is very satisfied with the results.

J.D. is the chief bass player for a major symphony orchestra. She never misses a concert, is considered one of the best musicians in the orchestra, and has been known to solo at performances. How handicapped is she by her hearing loss? Obviously the audiogram does not tell all.

CASE STUDY 12-1: MODERATELY IMPAIRED WOMAN
PURE TONE AUDIOGRAM

RIGHT EAR

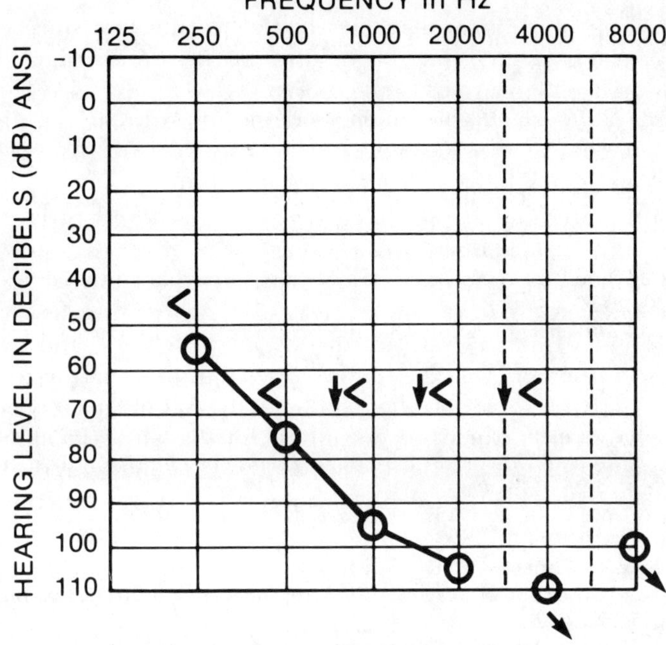

LEFT EAR

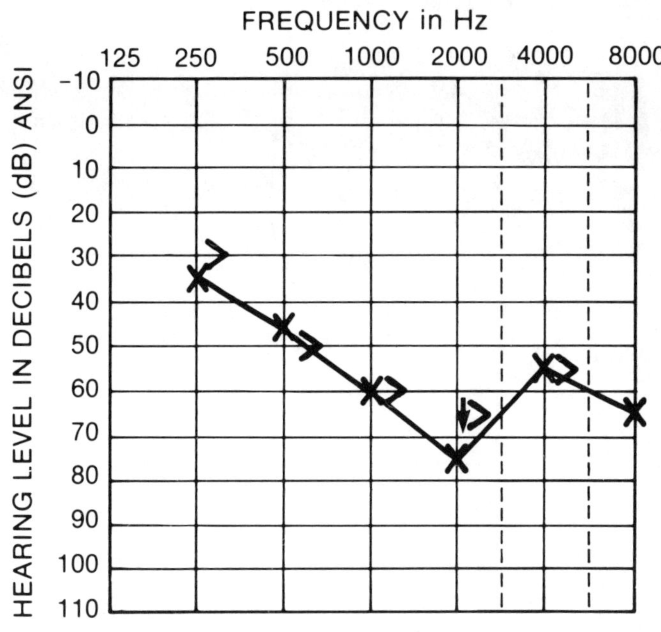

REFERENCES

AAOO Committee on Conservation of Hearing 1959. Guide for the evaluation of hearing impairment. *Trans. Am. Acad. Ophthalmol. Otolaryngol.* 63:236-238.

American Academy of Otolaryngology and the American Council of Otolaryngology 1979. Guide for the evaluation of hearing handicap. *JAMA* 241: 2055-2059.

Davis, H. 1948. The articulation area and the social adequacy index for hearing. *Laryngoscope* 58:761-778.

Derbyshire, A.J. 1970. Personal correspondence.

Downs, M.P. 1976. Early identification of hearing loss: Where are we: Where do we go from here? In *Early identification of hearing loss,* ed. G.T. Mencher. Basel: S. Karger.

Downs, M.P. 1978. The handicap of deafness. In *Hearing disorders,* ed. J.L. Northern. Boston: Little, Brown and Co.

Edwards, J. 1979. Unpublished manuscript.

Ewertsen, H. and Birk-Nielsen, H. 1973. Social hearing handicap index. *Audiology* 12:180-187.

Giolas, T.G., Owens, E., Lamb, S., and Schubert, E. 1979. Hearing performance inventory. *J. Speech Hear. Dis.* 44:169-195.

Newby, H.A. 1979. *Audiology.* 4th ed. Englewood Cliffs: Prentice-Hall, Inc.

Noble, W. and Atherley, G. 1970. The hearing measurement scale: A questionnaire for the assessment of auditory disability. *J. Auditory Res.* 10:229-250.

Northern, J.L. and Downs, M.P. 1978. *Hearing in children.* 2d ed. Baltimore: Williams & Wilkins Co.

Schein, J.D. and Delk, J.H. 1974. *The deaf population of the United States.* Silver Springs, MD.: Nat'l. Assoc. of the Deaf.

Silverman, S.R., Thurlow, W.R., Walsh, T.E., and Davis, H. 1948. Improvement in the social adequacy of hearing following the fenestration operation. *Laryngoscope* 58:607-620.

Ward, W.D. 1976. Public hearings on noise abatement and control. In *Effects of noise on hearing,* eds. D. Henderson, R.D. Hamernik, D.S. Dosanjh, and J.H. Mills. New York: Academic Press.

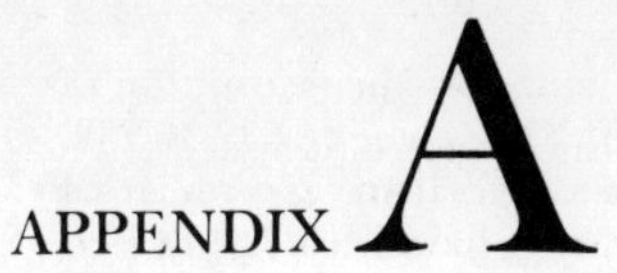

APPENDIX A

Hearing

Performance

Inventory

Stanford H. Lamb
San Francisco State University

Elmer Owens
University of California
School of Medicine

Earl D. Schubert
Stanford University

Thomas G. Giolas
University of Connecticut

We are interested in knowing how your hearing problem has affected your daily living. Below you will find a series of questions which describe a variety of everyday listening situations and ask you to judge how much difficulty you would have hearing in these situations.

Some of the questions ask you to judge how well you can understand what people are saying when their voices are loud enough. The term understand means hearing the words a person is saying clearly enough to be able to participate in the conversation. Other questions ask whether you can hear enough of a particular sound (doorbell, speech, etc.) to be aware of its presence. Other questions concern occupational, social or personal situations. Still others ask what you do when you miss something. Always assume you are interested in what is being said.

To answer each question, you are asked to check the phrase that best describes how often you experience the situation being described:

> Practically always . . . . . . (or always)
>
> Frequently . . . . (about three-quarters of the time)
>
> About half the time
>
> Occasionally . . . . (about a quarter of the time)
>
> Almost never . . . . (or never)

> For example, if you can understand what a person is saying on the telephone about 100% of the time, then you should check practically always. On the other hand, if you can understand almost nothing of what a person is saying on the telephone, then you should check almost never. If you can understand what a person is saying on the telephone about 50% of the time, then you should check about half the time.

Your answers to the questions should describe your present hearing ability as it is on the average rather than from a single instance.

If you wear a hearing aid in the situation described, answer the question accordingly.

Please check one, and only one, phrase for each question. You should check Does not apply only if you have not experienced a particular situation or one similar to it.

Questions that appear identical do differ in at least one important detail. Please read each question carefully before checking the appropriate phrase.

We know that people talk differently. Some mumble, others talk too fast, and others talk without moving their lips very much. Please answer the questions according to the way most people talk to you.

If the question does not specify whether the person speaking is male or female, answer according to which sex you have the most difficulty hearing.

Asterisks on the score sheet are for scoring purposes and should be ignored.

1. You are watching your favorite news program on television. Can you
    understand the news reporter (female) when her voice is loud enough for you?

2. You are reading in a room with music or noise in the background. Can you
    hear a person calling you from another room?

3. You are with a male friend or family member in a fairly quiet room. Can you
    understand him when his voice is loud enough for you and you can see his
    face?

4. Can you hear an airplane in the sky when others around you can hear it?

5. You are watching a drama or movie on television. Can you understand what is
    being said when the speaker's voice is loud enough for you and there is
    music in the background?

6. Can you understand what a woman is saying on the telephone when her voice is
    loud enough for you?

7. You are at a restaurant and you hear only a portion of something the
    waitress/waiter said. Do you repeat the portion when asking him/her for a
    repetition?

8. You are with a child (6 to 10 years old) in a fairly quiet room. Can you
    understand the child when his/her voice is loud enough for you and you can
    see his/her face?

9. You are the driver in an automobile with several friends or family members.
    One or more of the windows are open. Can you understand the passenger
    behind you when his/her voice is loud enough for you?

10. You are at a restaurant and there is background noise such as music or a
    crowd of people. Can you understand the waiter/waitress when his/her voice
    is loud enough for you and you can see his/her face?

11. You are talking with a close friend. When you miss something important that
    was said, do you immediately adjust your hearing aid to help you hear better?

12. You are with five or six strangers at a gathering of more than twenty people
    and there is background noise such as music or a crowd of people. One
    person talks at a time. When you are aware of the subject, can you
    understand what is being said when the speaker's voice is loud enough for
    you and you can see his/her face?

13. You are at a play or movie, or listening to a speech. When you miss
    something important that was said, do you ask the person with you?

14. You are with a child (6 to 10 years old) and several people are talking
    nearby. Can you understand the child when his/her voice is loud enough
    for you and you can see his/her face?

15. You are playing cards, monopoly or some similar game with several people
    and there is background noise such as music or a crowd of people. Can you
    understand what a friend or family member is saying to you when his/her
    voice is loud enough for you and you can see his/her face?

16. Does your hearing problem discourage you from attending lectures?

17. You are talking with five or six friends. When you miss something that
    was said, do you ask the person talking to repeat it?

18. You are in an auditorium listening to a lecturer (female) who is using
    a microphone. Can you understand what she is saying when her voice is
    loud enough for you and you can see her face?

19. Can you hear water running in another room when others around you can
    hear it?

20. You are with a friend or family member and you hear only a portion of what was said.' Do you repeat that portion when asking him/her for a repetition?

21. You are at a party or gathering of less than ten people and the room is fairly quiet. Can you understand what a friend or family member is saying to you when his/her voice is loud enough for you, but you can <u>not</u> see his/her face?

22. Does your hearing problem lower your self confidence?

23. You are in a fairly quiet room with five or six strangers. One person talks at a time. When you are aware of the subject, can you understand what is being said when the speaker's voice is loud enough for you, but you can <u>not</u> see his/her face?

24. You are with five or six friends or family members at a gathering of more than twenty people and several people are talking near by. One person talks at a time and the subject of conversation changes from time to time. Can you understand what is being said when the speaker's voice is loud enough for you and you can see his/her face?

25. When an announcement is given over a public address system in a bus station or airport, is it <u>loud enough</u> for you to hear?

26. You are talking with a stranger. When you miss something important that was said, do you ask for it to be repeated?

27. You are talking with a friend or family member. When you miss something that was said, do you pretend you understood?

28. You are at a fairly quiet restaurant. Can you understand the waiter/waitress when his/her voice is loud enough for you and you can see his/her face?

29. You are seated with five or six strangers around a table or in a living room. Often two persons are talking at once and one person frequently interrupts another. When you miss something important that was said, do you pretend you understood?

30. **You are playing cards, monopoly or some similar game and the room is fairly quiet. The subject of conversation changes from time to time. Can you understand what is being said when the speaker's voice is loud enough for you, but you can <u>not</u> see his/her face?**

31. You are at a party or gathering of less than ten people and the room is fairly quiet. Can you understand what a friend or family member is saying to you when his/her voice is loud enough for you and you can see his/her face?

32. Does your hearing problem discourage you from going to concerts?

33. Do you find that children (6 to 10 years old) speak loudly enough for you?

34. When an announcement is given over a public address system in a bus station or airport, can you understand what is being said when the speaker's voice is loud enough for you?

35. You are seated with five or six strangers around a table or in a living room. Often two persons are talking at once and one person frequently interrupts another. Can you understand what is being said when the speaker's voice is loud enough for you and you can see his/her face?

36. You are seated with five or six friends around a table or in a living room. Often two persons are talking at once and one person frequently interrupts another. When you miss something that was said, do you ask the person talking to repeat it?

37. You are with a female stranger in a fairly quiet room. Can you understand her when her voice is loud enough for you and you can see her face?

38. You are with a stranger and there is background noise such as music or a
     crowd of people. Can you understand the person when his/her voice is loud
     enough for you, but you can <u>not</u> see his/her face?

39. Does your hearing problem tend to make you impatient?

40. You are talking with five or six strangers. When you miss something
     important that was said, do you let the person talking know -- at least
     one time -- that you have a hearing problem?

41. You are at a party or gathering of less than ten people and several people
     are talking near by. Can you understand what a friend or family member
     (female) is saying to you when her voice is loud enough for you and you
     can see her face?

42. Does your hearing problem discourage you from going to plays?

43. You are having dinner with five or six friends and you hear only a portion
     of what was said. Do you repeat that portion when asking the speaker for
     a repetition?

44. You are at a restaurant with a friend or family member and there is
     background noise such as music or a crowd of people. Can you understand
     the person when his/her voice is loud enough for you and you can see
     his/her face?

45. When you have difficulty understanding a person who speaks quite rapidly,
     do you ask him/her to speak more slowly?

46. You are talking to a woman sitting in a ticket or information booth and
     it is fairly noisy. She is giving directions or information. Can you
     understand her when her voice is loud enough for you and you can see
     her face?

47. You are having dinner with five or six friends. When you miss something
     important that was said, do you ask the person talking to repeat it?

48. When others are listening to speech on the television or radio, is it
     loud enough for you?

49. Does your hearing problem discourage you from going to the movies?

50. You are riding in an automobile with several friends or family members.
     One or more of the windows are open and you are sitting in the front
     seat. Can you understand the driver when his/her voice is loud enough
     for you and you can see his/her face?

51. You are at home watching television or listening to the radio. Can you
     hear the doorbell ring when it is located in the same room?

52. You are in a fairly quiet room talking with five or six strangers. One
     person talks at a time and the subject of conversation changes from time
     to time. Can you understand what is being said when the speaker's voice
     is loud enough for you and you can see his/her face?

53. You are seated with five or six friends or family members around a table
     or in a living room. Often two persons are talking at once and one person
     frequently interrupts another. When you miss something important that
     was said, do you remind the person talking, at least once, that you have
     a hearing problem?

54. You are attending a stage play. Can you understand what the
     actors/actresses are saying when their voices are loud enough for you
     and you can see their faces?

55. You are with a friend or family member in a fairly quiet room. Can you
     understand him/her when his/her voice is loud enough for you, but you can
     <u>not</u> see his/her face?

56. A person is talking to you from a distance of no more than six feet.
     There is music or noise in the background. Would you be aware that
     he/she is talking if you did not see his/her face?

57. You are having dinner with five or six friends or family members at home
     and there is background noise such as music or a crowd of people. Can
     you understand what is being said when the speaker's voice is loud enough
     for you, but you can not see his/her face?

58. When you have difficulty understanding a person with a pipe, toothpick or
     similar object in his/her mouth, do you ask him/her to remove the object.

59. You are the driver in an automobile with several friends or family
     members. The windows are closed. Can you understand the passenger
     behind you when his/her voice is loud enough for you?

60. When you have difficulty understanding a person because he is holding
     his hand in front of his mouth, do you ask him to lower his hand?

61. You are at a party or gathering of more than twenty people and there is
     background noise such as music or a crowd of people. Can you understand
     what a stranger is saying to you when his/her voice is loud enough for
     you and you can see his/her face?

62. Do you feel that others cannot understand what it is to have a hearing
     problem?

63. You are at a movie. Can you understand what the actors/actresses are
     saying when their voices are loud enough for you and you can see their
     faces?

64. You are talking with five or six strangers. When you miss something
     important that was said, do you ask the person talking to repeat it?

65. You are at a party or gathering of more than twenty people and several
     people are talking near by. Can you understand what a friend or family
     member (male) is saying to you when his voice is loud enough for you and
     you can see his face?

66. You are in a fairly quiet room. Can you carry on a conversation with a
     man in another room if his voice is loud enough for you?

67. You are with a male friend or family member and several people are
     talking near by. Can you understand him when his voice is loud enough
     for you and you can see his face?

68. You are with five or six friends or family members. One person talks at
     a time. When you miss something important that was said, do you pretend
     you understood?

69. You are watching a drama or movie on television. Can you understand what
     is being said when the speaker's voice is loud enough for you and there
     is no music in the background?

70. You are with five or six friends or family members and there is background
     noise such as music or a crowd of people. One person talks at a time.
     When you are aware of the subject, can you understand what is being said
     when the speaker's voice is loud enough for you, but you can not see
     his/her face?

71. You are at a lecture. If you have difficulty hearing what is being said,
     do you move to a place where you can hear better?

72. Does your hearing problem tend to make you feel nervous or tense?

73. You are with a female stranger and there is background noise such as
     traffic, music, or a crowd of people. Can you understand her when her
     voice is loud enough for you and you can see her face?

226

74. You are in a quiet place and the person seated on the side of your better
    ear whispers to you. Can you hear the whisper?

75. You are at a small social gathering. If you have difficulty hearing what
    is being said, do you move to a place where you can hear better?

Occupational Items

76. You are with a male co-worker at work in a fairly quiet room. Can you
    understand him when his voice is loud enough for you and you can see
    his face?

77. You are with five or six co-workers at work. One person talks at a time.
    When you miss something important that was said, do you pretend you
    understand?

78. Does your hearing problem interfere with helping or instructing others on
    the job?

79. You are with a female co-worker at work and there is background noise such
    as traffic, music, or a crowd of people. Can you understand her when her
    voice is loud enough for you and you can see her face?

80. You are with a co-worker at work and you hear only a portion of what was
    said. Do you repeat that portion when asking the speaker for a
    repetition?

81. You are talking with a co-worker at work. When you miss something
    important that was said, do you ask for it to be repeated?

82. You are talking with your employer (foreman, supervisor, etc.) and
    several people are talking near by. Can you understand him/her when
    his/her voice is loud enough for you and you can see his/her face?

83. You are with a female co-worker at work in a fairly quiet room. Can you
    understand her when her voice is loud enough for you and you can see her
    face?

84. You are talking with a co-worker or employer. When you miss something
    important that was said, do you   remind him/her that you have a hearing
    problem?

85. You are in a fairly quiet room at work with five or six co-workers. One
    person talks at a time and the subject of conversation changes from time
    to time. Can you understand what is being said when the speaker's voice
    is loud enough for you and you can see his/her face?

86. Does your hearing problem interfere with learning the duties of a new
    job easily?

87. You are seated with five or six co-workers around a table at work.
    Often two persons are talking at once and one person frequently interrupts
    another. Can you understand what is being said when the speaker's voice
    is loud enough for you and you can see his/her face?

88. You are talking with a co-worker at work. When you miss something
    important that was said, do you pretend you understood?

89. You are with a male co-worker at work and there is background noise such
    as traffic, music, or a crowd of people. Can you understand him when his
    voice is loud enough for you and you can see his face?

90. You are talking with a co-worker at work. When you miss something that
    was said, do you immediately adjust your hearing aid to help you hear
    better?

HEARING PERFORMANCE INVENTORY (EXPERIMENTAL FORM II)

NAME _____________ AGE _______ DATE _______

ADDRESS _____________ PHONE _______

TEST LOCATION _____________ MARITAL STATUS _______

SEX _______

EMPLOYED _______ EDUCATION _______

HEARING AID WEARER: Yes ☐ No ☐

PRIOR AURAL REHABILITATION COURSE EXPERIENCE? ___________ IF YES, WHEN? ___________

C. Answer Sheet

1 — Practically Always
2 — Frequently
3 — About Half The Time
4 — Occasionally
5 — Almost Never
6 — Does Not Apply

	1	2	3	4	5		6			1	2	3	4	5		6
1.	☐	☐	☐	☐	☐	—	☐	33.	☐	☐	☐	☐	☐	—	☐
2.	☐	☐	☐	☐	☐	—	☐	34.	☐	☐	☐	☐	☐	—	☐
3.	☐	☐	☐	☐	☐	—	☐	35.	☐	☐	☐	☐	☐	—	☐
4.	☐	☐	☐	☐	☐	—	☐	36.	☐	☐	☐	☐	☐	—	☐
5.	☐	☐	☐	☐	☐	—	☐	37.	☐	☐	☐	☐	☐	—	☐
6.	☐	☐	☐	☐	☐	—	☐	38.	☐	☐	☐	☐	☐	—	☐
7.	☐	☐	☐	☐	☐	—	☐	39.	☐	☐	☐	☐	☐	—	☐
8.	☐	☐	☐	☐	☐	—	☐	40.	☐	☐	☐	☐	☐	—	☐
9.	☐	☐	☐	☐	☐	—	☐	41.	☐	☐	☐	☐	☐	—	☐
10.	☐	☐	☐	☐	☐	—	☐	42.	☐	☐	☐	☐	☐	—	☐
11.	☐	☐	☐	☐	☐	—	☐	43.	☐	☐	☐	☐	☐	—	☐
12.	☐	☐	☐	☐	☐	—	☐	44.	☐	☐	☐	☐	☐	—	☐
13.	☐	☐	☐	☐	☐	—	☐	45.	☐	☐	☐	☐	☐	—	☐
14.	☐	☐	☐	☐	☐	—	☐	46.	☐	☐	☐	☐	☐	—	☐
15.	☐	☐	☐	☐	☐	—	☐	47.	☐	☐	☐	☐	☐	—	☐
16.	☐	☐	☐	☐	☐	—	☐	48.	☐	☐	☐	☐	☐	—	☐
17.	☐	☐	☐	☐	☐	—	☐	49.	☐	☐	☐	☐	☐	—	☐
18.	☐	☐	☐	☐	☐	—	☐	50.	☐	☐	☐	☐	☐	—	☐
19.	☐	☐	☐	☐	☐	—	☐	51.	☐	☐	☐	☐	☐	—	☐
20.	☐	☐	☐	☐	☐	—	☐	52.	☐	☐	☐	☐	☐	—	☐
21.	☐	☐	☐	☐	☐	—	☐	53.	☐	☐	☐	☐	☐	—	☐
22.	☐	☐	☐	☐	☐	—	☐	54.	☐	☐	☐	☐	☐	—	☐
23.	☐	☐	☐	☐	☐	—	☐	55.	☐	☐	☐	☐	☐	—	☐
24.	☐	☐	☐	☐	☐	—	☐	56.	☐	☐	☐	☐	☐	—	☐
25.	☐	☐	☐	☐	☐	—	☐	57.	☐	☐	☐	☐	☐	—	☐
26.	☐	☐	☐	☐	☐	—	☐	58.	☐	☐	☐	☐	☐	—	☐
27.	☐	☐	☐	☐	☐	—	☐	59.	☐	☐	☐	☐	☐	—	☐
28.	☐	☐	☐	☐	☐	—	☐	60.	☐	☐	☐	☐	☐	—	☐
29.	☐	☐	☐	☐	☐	—	☐	61.	☐	☐	☐	☐	☐	—	☐
30.	☐	☐	☐	☐	☐	—	☐	62.	☐	☐	☐	☐	☐	—	☐
31.	☐	☐	☐	☐	☐	—	☐	63.	☐	☐	☐	☐	☐	—	☐
32.	☐	☐	☐	☐	☐	—	☐	64.	☐	☐	☐	☐	☐	—	☐

	Practically Always	Frequently	About Half The Time	Occasionally	Almost Never		Does Not Apply
	1	2	3	4	5		6
65.	☐	☐	☐	☐	☐	—	☐
66.	☐	☐	☐	☐	☐	—	☐
67.	☐	☐	☐	☐	☐	—	☐
68.	☐	☐	☐	☐	☐	—	☐
69.	☐	☐	☐	☐	☐	—	☐
70.	☐	☐	☐	☐	☐	—	☐
71.	☐	☐	☐	☐	☐	—	☐
72.	☐	☐	☐	☐	☐	—	☐
73.	☐	☐	☐	☐	☐	—	☐
74.	☐	☐	☐	☐	☐	—	☐
75.	☐	☐	☐	☐	☐	—	☐
76.	☐	☐	☐	☐	☐	—	☐
77.	☐	☐	☐	☐	☐	—	☐
78.	☐	☐	☐	☐	☐	—	☐
79.	☐	☐	☐	☐	☐	—	☐
*80.	☐	☐	☐	☐	☐	—	☐
81.	☐	☐	☐	☐	☐	—	☐
82.	☐	☐	☐	☐	☐	—	☐
83.	☐	☐	☐	☐	☐	—	☐
84.	☐	☐	☐	☐	☐	—	☐
85.	☐	☐	☐	☐	☐	—	☐
*86.	☐	☐	☐	☐	☐	—	☐
87.	☐	☐	☐	☐	☐	—	☐
88.	☐	☐	☐	☐	☐	—	☐
89.	☐	☐	☐	☐	☐	—	☐
90.	☐	☐	☐	☐	☐	—	☐
91.	☐	☐	☐	☐	☐	—	☐
92.	☐	☐	☐	☐	☐	—	☐
93.	☐	☐	☐	☐	☐	—	☐
*94.	☐	☐	☐	☐	☐	—	☐
95.	☐	☐	☐	☐	☐	—	☐
96.	☐	☐	☐	☐	☐	—	☐

	Practically Always	Frequently	About Half The Time	Occasionally	Almost Never		Does Not Apply
	1	2	3	4	5		6
97.	☐	☐	☐	☐	☐	—	☐
98.	☐	☐	☐	☐	☐	—	☐
99.	☐	☐	☐	☐	☐	—	☐
100.	☐	☐	☐	☐	☐	—	☐
101.	☐	☐	☐	☐	☐	—	☐
102.	☐	☐	☐	☐	☐	—	☐
103.	☐	☐	☐	☐	☐	—	☐
104.	☐	☐	☐	☐	☐	—	☐
105.	☐	☐	☐	☐	☐	—	☐
106.	☐	☐	☐	☐	☐	—	☐
107.	☐	☐	☐	☐	☐	—	☐
108.	☐	☐	☐	☐	☐	—	☐
109.	☐	☐	☐	☐	☐	—	☐
110.	☐	☐	☐	☐	☐	—	☐
111.	☐	☐	☐	☐	☐	—	☐
112.	☐	☐	☐	☐	☐	—	☐
113.	☐	☐	☐	☐	☐	—	☐
114.	☐	☐	☐	☐	☐	—	☐
115.	☐	☐	☐	☐	☐	—	☐
116.	☐	☐	☐	☐	☐	—	☐
117.	☐	☐	☐	☐	☐	—	☐
118.	☐	☐	☐	☐	☐	—	☐
119.	☐	☐	☐	☐	☐	—	☐
120.	☐	☐	☐	☐	☐	—	☐
121.	☐	☐	☐	☐	☐	—	☐
122.	☐	☐	☐	☐	☐	—	☐
123.	☐	☐	☐	☐	☐	—	☐
*124.	☐	☐	☐	☐	☐	—	☐
*125.	☐	☐	☐	☐	☐	—	☐
*126.	☐	☐	☐	☐	☐	—	☐
*127.	☐	☐	☐	☐	☐	—	☐

*Items to be reversed before scoring.

	Practically Always	Frequently	About Half The Time	Occasionally	Almost Never		Does Not Apply
	1	2	3	4	5		6
*128.	☐	☐	☐	☐	☐	—	☐
*129.	☐	☐	☐	☐	☐	—	☐
*130.	☐	☐	☐	☐	☐	—	☐
*131.	☐	☐	☐	☐	☐	—	☐
132.	☐	☐	☐	☐	☐	—	☐
133.	☐	☐	☐	☐	☐	—	☐
134.	☐	☐	☐	☐	☐	—	☐
135.	☐	☐	☐	☐	☐	—	☐
136.	☐	☐	☐	☐	☐	—	☐
137.	☐	☐	☐	☐	☐	—	☐
138.	☐	☐	☐	☐	☐	—	☐
139.	☐	☐	☐	☐	☐	—	☐
140.	☐	☐	☐	☐	☐	—	☐
141.	☐	☐	☐	☐	☐	—	☐
142.	☐	☐	☐	☐	☐	—	☐
143.	☐	☐	☐	☐	☐	—	☐

	Practically Always	Frequently	About Half The Time	Occasionally	Almost Never		Does Not Apply
	1	2	3	4	5		6
144.	☐	☐	☐	☐	☐	—	☐
*145.	☐	☐	☐	☐	☐	—	☐
146.	☐	☐	☐	☐	☐	—	☐
147.	☐	☐	☐	☐	☐	—	☐
148.	☐	☐	☐	☐	☐	—	☐
*149.	☐	☐	☐	☐	☐	—	☐
150.	☐	☐	☐	☐	☐	—	☐
151.	☐	☐	☐	☐	☐	—	☐
*152.	☐	☐	☐	☐	☐	—	☐
153.	☐	☐	☐	☐	☐	—	☐
154.	☐	☐	☐	☐	☐	—	☐
155.	☐	☐	☐	☐	☐	—	☐
*156.	☐	☐	☐	☐	☐	—	☐
*157.	☐	☐	☐	☐	☐	—	☐
*158.	☐	☐	☐	☐	☐	—	☐

*Items to be reversed before scoring.

D. Index of Items by Numbers for HPI Sections and Categories

Within the categories, the Social items are underlined and Occupational items are in parentheses. Formats follow tables in the text.

Sections

Understanding Speech: 1-56; 109-123
                With visual cues: 1-7, 10-19, 23-51, 54-55
                With no visual cues: 8, 9, 20-22, 52-53, 56, 109-123
Intensity: 57-75
Response to Auditory Failure: 76-108
Social: 10-13, 36-53, 78, 82, 84, 86-89, 91-94, 96-97, 99-102, 106, 112-123
Personal: 124-131
Occupational: 132-158
  Understanding Speech: 132-144
  Response to Auditory Failure: 145-155
  Personal: 156-158

Categories

Understanding Speech
　*Talker (one to one): 1-7, 10-11, 14-15, 18-19, 25-42, 54-55, 132-134, 137-142.
　　Male: 1, 4, 14, 18, 25, 28, *36, 39,* 55, (133, 139, 140)
　　Female: 2, 3, 15, 19, 26-27, 29, *37-38,* 54, (132, 137, 138)
　　Child: 5, 30, 31
　　Friend/family member: 1, 2, 7, *10-11,* 25-27, 34-35, *36-39, 41-42*
　　Stranger: 3, 4, 28, 29, *40*
　　Co-worker: (132-133, 137-140)
　　Employer: (134, 141-142)
　　Waiter/waitress: 6, 32, 33
Communicative Situations
　One to one (alone): 1-5, 7, 25-29, 30-31, 34-35, (132-134, 137-142)
　One to one in group less than 10: *10, 36-37*
　One to one in group more than 20: *38-40*
　One to one in group playing cards, etc.: *11, 41-42*
　*Group conversation: *12-13, 43-48, 50-51,* (135-136, 143-144)
　　5 or 6 friends/family members: *12, 47*
　　　Within group > 20: *43, 45-46*
　　5 or 6 strangers: *13, 48*
　　　Within group > 20: *44*
　　5 or 6 co-workers: (135-136, 143-144)
　　Several friends (automobile): *50-51*
　　One talker at a time: *12, 13, 43-46,* (135-136, 143)
　　　Aware of subject: *12, 43-44,* (135)
　　　Subject changes: *13, 45-46,* (136, 143)
　　Talkers interrupting: *48,* (144)
Communication Systems
　Public address (microphone)
　　Auditorium: 18, 19
　Television
　　News: 14, 15
　　Drama or movie: 16, 17
　Movie: 23
　Stage Play: 24
Noise Environment
　Fairly quiet: 1-7, *10-13,* 16, *50,* (132-136)
　Music, etc.: 17, 27-29, 31, 33, 35, *40, 42-44, 46-47, 51,* 54-55, (138, 140)
　People talking nearby: 25-26, 30, 32, 34, *36-39, 41, 45, 49,* (137, 139, 141)
Miscellaneous Situations
　Restaurant: 6, 7, 32-35
　Ticket-information booth: 54-55
　Dinner: *47*
Understanding Speech—no visual cues: 8, 9, 20-22, 52-53, 56, 109-111, 112-123
　Talker (one to one)
　　Male: 8, 21
　　Female: 9, 22
　　Friend/family member: 109, *112-114*
　　Stranger: 110-111, *115*
　Communicative Situations
　　One to one: 109-111　　Other room: 8, 9, 56
　　One to one, group: *112-115*
　　*Group conversations: *52-53, 116-123*
　　　5-6 friends/family: *116-117, 120-121*
　　　5-6 strangers: *118-119*
　　　Automobile: *52-53*
　　　Games: *122-123*
　　　One talker: *116-120*

*Because items comprising the subheadings are not mutually exclusive, the items comprising the total category are provided.

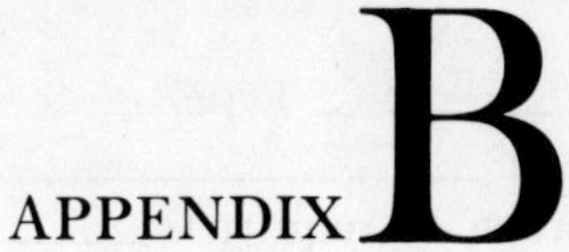

APPENDIX B

Auditory

Rehabilitation

Questionnaire

Dalhousie University
School of Human
Communication Disorders

Name:____

File:____

1. Statement of the problem by the hearing impaired person.

2. Does the hearing impaired person have difficulty in:
   (a) a person-to-person situation — facing?
   (b) a person-to-person situation — head turned?
   (c) groups as a whole?
   (d) using a telephone — hearing bell?
       using a telephone — hearing speech?
       using a telephone — without extra amplification?

3. Does the hearing impaired person have speech that is difficult for other people to understand:
   (a) person to person?
   (b) in group situations?
   (c) using telephone

4. Is a hearing aid worn? ______ Type?
   Needs repairs? ______ Needs Replacement?

   ____.

   Telephone attachment used? ______ Type?________________________.
   Public Announcement System helpful?
   _________________________. Type? ______ Is TTY used? ______

Own?____Type? ______

Is manual communication used? ______ System?__________________

_______________________ . Would an interpreter be required? ______

How often?

____ .

5. Does a hearing impaired person have difficulty with alerting systems?

____

____ .

6. Does the hearing impaired person have a tendency to ear infections, etc.
    (e.g., liable to frequent illness, has to be careful about environment?)

____

____ .

7. Does the hearing impaired person have a progressive problem?

____ .

8. Does the hearing impaired person attend remedial classes (e.g.,
    lipreading?)

____

____ .

Type?

____ .

9. Has past vocational training been affected by subsequent loss of hearing?

____

____ .

10. Does the hearing impaired person have a preferred vocational training
    other than received in the past?

____

____ .

11. Does the hearing impaired person need a vocational update?

____

____ .

Scoring of Questionnaire

(½ points given where no clear positive or negative was apparent)

1. The "statement" seemed to revolve around the desire to work, thus it was decided to score '0' for seeking a job and a '1' for being unable to do so.
2. This section relates to ability to comprehend the spoken word, including telephone without hearing aid. Separate points are given for a, b, c, d - if a person is able to communicate normally the result will be all zeros.
3. This section relates to the person's own speech ability.
4. This section relates to the actual use of a hearing aid and the ability to communicate by *either* aided telephone *or* T.T.Y.; this section also indicates the alternative use of manual communication and/or interpreter.

   The completely adequate use of hearing aid would thus give all zeros and constitute no handicap, but with each limitation one point is added - as being representative of the *work* situation.

5. This is given separate weighting because employers generally complain most of this "problem".
6. This question relates to possible problems in work attendance.
7. This is given separate weighting because it might mean a gradual change in score throughout the questionnaire.
8. This question is given separate weighting to accommodate sudden onset or progressive hearing loss.
9. This question relates to sudden onset or progressive loss.
10. This section relates to the fact that many deaf persons have had no choice of vocational training or perhaps would respond to further training.
11. This section relates to all, as it would to the normal hearing person.

   It will be seen that the questionnaire is both objective and subjective. The score indicates the extent of the problem only. The interpretation lies in the written answers, either given verbally to the interviewer, or through an Interpreter.

Joyce D. Edwards, Ph.D.
Assistant Professor

BIBLIOGRAPHY

AA00 Committee on Conservation of Hearing. 1959. Guide for the evaluation of hearing impairment. *Trans. Am. Acad. Ophthalmol. Otolaryngol.* 63:236-238.

Aballi, A.J. and Korones, S.B. 1963. The newborn infant. In *Synopsis of pediatrics,* ed. J.G. Hughes. St. Louis: The C.V. Mosby Co.

Abrams, I.F. 1977. Nongenetic hearing loss. In *Hearing loss in children,* ed. B.F. Jaffe. Baltimore: University Park Press.

Affias, S. and Embil, J.A. 1978. Congenital infections and the TORCH syndrome. *The Nova Scotia Medical Bulletin,* 57: 43-47.

Alport, A.C. 1927. Hereditary familial congenital haemorrhagic nephritis. *Brit. Med. J.* 1: 504-506.

American Academy of Otolaryngology and the American Council of Otolaryngology 1979. Guide for the evaluation of hearing handicap. *JAMA* 241: 2055-2059.

Amstey, M.S. 1977. Maternal viral infection with adverse results: cytomegalovirus and herpes virus. *Seminars in Perinatology* 1: 1-10.

Anderson, H., Barr, B. and Wedenberg, E. 1970. Genetic disposition as a prerequisite for maternal rubella deafness. *Arch. Otolaryngol.* 91: 141-174.

ANSI S3.6 1969. American National Standard Specifications for Audiometers.

Arnst, D.J. 1980. Personal communication.

Baldursson, G., Bjarnason, O., Halldorsson, S., Juliusdottir, E., and Kjeld, M. 1972. Maternal rubella in Iceland 1963-1964. *Scandinavian Audiol.* 1:3-10.

Barr, B. 1965. Early primary screening. In The young deaf child, ed. H. Davis. *Acta Otolaryngol.* Supp., Stockholm, 206:45-47.

Bartram, J.B. 1975. Cerebral dysfunction (learning disorders). In *Nelson's textbook of pediatrics,* eds. V.C. Vaughn, R.J. McKay and W.E. Nelson. Philadelphia: W.B. Saunders, Co.

Batteau, D.W. 1967. The role of the pinna in human localization. *Proceedings of the Royal Society* (London), Ser. B. 168: 158-180.

Battin, R.R. 1979. The effects of early middle ear problems on later learning development revisited. *Corti's Organ* 4: 4.

Bergstrom, L. 1976. Congenital deafness. In *Hearing disorders,* ed. J.L. Northern. Boston: Little, Brown and Co.

Bergstrom, L. 1977. Viruses that deafen. In *Childhood deafness,* ed. F.H. Bess. New York: Grune and Stratton, Inc.

Bergstrom, L. and Thompson, P. 1976. Ototoxicity. In *Hearing disorders,* ed. J.L. Northern. Boston: Little, Brown and Co.

Berkow, R. 1977. *The Merck manual.* 13 ed. Rahway: Dohme Research Laboratories.

Bocca, E. and Calearo, C. 1963. Central hearing processes. In *Modern developments in audiology,* ed. J. Jerger. New York: Academic Press.

Boedts, D. 1967. La surdité dans la dysostose craniofaciale ou maladie de Crouzon. *Acta Otolaryngol. Belg.* 21: 143-155.

Bohne, B.A. 1976. Mechanisms of noise damage in the inner ear. In *Effects of noise on hearing,* eds. D. Henderson, R.P. Hamernik, D.S. Dosanjh, and J. Mills. New York: Raven Press.

Bordley, J.E., Brookhouser, P.E., Hardy, J., et al. 1967. Observations on the effect of prenatal rubella in hearing. In *Deafness in childhood,* eds. F. McConnell and P.H. Ward. Nashville: Vanderbilt Univ. Press.

Bordley, J.E., Brookhouser, P.E. and Worthington, E.L. 1971. Viral infections and hearing: a critical review of the literature. *Laryngoscope* 81: 557-579.

Brazelton, T.B. 1969. *Infants and mothers: differences in development.* New York: Delacorte.

Brookhouser, P.E. and Bordley, J.E. 1973. Congenital rubella deafness. *Arch. Otolaryngol.* 98: 252-256.

Bryarly, R.C., Veach, S.R., and Kornblut, A.D. 1980. Metastatsizing auricular basal cell carcinoma. *Otolaryngol. Head Neck Surg.* 88: 40-43.

Burns, W. 1969. *Noise and man.* Philadelphia: J.B. Lippincott.

Carhart, R. 1950. The clinical application of bone conduction audiometry. *Arch. Otolaryngol.* 51: 789-807.

Carrel, R.J. 1977. Epidemiology of hearing loss. In *Audiometry in infancy,* ed. S.E. Gerber. New York: Grune and Stratton, Inc.

Catlin, F.I. 1978. Etiology and pathology of hearing loss in children. In *Pediatric audiology,* ed. F. Martin. Englewood Cliffs: Prentice-Hall, Inc.

Cherry, E.C. 1966. *On human communication.* 2d ed. Cambridge: The M.I.T. Press.

Cody, D.T.R. 1978. Otologic assessment and treatment. In *Audiological assessment.* 2nd ed., ed. D.E. Rose. Englewood Cliffs: Prentice-Hall, Inc.

Corso, J.F. 1963. Age and sex differences in pure-tone thresholds. *Arch. Otolaryngol.* 77: 398-399.

Cotton, R. 1977. Progressive hearing loss. In *Hearing loss in children,* ed. B.F. Jaffe. Baltimore: University Park Press.

Dahle, A.J., McCollister, F.P., Hamner, B.A., et al. 1974. Subclinical congenital cytomegalovirus infection and hearing impairment. *J. Speech Hear. Dis.* 39: 320-329.

Dahle, A.J., McCollister, F.P., Stagno, S., et al. 1979. Progressive hearing impairment in children with congenital cytomegalovirus infection. *J. Speech Hear. Dis.* 44: 220-229.

Dallos, P. 1964. Dynamics of the acoustic reflex: phenomenological aspects. *J. Acoust. Soc. Amer.* 36: 2175-2183.

Davis, H. 1948. The articulation area and the social adequacy index for hearing. *Laryngoscope* 58: 761-778.

Davis, H. 1976. Principles of electric response audiometry. *Ann. Otol. Rhinol. Laryngol.* Suppl. 28, 85: No. 3, part 3.

Davis, H. 1978. Audiometry: other auditory tests. In *Hearing and deafness.* 4th ed., eds. H. Davis and S.R. Silverman. New York: Holt, Rinehart and Winston.

Davis, H., Gernardt, B.E., Riesco-MacClure, J.S., and Covell, W.P. 1949. Aural microphonics in the cochlea of the guinea pig. *J. Acoust. Soc. Amer.* 21:502-510.

Davis, H. and Silverman, S.R. 1978. *Hearing and deafness.* 4th ed. New York: Holt, Rinehart and Winston.

DeBoer, E. 1967. Correlation studies applied to the frequency resolution of the cochlea. *J. Auditory Res.* 7: 209-217.

DeBoer, E. and Bouwmeester, J. 1975. Clinical psychophysics illustrated by the problem of auditory overload. *Audiology* 14: 274-299.

Derbyshire, A.J. 1970. Personal correspondence.

Derlacki, E. 1976. Otosclerosis. In *Hearing disorders,* ed., J.L. Northern. Boston: Little, Brown and Co.

DiBartolomeo, J.R. 1979. Exostoses of the external auditory canal. *Ann. Otol. Rhinol. Laryngol.* Suppl. 61, 88: 1-20.

DiBartolomeo, J.R. and Gerber, S.E. 1977. Pathology of hearing loss. In *Audiometry in infancy,* ed. S.E. Gerber. New York: Grune & Stratton, Inc.

Downs, M.P. 1976. Early identification of hearing loss: Where are we? Where do we go from here? In *Early identification of hearing loss,* ed. G.T. Mencher. Basel: S. Karger.

Downs, M.P. 1978. The handicap of deafness. In *Hearing disorders,* ed. J.L. Northern. Boston: Little, Brown and Co.

Downs, M.P. 1978. The interaction of critical periods with conductive losses. Presented to sixth annual meeting of Society for Ear, Nose and Throat Advances In Children. Santa Barbara.

Downs, M.P. and Silver, H.K. 1972. The A.B.C.D.'s to H.E.A.R. Early identification in nursery, office and clinic of the infant who is deaf. *Clin. Pediatr.* 11: 563-566.

Duane, D.D. 1977. A neurologic perspective of central auditory dysfunction. In *Central auditory dysfunction*, ed. R.W. Keith. New York: Grune & Stratton, Inc.

Dublin, W.B. 1976. *Fundamentals of sensorineural auditory pathology*. Springfield, IL: Charles C. Thomas.

Durrant, J.D. 1978. Anatomical and physiologic correlates of the effects of noise on hearing. In *Noise and audiology*, ed. D. Lipscomb. Baltimore: University Park Press.

Eames, B.L., Hamernik, R., Henderson, D., and Feldman, A. 1975. The role of the middle ear in acoustic trauma from impulses. *Laryngoscope* 85: 1582-1592.

Edwards, J.D. 1979. Unpublished manuscript.

Eichenwald, H. 1979. Rationale and efficacy of antibiotics use in ear, nose and throat practice. Presented to the Seventh Annual Meeting of the Society for Ear, Nose and Throat Advances in Children. Cincinnati.

Evans, E.F. and Wilson, J.P. 1977. *Psychophysics and physiology of hearing*. London: Academic Press.

Ewertsen, H. and Birk-Nielsen, H. 1973. Social hearing handicap index. *Audiology* 12: 180-187.

Feinmesser, M. and Tell, L. 1976. Evaluation of methods for detecting hearing impairment in infancy and early childhood. In *Early identification of hearing loss*, ed. G.T. Mencher. Basel: S. Karger.

Feldman, A.S. 1978. Acoustic impedance-admittance battery. In *Handbook of clinical audiology*, 2d ed., ed. J. Katz. Baltimore: Williams & Wilkins Co.

Feldman, A.S. and Wilber, L.A. 1976. *Acoustic impedance and admittance - the measurement of middle ear function*. Baltimore: Williams & Wilkins Co.

Fraser, G.R. 1971. The genetics of congenital deafness. *Otolaryngol. Clin. N. Amer.* 4: 227-247.

Fraser, G.R. 1976. *The causes of profound deafness in childhood*. Baltimore: The Johns Hopkins University Press.

Friedman, H. and Prier, J.E., eds. 1973. *Rubella*. First Annual Symposium of the Eastern Pennsylvania Branch, American Society for Microbiology. Springfield, IL: Charles C. Thomas Publisher.

Gerber, S.E. 1965. *Evaluation of air force hearing data*. Fullerton: Hughes Aircraft Co., Ground Systems Group.

Gerber, S.E. ed. 1974. *Introductory hearing science*. Philadelphia: W.B. Saunders Co.

Gerber, S.E. 1975. Will cochlear implants aid childhood deafness? *Clin. Pediatr.* July, p. 623.

Gerber, S.E. 1977. Prevention of handicap by early detection. Presented to Interprofessional Forum on Learning. University of Santa Clara.

Gerber, S.E. 1977. High-risk conditions. In *Audiometry in infancy*, ed. S.E. Gerber. New York: Grune & Stratton, Inc.

Gerber, S.E. and Mencher, G.T. eds. 1978. *Early diagnosis of hearing loss*. New York: Grune & Stratton, Inc.

Gerber, S.E., Mendel, M.I., and Goller, M. 1979. Progressive hearing loss subsequent to congenital cytomegalovirus infection. *Human Communication* 4: 231-234.

Giolas, T.G., Owens, E., Lamb, S., and Schubert, E. 1979. Hearing performance inventory. *J. Speech Hear. Dis.* 44: 169-195.

Glattke, T.J. 1978. Electronystagmography. In *Handbook of clinical audiology*, 2d ed., ed. J. Katz. Baltimore: Williams & Wilkins Co.

Glorig, A. 1953. Noise in industry. *Amer. Industrial Hygiene Assoc. Quart.* 14: No. 3.

Glorig, A., Wheeler, D., Quiggle, R., Grings, W., and Summerfield, A., 1957. 1954 Wisconsin State Fair hearing survey. *Amer. Acad. Ophthalmol. Otolaryngol. Monograph.*

Glorig, A., Ward, W.D., and Nixon, J. 1961. Damage risk criteria and noise induced hearing loss. *Arch. Otolaryngol.* 74: 413-23.

Goin, D.W. 1976. Otospongiosis. In *Otolaryngology: A textbook,* ed. G. English. New York: Harper & Row, Inc.

Goodhill, V. 1979. Otologic relationships with audiology. In *Hearing and hearing impairment,* eds. L.J. Bradford and W.G. Hardy. New York: Grune & Stratton, Inc.

Goodhill, V. ed. 1979. *Ear diseases, deafness, and dizziness.* New York: Harper and Row, Inc.

Goodhill, V. and Brockman, S.J. 1979. Secretory otitis media. In *Ear diseases, deafness, and dizziness,* ed. V. Goodhill. New York: Harper & Row, Inc.

Goodhill, V. and Harris, I. 1979. Examination of the dizzy patient. In *Ear diseases, deafness, and dizziness,* ed. V. Goodhill. New York: Harper and Row, Inc.

Goodhill, V. and Harris, I. 1979. Peripheral vertigo, labyrinthitis, and Ménière's Disease. In *Ear diseases, deafness, and dizziness,* ed. V. Goodhill. New York: Harper and Row, Inc.

Goodhill V. and Harris, I. 1979. Sudden hearing loss syndrome. In *Ear diseases, deafness and dizziness,* ed. V. Goodhill. New York: Harper & Row, Inc.

Gregg, N.M. 1941. Congenital cataract following German measles in the mother. *Trans. Ophthal. Soc. Aust. 3:35-46.*

Gregson, A.E., and LaTouche, C.J. 1961. Otomycosis: a neglected disease. *J. Laryngol. Otol.* 75:45-69.

Gulick, W.L. 1971. *Hearing: physiology and psychophysics.* New York: Oxford University Press.

Hanshaw, J.B. 1979. Cytomegaloviral infection. In *Textbook of pediatrics,* eds. V.C. Vaughan, R.J. McKay, and R.E. Behrman. Philadelphia: W.B. Saunders Co.

Hanshaw, J.B. and Dudgeon, J.A. 1978. Viral diseases of the fetus and newborn. *Major problems in clin. pediatr.* 17:1-9.

Hanshaw, J.B., Scheiner, A.P., Moxley, A.W., Gaev, L., Abel, V. and Scheiner, B. 1976. School failure and deafness after "silent" CMV infection. *New Engl. J. Med.* 295:468-470.

Hanson, D.G. and Ulvestad, R.F. 1979. Otitis media and child development. *Ann. Otol. Rhinol. and Laryngol.* Suppl. 60, 88:1-112.

Hardy, J.B. 1973. Fetal consequences of maternal virus infections in pregnancy. *Arch. Otolaryngol.* 98:218-27.

Hardy, J.B., Sever, J.L., and Gilkeson, M.R. 1969. Declining antibody titers in children with congenital rubella. *J. Pediatr.* 75:213-220.

Hardy, W.G. and Bordley, J.E. 1973. Problems in diagnosis and management of the multiply handicapped deaf child. *Arch. Otolaryngol.* 98:269-274.

Hawkins, J.E. 1975. Drug ototoxicity. In *Differential diagnosis in pediatric otolaryngology,* ed. M. Strome. Boston: Little, Brown and Co.

Hawkins, J.E., Johnsson, L.G. and Aran, J.M. 1969. Comparative tests of gentamycin ototoxicity. *J. Infect. Dis.* 119:417-431.

Holvey, D.N. 1972. *The Merck manual.* Rahway: Merck & Co., Inc.

House, W.F. 1975. Ménières Disease: management and theory. In Symposium on fluctuant hearing loss, ed. J.J. Shea. *The Otol. Clinics of N. Amer.* 8:505-535.

Howie, V.M. 1975. Natural history of otitis media. *Ann. Otol. Rhinol. Laryngol.* Suppl. 19, 85:67-72.

Howie, V.M. 1977. Acute and recurrent acute otitis media. In *Hearing loss in children,* ed. B.F. Jaffe. Baltimore: University Park Press.

Howie, V.M. 1978. The effect of early onset of otitis media on educational achievement. Presented to sixth annual meeting of the Society for Ear, Nose and Throat Advances in Children. Santa Barbara.

Hull, R.H. 1978. Assisting with elderly client. In *Handbook of clinical audiology,* 2d. ed. J. Katz. Baltimore: Williams & Wilkins Co.

Ivey, R.G. 1969. *Tests of CNS auditory function.* Unpublished Masters Thesis, Colorado State University, Fort Collins.

Jaffe, B.F. 1976. Pinna anomalies associated with congenital conductive hearing loss. *Pediatr.* 57:332-341.

Jaffe, B.F. ed. 1977. *Hearing loss in children.* Baltimore: University Park Press.

Jaffe, B.F. 1978. Topographical signs associated with congenital hearing loss. In *Early diagnosis of hearing loss,* eds. S.E. Gerber and G.T. Mencher. New York: Grune & Stratton, Inc.

Jaffe, B.F. 1979. The life cycle of middle ear disease in cleft palate children. Presented to seventh annual meeting of Society for Ear, Nose and Throat Advances in Children. Cincinnati.

Jerger, J. 1973. Audiological findings in aging. *Adv. Otorhinolaryngol.* 20:115-124.

Jerger, J.F. and Carhart, R.T. 1956. Temporary threshold shift as an index of noise susceptibility. *J. Acoust. Soc. Amer.* 28:611-613.

Johnson, E.W. 1968. Confirmed retrocochlear lesions. *Arch. Otolaryngol.* 88:598-603.

Karmody, C.S. 1969. Asymptomatic maternal rubella and congenital deafness. *Arch. Otolaryngol.* 89:720.

Katz, J. 1977. The staggered spondaic word test. In *Central auditory dysfunction,* ed. R.W. Keith. New York: Grune & Stratton, Inc.

Katz, J. 1978. The effects of conductive hearing loss on auditory function. *Asha* 20:879-886.

Katz, J. ed. 1978. *Handbook of clinical audiology.* 2d ed. Baltimore: Williams & Wilkins.

Keith, R.W. ed. 1977. *Central auditory dysfunction.* New York: Grune & Stratton, Inc.

Kelemen, G. 1977. Morquio's Disease and the hearing organ. *ORL* 39:233-240.

Kirikae, I. 1973. Physiology of the middle ear including eustachian tube. In *Otolaryngology,* vol. 1, eds. M.M. Paparella and D.A. Schumrick. Philadelphia: W.B. Saunders Co.

Kohji, U., Yukiaki, N., Kenji, O. and Sheppard, T.H. 1979. Congenital rubella syndrome: correlation of gestational age at time of maternal rubella with type of onset. *J. Pediatr.* 94:763-765.

Konigsmark, B.W. 1971. Hereditary and congenital factors affecting newborn sensorineural hearing. In *Conference on newborn hearing screening,* ed. G.C. Cunningham. Berkeley: California Department of Health.

Konigsmark, B.W. 1972. Genetic hearing loss with no associated abnormalities: A review. Part II. *J. Speech Hear. Dis.* 37:89-99.

Konigsmark, B.W. and Gorlin, R.J. 1976. *Genetic and metabolic deafness.* Philadelphia: W.B. Saunders Co.

Kramer, R.I. 1978. Miniseminar on chronic otitis media. Presented to the Annual Convention of the American Speech and Hearing Assn. San Francisco.

Kryter, K.D. 1970. *Effects of noise on man.* New York: Academic Press.

Lempert, J. 1938. Improvement of hearing in cases of otosclerosis: A new one-stage surgical technic. *Arch. Otolaryngol.* 28:42-97.

Leopold R.E. 1979. *A retrospective study of the relationship between preinatal anoxia and communicative disorders.* Unpublished Masters Thesis, University of California, Santa Barbara.

Leroy, J.G. and Crocker, A.C. 1966. Clinical definition of Hunter-Hurler phenotypes. A review of 50 patients. *Am. J. Dis. Child* 112:518-530.

Lindsay, J.R. 1973. Otosclerosis. In *Otolaryngology*, vol. 2 eds. M.M. Paparella and D.A. Shumrick.Philadelphia: W.B. Saunders Co.

Lindsay, J.R. and Matz, G. 1966. The differentiation of acquired congenital from genetically determined inner ear deafness. *Ann. Otol. Rhinol. Laryngol.* 75:830-843.

McCabe, B.F. 1963. The etiology of deafness. *Volta Rev.* 65:471-477.

MacKenzie, I. 1965. Consequences of removing an acoustic neuroma by conventional surgical means. *Proc. R. Soc. Med.* 58:1071.

Manson, M.M., Logan, W.P.D. and Loy, R.M. 1960. *Rubella and other virus infections during pregnancy.* London: H.M. Stationery Office.

Marx, J.L. 1977. Cytomegalovirus: A major cause of birth defects. *Science,* 190:1184-1186.

Matzker, J. 1959. Two new methods for the assessment of central auditory functions in cases of brain disease. *Ann. Otol. Rhinol. Laryngol.* 68:1185-1197.

Mawson, S.R. 1967. *Diseases of the ear.* London: Edward Arnold.

Mencher, G.T., ed. 1976. *Early identification of hearing loss.* Basel: S. Karger.

Mencher, G.T. 1976. Personal communication.

Mencher, G.T., Baldursson, M.S., Tell, L. and Levi, C. 1978. Mass behavioral screening and follow-up. Presented to the meeting of the National Research Council-National Academy of Sciences. Assembly of Behavioral and Social Sciences Meeting of the Committee on Hearing, Bioacoustics and Biomechanics. Omaha.

Mencher, G.T. and Stick, S.L. 1976. On beyond the cochlea: auditory perceptual disorders. In *Early identification of hearing loss,* ed. G.T. Mencher. Basel: S. Karger.

Mendel, M.I. 1977. Electroencephalic tests of hearing. In *Audiometry in infancy,* ed. S.E. Gerber. New York: Grune & Stratton, Inc.

Monif, G. and Jordon, P.A. 1977. Rubella virus and rubella vaccine. *Seminars in Perinatology,* 1:41-49.

Myers, E.N. and Stool, S. 1968. Cytomegalic inclusion disease of the inner ear. *Laryngoscope* 78:1904-1915.

Nager, G.T. 1973. Congenital aural atresia: anatomy and surgical management. In *Otolaryngology*, vol. 2, eds. M.M. Paparella and D.A. Shumrick. Philadelphia: W.B. Saunders Co.

Naunton, R.F. 1973. Presbycusis. In *Otolaryngology*, vol. 2, eds. M.M. Paparella and D.A. Shumrick. Philadelphia: W.B. Saunders Co.

Newby, H.A. 1979. *Audiology.* 4th ed. Englewood Cliffs: Prentice-Hall, Inc.

Newman, M.H. 1975. Hearing loss. In *Differential diagnosis in pediatric otolaryngology,* ed. M. Strome. Boston: Little, Brown and Co.

Noble, W. and Atherley, G. 1970. The hearing measurement scale: a questionnaire for the assessment of auditory disability. *J. Aud. Research* 10:229-250.

Northern, J.L. 1979. Tinnitus — a continuing enigma. *Hearing Inst.* 30:11, 46.

Northern, J.L. 1977. Acoustic impedance in the pediatric population. In *Childhood deafness: causation, assessment, and management,* ed. F. Bess. New York: Grune & Stratton, Inc.

Paparella, M.M. 1973. Cysts and tumors of the external ear. In *Otolaryngology,* vol. 2, eds. M.M. Paparella and D.A. Shumrick. Philadelphia: W.B. Saunders Co.

Paparella, M.M. 1973. Surgery of the middle ear, eustachian tube and mastoid. In *Otolaryngology* vol. 2, eds. M.M. Paparella and D.A. Shumrick. Philadelphia: W.B. Saunders Co.

Paparella, M.M. and Capps, M.J. 1973. Sensorineural deafness in children-nongenetic. In *Otolaryngology*, vol. 2, eds. M.M. Paparella and D.A. Shumrick. Philadelphia: W.B. Saunders Co.

Payne, E.E. and Paparella, M.M. 1976. Otitis media. In *Hearing disorders*, ed. J.L. Northern. Boston: Little, Brown and Co.

Penfield, W. and Roberts, L. 1959. *Speech and brain mechanisms.* Princeton: Princeton University Press.

Perkins, R. 1975. Ear bank of project HEAR. *Trans. Amer. Acad. Ophthalmol. and Otolaryngol.* 80:23-29.

Potsic, W. 1978. Miniseminar on chronic otitis media. Presented to the annual convention of the American Speech and Hearing Assn. San Francisco.

Prescod, S.V. 1978. *Audiological handbook of hearing disorders.* New York: Van Nostrand Reinhold Co.

Proctor, C. 1977. Congenital rubella and sensorineural hearing loss. *Laryngoscope.* Suppl. 7, 87:1-60.

Pulec, J.L. 1973. Surgery of the inner ear and retrocochlear region. In *Otolaryngology*, vol. 2, eds. M.M. Paparella and D.A. Shumrick. Philadelphia: W.B. Saunders Co.

Pulec, J.L. 1976. Ménière's Disease. In *Hearing disorders*, ed. J.L. Northern. Boston: Little, Brown and Co.

Quick, C.A. 1973. Chemical and drug effects on the inner ear. In *Otolaryngology*, vol. 2, eds. M.M. Paparella and D.A. Shumrick. Philadelphia: W.B. Saunders Co.

Rapin, I., and Ruben, R.J. 1979. Clinical appraisal of auditory function. Presented to the symposium on Developmental Disabilities in the Preschool Child, Chicago.

Robertson, C. 1978. Pediatric assessment of the infant at risk for deafness. In *Early diagnosis of hearing loss*, eds. S.E. Gerber and G.T. Mencher. New York: Grune & Stratton, Inc.

Rosen, S. 1953. Mobilization of the stapes to restore hearing in otosclerosis. *New York State J. Med.* 53:2650-2653.

Rosen, S., Bergman, M., Plester, D., et al. 1962. Presbycusis study of a relatively noise free population in the Sudan. *Ann. Otol. Rhinol. Laryngol.* 71:727-743.

Ruben, R.J. 1972. The external ear. In *Pediatric otolaryngology*, vol. 2, eds. C. Ferguson & E. Kendig. Philadelphia: W.B. Saunders Co.

Rubin, W. 1968. Sudden hearing loss. *Laryngoscope 78: 829-833.*

Salomon, G. and Starr, A. 1963. Electromyography of middle ear muscles in man during motor activities. *Acta Neuro. Scand.* 39:161.

Sataloff, J. 1966. *Hearing loss.* Philadelphia: J.B. Lippincott Co.

Schein, J.B. and Delk, J.T., Jr. 1974. *The deaf population of the United States.* Silver Springs, MD : Nat'l. Assoc. of the Deaf.

Schuell, H. 1965. *Differential diagnosis of aphasia with the Minnesota test.* Minneapolis: University of Minnesota Press.

Schuknecht, H.F. 1964. Further observations on the pathology of presbycusis. *Arch. Otolaryngol.* 80:369-382.

Schuknecht, H.F. 1974. *Pathology of the ear.* Cambridge: Harvard University Press.

Schuknecht, H.F. 1975. Pathophysiology of Ménière's Disease. In Symposium on fluctuating hearing loss, ed. J.J. Shea, *Otolaryngol. Clin. N. Amer.* 8:507-514.

Sever, J.L. and Bethesda, M.D. 1973. Present status of vaccines for rubella. *Arch. Otolaryngol.* 98:265-268.

Shambaugh, G.E., Jr. 1966. Therapy of cochlear otology. *Ann. Otol. Rhin. Laryng.* 75:579.

Shambaugh, G.E., Jr. 1967. *Surgery of the ear.* 2d ed. Philadelphia: W.B. Saunders Co.

Shulman, J.B. 1979. Ototoxicity. In *Ear diseases, deafness and dizziness*, ed. V. Goodhill. New York: Harper & Row, Inc.

Shulman, J.B. 1979. Traumatic diseases of the ear and temporal bone. In *Ear diseases, deafness and dizziness*, ed. V. Goodhill. New York: Harper & Row, Inc.

Shulman, J.B. 1979. Syphilis of the temporal bone. In *Ear diseases, deafness, and dizziness*, ed. V. Goodhill. New York: Harper & Row, Inc.

Silverman, S.R., Thurlow, W.R., Walsh, T.E., and Davis, H. 1948. Improvement in the social adequacy of hearing following the fenestration operation. *Laryngoscope* 58:607-620.

Simmons, F.B. and Russ, F.N. 1974. Automated newborn hearing screening, the crib-o-gram. *Arch. Otolaryngol.* 100:1-7.

Simons, M.R. 1979. Acoustic impedance tests. In *Ear diseases, deafness, and dizziness*, ed. V. Goodhill. New York: Harper & Row, Inc.

Snow, J.B. 1973. Sudden deafness. In *Otolaryngology*, vol. 2, eds. M.M. Paparella and D.A. Shumrick. Philadelphia: W.B. Saunders Co.

Spoendlin, H. 1976. Anatomical changes following various noise exposures. In *Effects of noise on hearing*, eds. D. Henderson, R. Hamernik, D.S. Dosanjh, and J. Mills. New York: Raven Press.

Strome, M. 1977. Sudden fluctuating hearing losses. In *Hearing loss in children*, ed. B.F. Jaffe. Baltimore: University Park Press.

Tell, L. 1976. Personal communication.

Theissing, G. and Kittel, G. 1962. Die Bedeutung der Toxoplasmose in der Atiologie der connatalen und fruh erworbenen Hörstorungen. *Arch. Ohr. -Nas. -u. Kehlk.-heilk.* 180:219.

Thomsen, J., Terkildsen, K., and Osterhammel, P. 1978. Auditory brain stem responses in patients with acoutic neuromas. *Scand. Audiol.* 7:179-183.

Tietz, W. 1963. A syndrome of deaf-mutism associated with albinism showing dominant autosomal inheritance. *Amer. J. Hum. Genet.* 15:259-264.

Tooley, W. 1973. *Hyperbilirubinemia and respiratory distress syndrome.* 65th Ross Conference. Columbus: Ross Laboratories.

Top, F.H. and Wehrle, P.E. 1976. *Communicable and infectious diseases.* 8th ed. St. Louis: C.V. Mosby Co.

Uziel, A., Romand, R., and Marot, M. 1979. Electrophysiological study of the otoxicity of kanamycin during development in guinea pigs. *Hearing Research* 1:203-212.

Vernon, M. 1969. Usher's Syndrome-deafness and progressive blindness. *J. Chron. Dis.* 22:133-151.

Visencio, L.H. and Gerber, S.E. 1979. Effects of hemodialysis on pure-tone thresholds and blood chemistry measures. *J. Speech Hear. Res.* 22:756-764.

Von Békésy, G. 1956. Current status of theories of hearing. *Science* 123:779-783.

Waardenburg, P.J. 1951. A new syndrome combining developmental anomalies of the eyelids, eyebrow, and nose root with pigmentary defects of the iris and head hair and with congenital deafness. *Amer. J. Human Gen.* 3:195-253.

Wada, J. and Rasmussen, T. 1960. Intracarotid injection of sodium amytal for the lateralization of cerebral speech dominance. Experimental and clinical observations. *J. Neurosurg.* 17:266-282.

Ward, W.D. 1973. Adaptation and fatigue. In *Modern developments in audiology*, 2d ed., ed. J. Jerger. New York: Academic Press.

Ward, W.D. 1976. Public hearings on noise abatement and control. In *Effects of noise on hearing*, eds. D. Henderson, R.D. Hamernik, D.S. Dosanjh, and J.H. Mills. New York: Raven Press.

Weaver, M. and Northern, J.L. 1976. The acoustic nerve tumor. In *Hearing disorders*, ed. J.L. Northern. Boston: Little, Brown and Co.

Weller, T.H. and Hanshaw, J.B. 1962. Virologic and clinical observations on cytomegalic inclusion disease. *N. Engl. J. Med.* 266:1233.

Willeford, J. 1977. Assessing central auditory behavior in children: a test battery approach. In *Central auditory dysfunction*, ed. R.W. Keith. New York: Grune & Stratton, Inc.

World Health Organization 1967. *The early detection and treatment of handicapping defects in young children.* Report on a working group convened by the Regional Office for Europe of the World Health Organization.

Subject Index

Author Index